SpringerWienNewYork

Sponsored by the
European Association of Neurosurgical Societies

Advances and Technical Standards in Neurosurgery

Vol. 32

Edited by
J. D. Pickard, Cambridge (Editor-in-Chief),
N. Akalan, Ankara, C. Di Rocco, Roma,
V. V. Dolenc, Ljubljana, J. Lobo Antunes, Lisbon,
J. J. A. Mooij, Groningen, J. Schramm, Bonn,
M. Sindou, Lyon

SpringerWienNewYork

With 95 Figures (thereof 50 coloured)

Printed in Austria

SpringerWienNewYork is part of Springer Science Business Media
springeronline.com

Printed on acid-free and chlorine-free bleached paper

ISSN 0095-4829

ISBN 978-3-211-99890-8
e-ISBN 978-3-211-47423-5

Preface

As an addition to the European postgraduate training system for young neurosurgeons, we began to publish in 1974 this series of *Advances and Technical Standards in Neurosurgery* which was later sponsored by the European Association of Neurosurgical Societies.

This series was first discussed in 1972 at a combined meeting of the Italian and German Neurosurgical Societies in Taormina, the founding fathers of the series being Jean Brihaye, Bernard Pertuiset, Fritz Loew and Hugo Krayenbuhl. Thus were established the principles of European co-operation which have been born from the European spirit, flourished in the European Association, and have been associated throughout with this series.

The fact that the English language is now the international medium for communication at European scientific conferences is a great asset in terms of mutual understanding. Therefore we have decided to publish all contributions in English, regardless of the native language of the authors.

All contributions are submitted to the entire editorial board before publication of any volume for scrutiny and suggestions for revision.

Our series is not intended to compete with the publications of original scientific papers in other neurosurgical journals. Our intention is, rather, to present fields of neurosurgery and related areas in which important recent advances have been made. The contributions are written by specialists in the given fields and constitute the first part of each volume.

In the second part of each volume, we publish detailed descriptions of standard operative procedures and in depth reviews of established knowledge in all aspects of neurosurgery, furnished by experienced clinicians. This part is intended primarily to assist young neurosurgeons in their postgraduate training. However, we are convinced that it will also be useful to experienced, fully trained neurosurgeons.

We hope therefore that surgeons not only in Europe, but also throughout the world, will profit by this series of *Advances and Technical Standards in Neurosurgery.*

The Editors

Contents

Advances

Conflicts of interest in medical practice. J. LOBO ANTUNES, Department of Neurosurgery, University of Lisbon, Lisbon, Portugal

Neurosurgical treatment of perineal neuralgias. R. ROBERT[1], J. J. LABAT[2], T. RIANT[1], M. KHALFALLAH[3], and O. HAMEL[1], [1] Service de Neurotraumatologie, Nantes, France, [2] Service d'Urologie, Nantes, France, [3] Service de Neurochirurgie, Centre Hospitalier de la côte Basque, Bayonne, France

Spinal cord stimulation for ischemic heart disease and peripheral vascular disease. J. DE VRIES[1], M. J. L. DE JONGSTE[1], G. SPINCEMAILLE[2], and M. J. STAAL[3], [1] Department of Cardiology, Thoraxcenter, University Medical Center Groningen, Groningen, The Netherlands, [2] Department of Neurosurgery, University Medical Center Maastricht, Maastricht, The Netherlands, [3] Department of Neurosurgery, University Medical Center Groningen, Groningen, The Netherlands

Surgical anatomy of the petrous apex and petroclival region. H.-D. FOURNIER[2], P. MERCIER[2], and P.-H. ROCHE[1], [1] Departement de Neurochirurgie, Hôpital Saint Marguerite, Marseille, France, [2] Departement de Neurochirurgie, Laboratoire d'Anatomie, Faculté de Médecine, Angers, France

Percutaneous destructive pain procedures on the upper spinal cord and brain stem in cancer pain: CT-guided techniques, indications and results. Y. KANPOLAT, Department of Neurosurgery, School of Medicine, Ankara University, Ankara, Turkey

List of Contributors

De Jongste, M. J. L., Department of Cardiology, Thorax Center, University Medical Center Groningen, PO Box 3001, 9700 RB Groningen, The Netherlands

De Vries, J., University Hospital Groningen, PO Box 30001, 9700 RB Groningen, The Netherlands

Dhellemmes, P., Clinique de Neurochirurgie, Unite Pediatrique, Hopital Roger Salengro, CHRU, 59037 Lille-Cedex, France

Fournier, H.-D., Laboratoire d'Anatomie, Faculté de Médecine, rue haute de reculée, 49100 Angers, France

Haase, J., Department of Neurosurgery, Aalborg University, Frederik Bajers vej 7D1, 9220 Aalborg, Denmark

Hamel, O., Service de Neurotraumatologie, Hôtel Dieu 2 place Alexis Ricordeau, CHU Nantes, 44035 Nantes Cedex 01, France

Kanpolat, Y., Department of Neurosurgery, School of Medicine, University of Ankara, Inkilap Sokak No. 24/4 Kizilay, 06640 Ankara, Turkey

Khalfallah, M., Service de Neurochirurgie, Centre Hospitalier de la côte Basque 14, Avenue Jacques Loeb, BP8 64109 Bayonne, France

Labat, J. J., Service d'Urologie, Hôtel Dieu 2 place Alexis Ricordeau, CHU Nantes, 44035 Nantes Cedex 01, France

Lobo Antunes, J., Hospital de Santa Maria, Univ. de Lisboa Neurocirurgia, Av. Prof. Egas Moniz, 1699 Lisboa Codex, Portugal

Mercier, P., Laboratoire d'Anatomie, Faculté de Médecine, rue haute de reculée, 49100 Angers, France

Riant, T., Service de Neurotraumatologie, Hôtel Dieu 2 place Alexis Ricordeau, CHU Nantes, 44035 Nantes Cedex 01, France

Robert, R., Service de Neurotraumatologie, Hôtel Dieu 2 place Alexis Ricordeau, CHU Nantes 44035 Nantes Cedex 01, France

Roche, P.-H., Service de neurochirurgie, Hospital Sainte Marguerite, 270 Boulevard Sainte Marguerite, 13274 Marseille Cedex 2, France

Spincemaille, G., University Hospital Maastricht, PO Box 5800, 6202 AZ Maastricht, The Netherlands

Staal, M. J., Department of Neurosurgery, University Medical Center Groningen, PO Box 30001, Groningen, The Netherlands

Vinchon, M., Pediatric Neurosurgery, Lille University Hospital, Lille-Cedex, France

Advances

Offprint from
Advances and Technical Standards in Neurosurgery, Vol. 32
Edited by J.D. Pickard

The transition from child to adult in neurosurgery

M. Vinchon and P. Dhellemmes

Pediatric Neurosurgery, Lille University Hospital, Lille-Cedex, France

With 8 Figures

Contents

Abstract

The transition from child to adult is a growing concern in neurosurgery. Data documenting long-term follow-up are necessary to define this population's healthcare needs. In order to evaluate the problems posed by the child-to-adult transition in neurosurgery, we have studied the neurological, functional and social outcome of patients treated in our department for tumor of the central nervous system, hydrocephalus or myelomeningocele, and followed beyond the age of eighteen years. A large number of patients suffered from chronic ailments, either sequelae of their initial disease, or delayed complications of their initial treatment, with significant morbidity. The mortality during adulthood was 4.6% in the tumor group, 1.1% in the hydrocephalus group, and zero in the spina bifida group. The proportion of patients employed in normal jobs was 35.6, 18.7 and 11.5% for tumors, hydrocephalus and myelomeningocele respectively. IQ score and performance at school generally overestimated the capacity for social integration. Based on these data and on the available literature, we tried to identify the problems and devise solutions for the management of the transition from child-to-adulthood transition. Many problems present during childhood persist to adulthood, some of which are made more acute because of a more competitive environment, the lack of structures and inadequate medical follow-up. The transition from child to adult must be managed jointly by pediatric and adult neurosurgeons. More clinical research is required in order to precisely evaluate the problems posed by adult patients treated during childhood for the different neurosurgical diseases. Based on these data, a concerted trans-disciplinary approach is necessary, tailored to the specific needs of patients suffering from different diseases.

Keywords: Myelomeningocele; cerebral neoplasms; hydrocephalus; outcome; age.

Introduction

With recent advances in pediatric neurosurgery and the resulting increase in survival, the care of adult patients treated for pediatric neurosurgical disease during childhood has become a new field of activity. In many of these patients, although the initial disease is cured, or at least well controlled by various treatments, several problems are present in adulthood. In some patients, these problems become worse with advancing age because of premature degenerative ailments, e.g. patients with spina bifida loosing ambulation. In other diseases, like hydrocephalus, the initial problem is only temporarily settled by a prosthetic device (the valve) or a palliative procedure (endoscopic third ventriculostomy), both of which may present with delayed failure. Finally new problems may arise as a delayed consequence of the initial treatments, such as brain lesions after irradiation for brain tumors, or as complications of initial treatment, like meningeal infection, or because of an inborn defect predisposing to disease, like the phakomatoses.

Adult patients with pediatric neurosurgical antecedents pose difficult management problems: their medical history is often complicated, and may be difficult to reconstruct because of missing records. Another problem is that neurosurgical subspecialties tend to separate from each other, and in particular, pediatric neurosurgery tends to become the exclusive field of pediatric neurosurgeons. As a result, many adult neurosurgeons do not have any longer the necessary experience to treat specific diseases, e.g. the dysraphisms. The management of the child-to-adult transition poses thus several problems regarding medical competence, training, and availability of care for these patients.

Recently, the American academy for pediatrics has issued recommendation for the transition from child to adult, to be implemented and adapted to the different fields of child-oriented care [1]. Neurologists have begun to show concern over this problem [35]; however, we were unable to find any neurosurgical literature dealing with this subject.

By focusing on adult patients treated during childhood for three categories of diseases – myelomeningocele (MM), tumors, and hydrocephalus – we have tried to evaluate the magnitude of the problem and explore some possible solutions.

Example of three groups of patients

We selected the cases of patients with tumors of the central nervous system, myelomeningocele and hydrocephalus (the latter group overlapping widely with the other two) treated in our department, who had reached the age of eighteen. We chose to study the adult outcome of these three groups because they represent large shares of the accrual of pediatric neurosurgical departments, and their medical follow-up is prolonged into adulthood because of specific problems.

In our institution, we are in a situation of virtual monopoly for pediatric neurosurgical diseases for a four-million population, and we have the opportunity to follow these patients beyond their entry into adulthood. Medical data have been stored in a quasi-prospective fashion for more than three decades; our medical database includes now over 5,000 patients with pediatric neurosurgical diseases, of which over 800 were followed beyond child age.

We evaluated the overall functional outcome using the semi-quantitative Glasgow Outcome Score for hydrocephalus and MM patients, and with the Karnofsky independence scale for tumor cases; more specific ailments (like endocrine disorders) were rated in a binary fashion (present or absent). The social outcome of the patients having completed their training was rated as "normal employment" (which includes child-rearing for mothers-at-home); "sheltered employment" (when the job was obtained by legal protection for the handicapped); "occupational activity" (when the job was part of a therapeutic

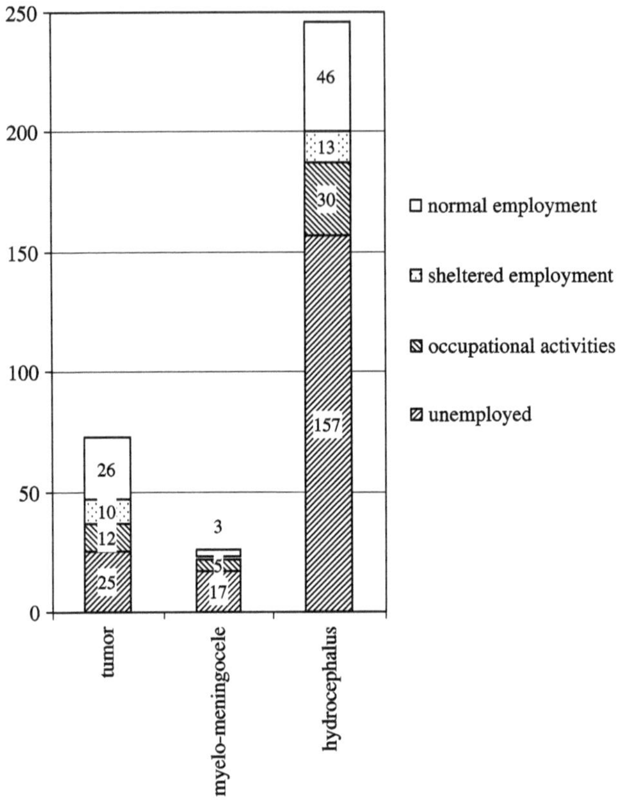

Fig. 1. Diagram showing the proportion of patients normally employed, employed in a sheltered environment, having occupational activities, and unemployed, in the three diseases studied. The particularly low employment rate among patients with myelomeningocele can be explained by the disturbance of schooling due to repeated hospitalizations during childhood, in addition to their neurological handicap

program rather than market-driven); and unemployed. The social outcome in the three groups of patients studied is summarized in Fig. 1.

Tumors

Personal series

From our series of 1065 children treated for tumors of the central nervous system since the advent of CT scanner, we selected 213 cases followed beyond the age of 18; 277 patients had died before reaching that age, and the rest are either still of child age, or lost to follow-up. For the purpose of this study, tumors were regrouped: cerebellar astrocytoma (34); lobar low-grade glioma

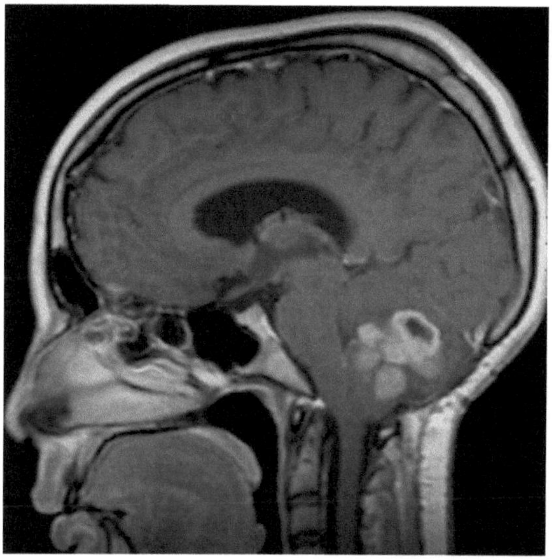

Fig. 2. 21-year old female, treated age 18 months for medulloblastoma with total removal and external irradiation (45 Gy); she developed a cerebellar high-grade astrocytoma, which was excised and treated with chemotherapy, but recurred after five months, and was the cause of demise 10 months after surgery

(22); optic pathway glioma (21); diencephalic low-grade glioma (19); brainstem low-grade glioma (18); malignant glioma (10); medulloblastoma (34); ependymoma (19); craniopharyngioma (14); pineal tumor (13); subependymal giant-cell astrocytoma (6); and schwannomas (3). The mean age at diagnosis was 10.0 years, and the mean duration of follow-up was 134 months.

Twelve patients (5.6%) died after having reached adult age: 9 because of tumor progression, one after surgery for recurrent craniopharyngioma, one because of a radio-induced malignant glioma (Fig. 2), and one because of radiation-induced vasculitis (Fig. 3). The overall clinical outcome at the last visit was evaluated with the Karnofsky independence score: 75 patients (35.2%) had a score of 100 (asymptomatic), 33 (15.5%) had a score of 90 (some symptoms but normal activity), 36 (16.4%) had a score of 80 (some symptoms but able to go to work or school), 20 (9.4%) had a score of 70 (independent at home but no outdoor activity), and 12 (5.6%) had KNK scores between 60 and 10 (diverse degrees of dependence on a third person and altered health status). In Fig. 4, we report the number of patients having behavioral, cognitive, memory, motor, endocrine, sensory deficit, as well as the presence or absence of obesity, epilepsy, spinal or shunt problem; those patients who had none of these afore-mentioned ailments were rated as having "no problem": only 37 patients (17.4%) were thus completely normal. The discrepancy between 37 "completely normal" patients and 75 patients with a Karnofsky score of

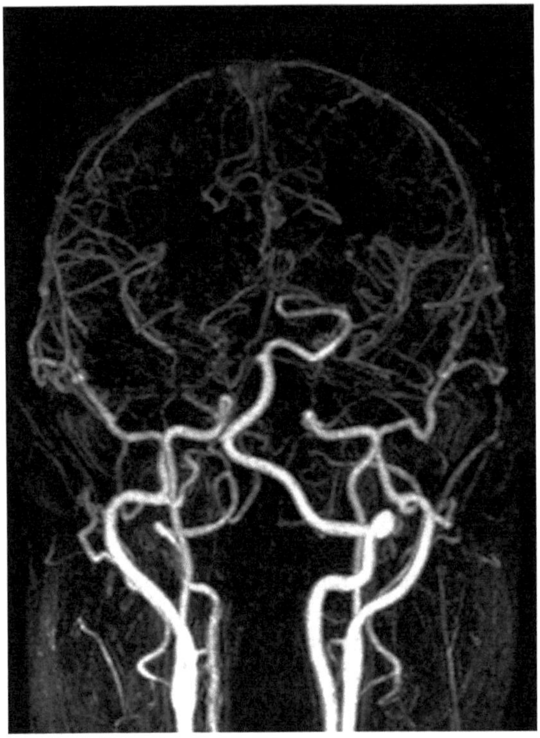

Fig. 3. 23-year old male, treated age 11 months for optic glioma, with subtotal resection followed by irradiation at the age of 18 months. He has severe visual loss and pursues occupational activities (upholstery). His MRI shows severe post-irradiation angiopathy with complete occlusion of the left posterior cerebral and both internal carotid arteries

100 was explained by patients having mild clinical signs (like ataxia) but no awareness of it, or patients with epilepsy well controlled under medication. Figure 5 summarizes the number of patients in each group of tumors, with the number of patients having "no problem" in each group: totally asymptomatic patients were found mostly in the cerebellar astrocytoma and low-grade lobar glioma groups.

Formal IQ testing was performed in 76 patients: the mean full-IQ score was 81.9, and 46 patients (59.7%) had full-IQ scores at or above 80. At the time of evaluation, 34% of the patients had completed high school, and 13% were or had been in university. Among 73 patients having completed their training, 36% were employed on a normal job, 14% were employed in a sheltered environment, 16% had occupational activities, and 34% were unemployed (the present official unemployment rate in the normal population is around 9% in our country).

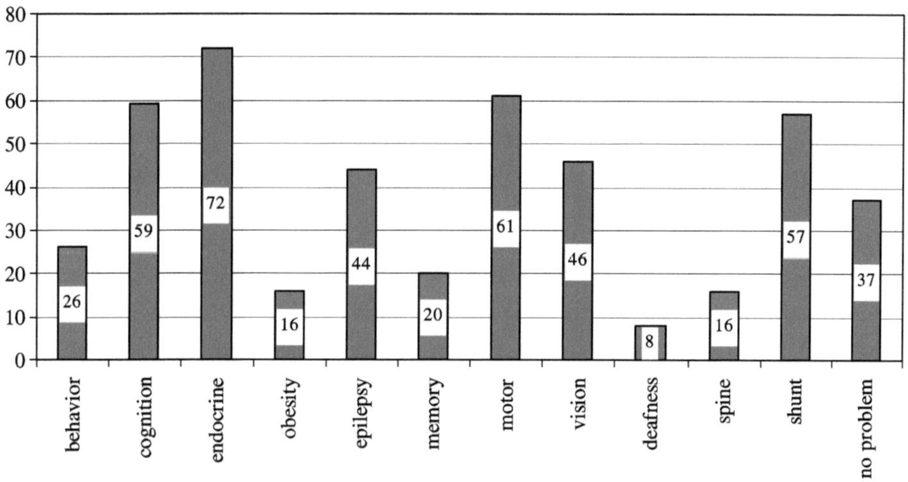

Fig. 4. Prevalence of the different sequelae in adult survivors of childhood tumors of the nervous system. The patients having "no problem" were the group of patients having none of the different ailments detailed here

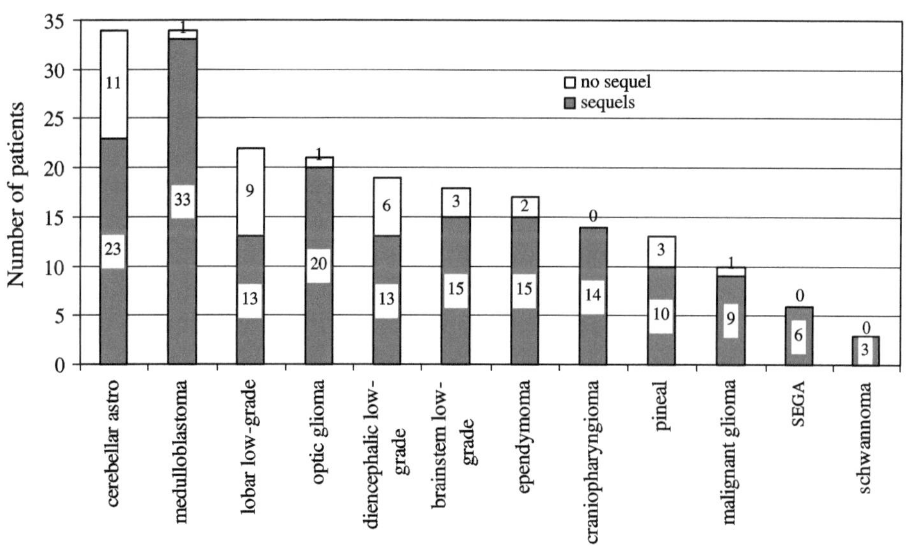

Fig. 5. Presentation of the different groups of tumors, with the proportion of patients having or having not neurological sequels. As expected, medulloblastoma, optic pathway glioma and craniopharyngioma were associated with the highest morbidity. However, contrary to common wisdom, cerebellar astrocytomas and low-grade lobar gliomas left sequels in more than half of cases, although generally not severe enough to impede normal life. (*SEGA* subependymal giant-cell astrocytoma)

Survival and oncological outcome

The long-term outlook of patients treated during childhood for brain tumor is characterized by an «appreciable burden of morbidity», with higher morbidity and poorer quality of life, compared with other childhood malignancies [10]. Nicholson calculated that mortality during the fourth decade of life was increased four-fold for patients with a history of brain tumor during childhood [24]. Although late tumor progression is the most likely cause of death, other causes, mostly treatment-related, are to be expected. Second tumors can be radio-induced, or due to a genetic predisposition (phakomatosis). In our experience, among 419 children irradiated for brain tumor, 14 developed tumors or cavernomas, and survival analysis showed that the prevalence of radio-induced tumors was 4.2% after ten years (unpublished data); this means that many of these tumors occurred in adults. The risk of radio-induced tumors could be higher when patients are irradiated at a younger age, because of a higher number of pluripotent cells [21]. Some diseases appear to predispose patients to develop radio-induced lesions, like neurofibromatosis type 1 [6] and Gorlin disease [2].

Functional outcome

Our data show that even among fully functional patients, many are not asymptomatic. The chief causes of this morbidity are the tumor itself, surgery, and irradiation. The most prominent sequels are neurological, neuropsychological, endocrine and sensory disturbances [25]; however, as shown in our Fig. 4, every facet of the functions of the nervous system can be more or less severely affected.

Neuropsychological sequels vary in severity according to tumor location, patient's age, and irradiation [23]. These results can be ascribed to progressive lesions of the central nervous system, as well as to difficulty increasing with age, as the school environment becomes more demanding. Hope-Hirsch and coworkers have alerted about the occurrence of progressive loss of IQ after irradiation for medulloblastoma [17]. Palmer calculated that the mean loss of full-scale IQ adjusted for age was 2.55 point per year in patients irradiated for medulloblastoma; the effect was especially marked for children who were younger at the time of irradiation, and for those who received higher irradiation doses [26]. This prolonged and sustained decline in intellectual function implies that a prolonged follow-up is necessary to evaluate its full extent [20]. Cognitive deficits are also related to the location of the tumor, and to the cerebral damage caused by the tumor and its resection. Recently, the role of the cerebellum in cognitive functions has been highlighted; Grill has shown that a lower performance IQ in medulloblastomas was associated with splitting of the vermis and damage to the dentate nuclei of the cerebellum, whereas lower verbal IQ was associated with hydrocephalus [13]. Patients with supratentorial tumors often have dysfunctions of executive tasks like programming strategy and inhibition, amounting to a «deficit in social competence» [24]. IQ tests show their limits in predicting the patient's adult outlook, because these problems, which can represent a major handicap for adult life, are most difficult to assess [3, 20]. Long-term data on adult independence score and social achievement are rare in the literature. Our series show a wide gap between independence score (67% were autonomous for outdoor activities) and actual academic and social achievements (only 36% were normally employed). This can perhaps be explained in part by repeated hospital stays disturbing schooling, but also, more probably, by more subtle sequels of higher brain functions, which may constitute a major handicap in a competitive environment. The gap might be even wider if we could compare the patient's achievements to what could be expected from his familial background. Our dataset does not give access to such information, and more detailed studies would be necessary to precise this point.

Endocrine problems are another major group of complications in brain tumors, resulting from damage to the hypothalamic-pituitary axis caused by the tumor, surgery and irradiation [34]. After having complicated the patients' growth and pubertal development, hypopituitarism continues to represent a sizeable problem during adulthood. Growth hormone deficiency is almost universal after brain irradiation of more than 30 Gys [11], and puts patients at higher risk of osteoporosis, muscle wasting, obesity, cardiovascular and cerebrovascular diseases. The benefits of treatment with growth hormone during adulthood on health risk factors and general fitness have been demonstrated [16], however the financial cost as well as lack of motivation for a lifelong injected treatment have limited its spread. Obesity is associated with hypothalamic damage due to the tumor, surgery, or irradiation. It is considered to result

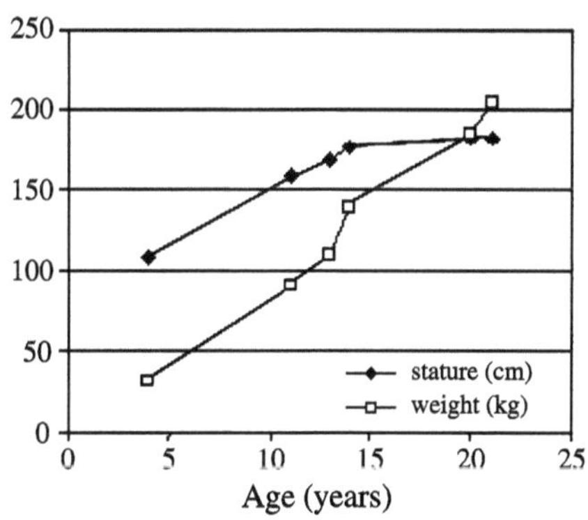

Fig. 6. Eighteen-year female treated since the age of four for craniopharyngioma, with surgery alone. At the time of the fourth tumor recurrence, her weight was 204 kg and rising

from lesions of the ventromedial nuclei, which mediate the blood-borne information from insulin, ghrelin and leptin [11]. The result of these lesions can be compounded with growth hormone deficiency and obesity-inducing treatments (like steroids or Valproate®) to produce morbid obesity. In craniopharyngiomas in particular, all these factors concur to make obesity a major concern, affecting up to 50% of patients [33]. We experienced a case of craniopharyngioma who reached a peak weight of 204 kg (450 lb), aged eighteen, at the time of her fourth recurrence (Fig. 6). Strategies seeking to avoid damage to the hypothalamus should be developed, and strict measures to contain weight gain should be enforced early during childhood, in order to avoid such nightmarish developments. Fertility problems are also common in adults treated for brain tumor during childhood, resulting from hypothalamic damage as well as gonadic toxicity due to chemotherapy [11]. Our series confirm a low fertility rate, only 14 of our 174 adult female patients (8.0%) having given birth to 16 children. Other possible obstacles to reproduction are teratogenic drugs (chief among them being antiepileptic drugs), genetic disorders like phakomatosis, and obstacles to delivery due to pelvic deformity or neurological deficits. However, the prevalence of inborn defects in offspring of patients treated for cancer during childhood (3.3%) does not appear different from that of the general population [12].

Implications for initial treatment of the tumor

The price tag of survival in brain tumor patients may look prohibitive. The elaboration of oncological protocols should include the evaluation of long-term morbidity [20]. The cause of long-term morbidity in tumor patients can generally be ascribed to one of the "three villains": the tumor, surgery, and irradiation. Radiotherapy is especially deleterious in infants, as well as patients predisposed to radio-induced lesions, like NF1 and Gorlin disease, and should thus be considered a last resort in these patients. Early recognition of morbidity related to radiotherapy and surgery has led to the development of alternative treatments with chemotherapy, for example for infiltrative low-grade astrocytomas (BBSFOP protocol) and germ-cell tumors. The quest for lower morbidity should not let forget, however, the first aim of treatment, which is the eradication (or at least stabilization) of the disease. In the long run, the risk of tumor recurrence, and the risks associated with the treatment for recurrent tumor, should be taken in account. For example, radical resection for craniopharyngiomas is known to be associated with a risk of severe morbidity, and subtotal resection followed by irradiation have been advocated [30]. Conversely, surgery for recurrent craniopharyngioma is technically demanding and risky, especially after irradiation, and our data show that operative morbidity was highest in case of surgery for tumor recurrence; this would incite to perform maximal initial resection whenever it can be done safely [8]. This question remains open, until more long-term data are available. In other tumors, like ependymomas, aggressive resection is recognized as the main factor influencing outcome [37]; in some cases however, resection cannot be carried out without unacceptable morbidity, and we have to rely on postoperative treatments. Because the decision to pursue or not complete resection has to be taken on-the-spot during surgery, it is important that we try to settle these questions in advance, based on long-term oncological and functional results.

Myelomeningocele

Personal series

Among 452 patients with MM treated in our department, we selected 38 patients (19 male and 19 female) aged between 21 and 23 years, and surveyed them with a detailed questionnaire and interview by phone call. The quality of life was studied using the SF-36 health survey, which is a validated scale based on a questionnaire regarding physical health, fitness, pain, mental health, social skills, and emotions [40], and has been translated and validated in French language [28].

Thirty-three patients (86.8%) had a CSF shunt. The average number of reoperations for shunt failure was 2.5 per shunted patient; 6 patients had undergone surgery for Chiari malformation, 14 patients (36.4%) for tethered spinal cord, and 5 (13.2%) for scoliosis. Overall, the average number of surgeries (including initial closure and shunt) was 10.2 per patient (1 to 28).

At last control, 14 patients were able to walk for more than 500 meters, four were able to walk between 50 and 500 meters, 9 were able to walk for less than 50 meters, and 11 were non-walking. Among 31 patients initially using walk as their regular mode of ambulation, 8 had lost walking between the age of 7 and 20 years (Fig. 7). Although loss of ambulation was often multifactorial, the chief cause was considered to be prolonged immobilization after orthopedic problems in four cases; obesity, spinal cord tethering, and degradation due to Chiari malformation, and accidental brain damage after drowning in one case each.

Among 16 patients who underwent formal neuropsychological testing, mean verbal IQ was 96.1, performance IQ was 85.8, and global IQ was 92.1. Eleven patients had no school degree, 5 had completed primary school, 14 were in high school, and 8 were at university. At last control, 12 patients were studying, 3 were working on a normal employment, one in a sheltered environment, 5 had occupational activitics, and 17 had no outdoor activities. The quality of life studied using the SF-36 health survey showed that although the health and vitality indices were as expected lower than in the controls; however, surprisingly, the indices relating to psychological and emotional domains scored on average better than in the control population published by Pergener [14].

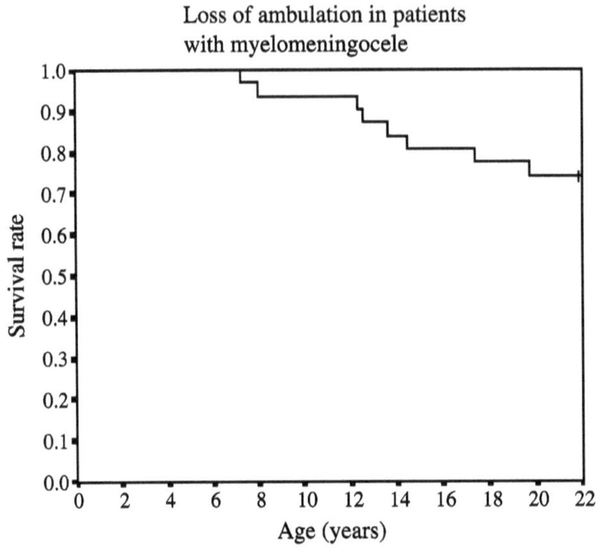

Fig. 7. Diagram showing the incidence of loss of ambulation among 36 patients with myelomeningocele surveyed: among 31 initially ambulating patients, 8 lost walking as their regular mode of ambulation between the age of 7 and 20 years. The 20-years actuarial survival rate was 74%

Discussion

Because of antenatal diagnosis and the common practice of termination of pregnancy, MM is a disappearing disease in pediatric neurosurgery; the bulk of patients with MM are now slowly but surely becoming adults, and their needs must be addressed. Adult patients with spina bifida are considered "the most neglected individuals in the population with neurosurgical disease" [22]. The population followed in the long term is biased compared to the initial population, because the most severe cases died before reaching adulthood, and the less severe, often not shunted, tend to abandon medical follow-up [18]. Even during adulthood, patients with MM have an excess mortality, mostly because of shunt failure [4].

Although the initial motor deficit is a direct function of the anatomical level of the MM, children who have managed to acquire walking can lose it lately because of tethered cord, syringomyelia, or neuro-orthopedic problems. Bowman considered that loss of ambulation occurred mostly during childhood and that "patients who remain mobile in their teens continue to ambulate . . . in their young adult years [4]. Our data do not concur, as shown in our Fig. 7. We have some reasons to fear that with increasing obesity and neuro-orthopedic problems, compounded with premature skeletal aging, loss of ambulation will become more and more prevalent in this group of patients.

Tethered cord is a delayed complication of MM occurring mostly during late childhood and adolescence [32]. However four patients in our experience underwent spinal cord untethering between 24 and 37 years. The rarity of this condition in adults may be due to the lack of information amid adult neurosurgeons, and the number of adult cases is likely to grow in the future. In order to be performed safely, spinal cord untethering requires careful indications, surgical skill and experience, and we think that pediatric neurosurgeons should continue to operate adult patients with tethered spinal cord.

Academic and social achievements are low in the MM population for several reasons. Their IQ is frequently low [27], especially performance IQ [15]. Lower IQ may be due to associated brain malformation, and/or hydrocephalus, with repeated episodes of raised intracranial pressure [18]; however the relation between the number of shunt revisions and social achievements has not been confirmed [15]. The correlation of hydrocephalus with schooling and social achievement in MM patients is blurred because patients with low-level MM are often doubly blessed with shunt-independence as well as autonomous walking. Even with a normal IQ, schooling may be difficult: our data show that the vast majority of patients underwent multiple surgical procedures during childhood. In addition, because of their motor deficiencies, these patients often had to attend schooling in rehabilitation centers. In itself, this hectic curriculum may be responsible for low achievements. Also, a sense of discouragement and lack of motivation when reaching adulthood often appears to be a potent obstacle to these patients' social life.

These data on MM are important for antenatal counseling, because the decision to continue or interrupt pregnancy must be assisted by medical evidence. An illustrative case is the only male MM patient in our experience who was able-bodied enough to sire a child; when it turned out that the fetus had spina bifida too, his decision to have the pregnancy terminated was immediate and final. On the other hand, our study found that SF-36 health survey indices relating to psychological and emotional domains were at least as high in MM patients as in healthy controls; this surprising result shows that in spite of their handicaps, a degree of well-being is undeniable in these patients.

Hydrocephalus

Personal series

We selected 450 patients shunted for hydrocephalus during childhood, and aged more than 18 years at last control. The median age at shunt insertion was 8 months. Overall 1188 shunt revisions were necessary, the mean number of shunt revisions being 2.6 per patient; only 65 patients (14.4%) had no shunt revision. In 15 patients, the first shunt revision was performed more than 20 years after insertion. Eighty-two episodes of shunt infection occurred in 70 patients; the rate of infection was thus 15.6% per patient and 5.0% per operation.

Ten patients died between 18 and 34 years: 4 of tumor progression, 2 of medical causes related to the cause of hydrocephalus, one of radio-induced lesions, one because of shunt infection, one of ascertained shunt failure, and one of unexplained sudden death (possibly caused by shunt failure). Five patients (1.1%) can thus be considered to have died of hydrocephalus-related causes. Overall evaluation following the GOS showed that 184 patients (40.9%) had normal activity, 70 (15.6%) had a mild handicap, 141 (31.3%) had a more severe handicap, and 5 (1.1%) were vegetative. Schooling had been; normal in 149 cases (33.1%); difficult in 70 (15.6%); delayed in 29 (6.4%); special schooling for the handicapped in 121 (26.9%); and no schooling had been possible in 32 (7.1%). At last control, among 246 patients having completed or abandoned school, 46 (18.7%) were working on a normal job, 13 (5.3%) were working in a sheltered environment, 58 (23.6%) had occupational activities, and 157 (52.4%) were unemployed or unable to have outdoor activities.

In a previous study [39], we determined in a binary logistic regression analysis which factors influenced independently the schooling and overall outcome of shunted patients. The results are shown on Table 1. Most of these factors pertained to the cause of hydrocephalus (post-hemorrhagic, post-meningitis, or due to spina bifida), but shunt infection was also a major independent factor influencing both schooling and overall outcome. These results highlight the fact that complications of treatment play a major role on adult outcome.

Table 1. *Determinants of schooling and overall outcome in hydrocephalus: binary logistic regression analysis [39]*

Variables in the model	Outcome (GOS = 1 or more)*	Schooling (normal or not)†
Post-meningitic hydrocephalus	<0.001	<0.001
Post-hemorrhagic hydrocephalus	0.004	NS
Myelomeningocele	<0.001	<0.001
Prematurity	NS	NS
Antenatal diagnosis	NS	NS
Shunt infection	0.002	0.009

* *and* † Significance of the model: $p<0.001$. *GOS* Glasgow Outcome Score; *NS* not statistically significant. These data show that the prognosis is mostly dependent on the cause of hydrocephalus, but also on complications of treatment like shunt infection.

Discussion

Shunt outcome

The risk of shunt obstruction is the main burden for shunted patients who otherwise do well. It may be the cause of sudden death, with a risk estimated as high as 1% a year [29]. Repeated episodes of shunt obstruction have also been deemed responsible for poor functional outcome [18]. We consider that the potentially devastating complications of shunt obstruction make a regular and life-long follow-up necessary for all hydrocephalus patients; whenever an asymptomatic shunt failure is detected, we perform elective shunt revision, unless the patient can be determined as shunt-independent [36]. Conversely, symptomatic shunt failure is proof that the patient is shunt-dependent. When a shunted patient has never presented with shunt failure, the question whether the shunt might have been blocked long ago but the patient has become shunt-independent may be legitimately raised. The actuarial survival curve after shunt insertion shows typically a binary curve, with early failure due to surgical causes, and delayed failure due to interactions between the shunt and the patient. However, close examination of the actuarial survival curve prolonged beyond 20 years

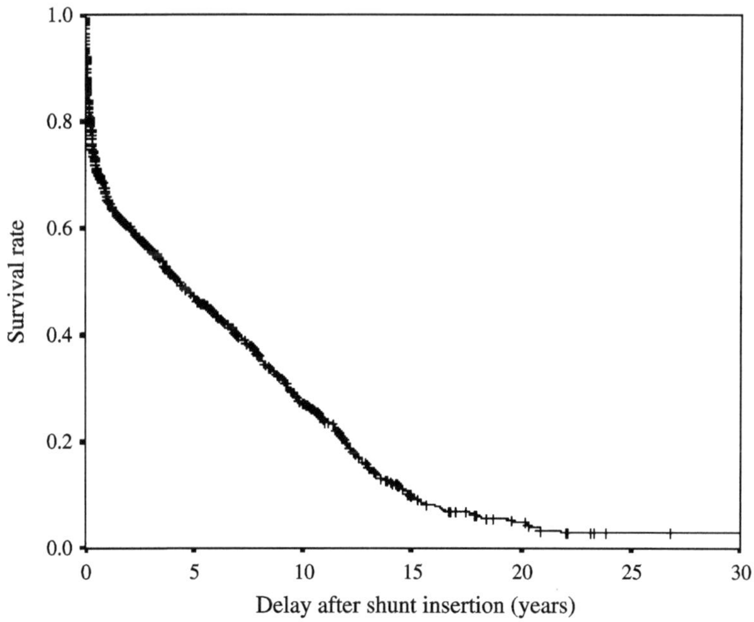

Fig. 8. Event-free survival after first shunt insertion: the curve shows that, although most cases of shunt obstruction occurred within the years following shunt insertion, the first shunt failure could occur after more than 20 years. Although very long follow-up introduces a selection bias, this diagram indicates that a long period of time without shunt failure cannot be equated with shunt independence

shows that shunt failure can occur very late (Fig. 8). In our experience, 15 patients had their first shunt revision performed more than 20 years after insertion. This shows that shunt-independence cannot be guessed from the absence of shunt failure, but has to be proved by a controlled procedure. Our routine procedure includes a shuntogram followed by shunt ligature, then shunt removal a month later if the ligature is well tolerated [36]. Regarding endoscopic third ventriculostomy (ETV), the risk of delayed obstruction appears more and more to pose problems similar to shunts, with catastrophic consequences in some cases; close radiological and clinical follow-up is warranted after ETV as well [9].

Although shunt infection is generally considered to result from intra-operative contamination, we found in a previous study that 12% of episodes of shunt infection occurred more than a year, and up to 15 years after previous surgery [39]. The causes of delayed shunt infection include hematogenous seeding, spontaneous bowel perforation, abdominal surgery, accidental penetrating trauma, but also possibly the prolonged persistence of dormant bacteria. We calculated that the incidence of spontaneous bowel perforation was 0.1% a year; we also found that it occurred more often in patients having walking difficulties, like spina bifida, which suggests that it might be facilitated by abnormal bowel motility [38].

Intellectual outcome

The impact of shunt obstruction on IQ has been suggested by Hunt, who noted that patients with more shunt revision had poorer achievements than patients with less shunt revisions, or without shunt; however the statistics backing this assertion were poor [18]. Most authors consider that the intellectual outcome depends on the cause of hydrocephalus rather than on the number of shunt revisions and the occurrence of shunt infection [5]. In particular, brain malformations, neonatal meningitis or ventricular hemorrhage have a major impact on development [29, 31]. Our opinion is that the number of shunt revisions does not necessarily indicate a high number of episodes of raised intracranial pressure, but may instead reflect the care with which patients are followed. A good illustration of this is provided in the series of patients with MM from Chicago, who underwent a high average number of shunt revisions (4.3 per patient), because shunt obstruction was systematically considered as a cause for neurological deterioration in these patients [4]. Shunt infection is classically associated with loss of IQ [19], although this view has been challenged by Casey [5]; in our series, we found that shunt infection had a major and independent impact on both schooling and quality of life of shunted patients [39]. Overall, we consider that IQ measurements overestimate the school abilities, which in turn overestimate the patients' professional achievement. Although Sgouros reported that 56% of shunted patients are normally employed [31], our results are much inferior, which might reflect differences in patient accrual or in toughness of the labor market.

Organization of the transition from child to adult in neurosurgery

In 2002, the American Academy of Pediatrics stated that « by the year 2010 all physicians who provide primary or subspecialty care to young people with special health care needs 1) understand the rationale for transition from child-oriented to adult-oriented health care; 2) have the knowledge and skills to facilitate that process; and 3) know if, how, and when transfer of care is indicated » [1]. These recommendations apply to all fields of child-oriented care, including pediatric neurosurgery; up to now, the literature dealing with the transition from child to adult in neurosurgery is conspicuously lacking. The present report aims at pointing out some of the problems regarding the necessary "knowledge and skills", and raising awareness of our responsibility in ensuring the transition from child to adult. In European healthcare systems, the financial aspect of the child-to-adult transition is not as large an issue as it may be in North America; with the current trend toward liberalization in our healthcare systems however, we must be wary that the rights of our patients for continued care are respected.

Relation of pediatric to adult neurosurgery

The treatment of many neurosurgical diseases often transforms an acute and deadly disease into a chronic, lifelong condition. Tuffrey stated that « diseases of childhood are becoming diseases that begin in childhood and continue into adult life » [35]. As is the case for many chronic diseases, the transition from child to adult has become a major problem in neurosurgery. In her paper on long-term follow-up of spina bifida, R. Bowman stated that "one of the greatest challenges in medicine today is to establish a network of care for these adults with spina bifida" [4]. Although the same can be said of many other pediatric diseases, we neurosurgeons must be part this endeavor.

In the majority of neurosurgical centers in France, neurosurgeons are not age-specialized. A commonly accepted view in neurosurgery is that, apart from a few specifically pediatric fields (craniofacial, dysraphism, and neurosurgery in infants and newborns), children are not much different from adults. We do not share that view for several reasons. First, many diseases which look similar behave completely differently in children and in adults (e.g. subdural hematomas), while others, which have marginal importance in adults are major issues in children (e.g. arachnoid cysts). Second, the clinical presentation in non-verbal or unreliable patients requires specific communication skills for the diagnosis and medical management. Third, the small body size and immaturity of tissues implies specific surgical and anesthetic techniques. Fourth, the patient's process of development and learning implies protracted follow-up and evaluation of long-term consequences. The downside of developing pediatric neurosurgery as an autonomous specialty is that it may easily lose contact with rapidly evolving fields (like spine or vascular surgery). Another problem is that pediatric neurosurgeons may become unable (because of limitations of resources or tight regulations), or unwilling (because of a busy schedule), to take care of patients becoming adults. The worst solution would be to simply discharge the patient to adult colleagues. Several halfway solutions have emerged in different places. In non-specialized centers, generally one adult neurosurgeon in the team is designated to take care of most pediatric cases (especially urgent cases), while more specifically pediatric (and non-urgent) cases are referred to another, more specialized centre. In specialized centers (like ours), the segregation is not complete, pediatric neurosurgeons having a "double citizenship" which allows them to continue to take care of their patients beyond their entry into adulthood, ensuring a relatively smooth transition.

Another possibility would be to subspecialize by disease instead of by age: this is already the case in some places for epilepsy surgery and for surgery of movement disorders; one can imagine that this concept could be extended to other fields, like the skull-base, spine, cerebrovascular, trauma, oncology, hydrocephalus . . . . However, a single patient's disease often encroaches on several subspecialties; CSF problems in particular are almost ubiquitous in their association with any other disease in pediatric neurosurgery. In addition, the problem of follow-up of the patient's development would require some form of centralization by a truly pediatric neurosurgeon, or a pediatrician dedicated to neurosurgery. The main obstacle to such an organization would be a shortage of manpower, because devoting one neurosurgeon (or ideally a team) to all the potential neurosurgical subspecialties would be beyond the reach of even in the largest centers.

Offer/demand of care

The offer of care for patients becoming adults is often insufficient. As mentioned above, adult neurosurgeons do not always have the necessary expertise for highly specific diseases, and pediatric neurosurgeons are not always available for adult follow-up. A major problem is the lack of adult structures for the care, professional training and employment of adults with handicaps. Grownup patients and their families are often dismayed when reaching the adult age limit, facing a medical and institutional vacuum they could hardly imagine while in the (relative) abundance and coziness of childhood care.

On the other hand, the demand for care from these patients is not always clear. The sense of discouragement often resulting from years of struggle against handicap often leads patients to abandon medical follow-up. In some cases, these patients come to us for motives like recognition of a handicapped status, or demands for social benefits, which we can hardly satisfy, and are not aware of possibilities of medical treatments that we can offer. This mismatch between demand and offer of care needs to be clarified by exchange of information in both directions between patients, notably through their associations, and physicians.

Networking

From the present state of neurosurgery in our country, we are convinced that progress can be made through the training of young neurosurgeons, who should devote some part of their curriculum to pediatric neurosurgery, and dialogue between pediatric and adult neurosurgeons for example during post-graduate sessions. We need to spare some time for this necessary dialogue, during which adult neurosurgeons, pediatric neurosurgeons, and above all the patients, have much to gain. Also, if we are to make some progress in this field, more clinical data should be gathered and published; some of the above-mentioned examples show that the transition from child to adult is a rich field for useful clinical research.

The transition from child to adult can be at least as chaotic in specialties neighboring neurosurgery. For example, neuropediatricians stem from a general pediatric training, whereas neurologists generally do not have any training in pediatrics. The same can be said for intensivists, oncologists, and physical therapists. Bridges between the pediatric and adults side of these many specialties often remain to be built. Neurosurgeons caring for pediatric patients becoming adult have to create their own network, and establish preferred relations with colleagues in these neighboring specialties. In so doing, neurosurgeons play, in its most valuable sense, the role of a general practitioner. Establishing and motivating such a network can be both arduous and rewarding.

Conclusion

The transition from child to adult is a crucial period of everybody's life; social and professional integration requires the best from an individual's highest intellectual functions, as well as physical fitness. Patients with a history of neurosurgical disease during childhood often have cognitive, sensory or endocrine sequels that make them especially vulnerable and result in inferior social and professional achievements.

The fact that so few of our patients become successful adults in a competitive environment may be somewhat sobering. Like many physicians dealing with children, we indulge in self-complacency, in the belief that the children we have saved will become fit and productive adults, and that our actions are profitable for society. Clearly, if healthcare planners caring only for profitability were to learn from these data, their reaction would be to cut down on the funding of pediatric neurosurgery. It should be stated loud and clear that the benefits of care for children as well as for handicapped adults should not be counted in economic terms. Its financing should thus be written in the losses column of the balance sheet; in the profit column however stands social equity and solidarity, the value of which is incalculable. How large a part of its gross domestic product our society is ready to spend on solidarity may be a vital choice for the future.

References

1. American Academy of Pediatrics (2002) A consensus statement on health care transitions for young adults with special health care needs. Pediatrics 100: 1304–1306
2. Amlashi SFA, Riffaud L, Brassier G, Morandi X (2003) Nevoid basal cell carcinoma syndrome: relation with desmoplastic medulloblastoma in infancy. Cancer 98: 618–624
3. Anderson CA, Wilkening GN, Filley CM, Reardon MS, Kleinschmidt-DeMasters BK (1997) Neurobehavioral outcome in pediatric craniopharyngioma. Pediatr Neurosurg 26: 255–260
4. Bowman RM, McLone DG, Grant JA, Tomita T, Ito JA (2001) Spina bifida outcome: a 25-year prospective. Pediatr Neurosurg 34: 114–120
5. Casey ATH, Kimmings EJ, Kleinlugtebeld AD, Taylor WAS, Hayward RD (1997) The long-term outlook for hydrocephalus in childhood. Pediatr Neurosurg 27: 63–70
6. Czech T, Slavc I, Aichholzer M, Haberler C, Dietrich W, Dieckmann K, Koos W, Budka H (1999) Proliferative activity as measured by MIB-1 labeling index and long-term outcome of visual pathway astrocytomas in children. J Neurooncol 42: 143–150
7. Defoort-Dhellemmes S, Moritz F, Bouacha I, Vinchon M (2006) Craniopharyngioma: ophthalmological aspects at diagnosis. J Pediatr Endocrinol Metab 19 Suppl 1: 322–324
8. Dhellemmes P, Vinchon M (2006) Radical resection for craniopharyngiomas in children: surgical technique and clinical results. J Pediatr Endocrinol Metab 19 Suppl 1: 329–335
9. Drake J, Chumas P, Kestle J, Pierre-Kahn A, Vinchon M (2006) Late Rapid Deterioration after endoscopic third ventriculostomy – additional cases and literature review. J Neurosurg 105 Suppl 2: 118–126
10. Foreman NK, Faestel PM, Pearson J, Disabato J, Poole M, Wilkening G, Arenson EB, Greffe B, Thorne R (1999) Health status in 52 long-term survivors of pediatric brain tumors. J Neurooncol 41: 47–53
11. Gleeson HK, Shalet SM (2004) The impact of cancer therapy on the endocrine system in survivors of childhood brain tumours. Endocrine-Related Cancer 11: 589–602
12. Green DM, Fiorello A, Zevon MA, Hall B, Seigelstein N (1997) Birth defects and childhood cancer in offspring of survivors of childhood cancer. Arch Pediatr Adolesc Med 151: 379–383
13. Grill J, Viguier D, Kieffer V, Bulteau C, Sainte-Rose C, Hartmann O, Kalifa C, Dellatolas G (2004) Critical risk factors for intellectual impairment in children with posterior fossa tumors: the role of cerebellar damage. J Neurosurg Pediatrics 101 Suppl 2: 152–158
14. Herbeau C (2004) Devenir à long terme de patients présentant une myéloméningocèle à la naissance nés entre 1981 et 1982 dans le nord de la France [Outcome of patients with myelomeningocele born between 1981 and 1982 in the north of France]. Dissertation for Medical Thesis, Lille

15. Hetherington R, Dennis M, Barnes M, Drake J, Gentili F (2006) Functional outcome in young adults with spina bifida and hydrocephalus. Child's Nerv Syst 22: 117–124
16. Hoffman AR, Kuntze JE, Baptista J, Baum HBA, Baumann GP, Biller BMK, Clark RV, Cook D, Inzucchi SE, Kleinberg D, Kliblanski A, Phillips LS, Ridgway EC, Robbins RJR, Schlechte JS, Sharma M, Thorner MO, Vance ML (2004) Growth hormone (GH) replacement therapy in adult-onset GH deficiency: effects on body composition in men and women in a double-blind, randomized, placebo-controlled trial. J Clin Endoc Metab 89: 2048–2056
17. Hoppe-Hirsch E, Renier D, Lellouch-Tubiana A, Sainte-Rose C, Pierre-Kahn A, Hirsch JF (1990) Medulloblastoma in childhood: progressive intellectual deterioration. Child's Nerv Syst 6: 60–65
18. Hunt GM, Oakeshot P, Kerry S (1999) Link between the CSF shunt and achievement in adults with spina bifida. J Neurol Neurosurg Psychiatr 67: 591–595
19. Kang JK, Lee IW (1999) Long-term follow-up of shunting therapy. Child's Nerv Syst 15: 711–717
20. Kennedy C, Glaser A (2004) Quality of survival. In: Walker DA, Perilongo G, Punt JAG, Taylor RE (eds) Brain and spinal tumors of childhood. Arnold, London, pp 493–500
21. Lonser RR, Walbridge S, Vortmeyer AO, Pack SD, Nguyen TT, Gobate N, Olson JJ, Bobo RH, Goffman T, Shunang Z, Oldfield EH (2002) Induction of glioblastoma in nonhuman primates after therapeutic doses of fractionated whole-brain radiation therapy. J Neurosurg 97: 1378–1389
22. McLone DG (1995) The adult with a tethered cord. Clin Neurosurg 43: 203–209
23. Mulhern RK, Kun LE (1999) Cognitive deficits. In: Berger MS, Wilson CB (eds) The gliomas. Saunders, Philadelphia, pp 741–749
24. Nicholson HS, Butler R (2001) Late effects of therapy in long-term survivors. In: Keating RF, Goodrich JT, Packer RJ (eds) Tumors of the pediatric central nervous system. Thieme, New York, pp 535–545
25. Packer RJ, Gurney JG, Punyko JA, Donaldson SS, Inskip PD, Stovall M, Yasui Y, Mertens AC, Sklar CA, Nicholson HS, Zeltzer LK, Neglia JP, Robison LL (2003) Long-term neurologic and neurosensory sequelae in adult survivors of a childhood brain tumor: childhood cancer survivor study. J Clin Oncol 21: 3255–3261
26. Palmer SL, Goloubeva O, Reddick WE, Glass JO, Gajjar A, Kun L, Merchant TE, Mulhern RK (2001) Patterns of intellectual development among survivors of pediatric medulloblastoma: a longitudinal analysis. J Clin Oncol 19: 2302–2308
27. Park TS (1999) Myelomeningocele. In: Albright AL, Pollack IF, Adelson PD (eds) Principles and practice of pediatric neurosurgery. Thieme, New York, pp 291–320
28. Pergener TV, Leplège A, Etter JF, Rougemont A (1995) Validation of a French-language version of the mos 36-item short form health survey (SF-36) in young healthy adults. J Clin Epidemiol 48: 1051–1060
29. Rekate HL (1999) Treatment of hydrocephalus. In: Albright AL, Pollack IF, Adelson PD (eds) Principles and practice of pediatric neurosurgery. Thieme, New York, pp 47–73
30. Sainte-Rose C, Puget S, Wray A, Zerah M, Grill J, Brauner R, Boddaert N, Pierre-Kahn A (2005) Craniopharyngioma: the pendulum of surgical management. Child's Nerv Syst 21: 691–695
31. Sgouros S, Mallucci C, Walsh AR, Hockley AD (1995) Long-term complications of hydrocephalus. Pediatr Neurosurg 23: 127–132

32. Shurtleff DB, Duguay S, Duguay G, Moskowitz D, Weinberger E, Roberts T, Loeser J (1997) Epidemiology of tethered cord with meningomyelocele. Eur J Pediatr Surg 7 Suppl 1: 7–11
33. Sklar CA (1994) Craniopharyngioma: endocrine sequelae of treatment. Pediatr Neurosurg 21 Suppl 1: 120–123
34. Sutton LN, Molloy PT, Sernyak H, Goldwein J, Phillips PL, Rorke LB, Moshang T Jr, Lange B, Packer RJ (1995) Long-term outcome of hypothalamic/chiasmatic astrocytomas in children treated with conservative surgery. J Neurosurg 83: 583–589
35. Tuffrey C, Pearce A (2003) Transition from pediatric to adult neurological services for young people with chronic neurological problems. J Neurol Neurosurg Psychiatr 74: 1011–1013
36. Vinchon M, Fichten A, Delestret I, Dhellemmes P (2003) Revision for asymptomatic shunt failure: surgical and clinical results. Neurosurgery 52: 347–356
37. Vinchon M, Leblond P, Noudel R, Dhellemmes P (2005) Intracranial ependymomas in childhood: recurrence, reoperation, and outcome. Child's Nerv Syst 21: 221–226
38. Vinchon M, Baroncini M, Thines L, Dhellemmes P (2006) Bowel perforation by peritoneal shunt catheters: diagnosis and treatment. Neurosurgery 58 Suppl 1: 76–82
39. Vinchon M, Dhellemmes P (2006) Cerebrospinal shunt infection: risk factors and long term follow-up. Child's Nerv Syst 22: 692–677
40. Ware JE, Gandek B (1998) Overview of the SF-36 health survey and the international quality of life assessment (IQOLA) project. J Clin Epidemiol 51: 903–912

Offprint from
Advances and Technical Standards in Neurosurgery, Vol. 32
Edited by J.D. Pickard

Conflicts of interest in medical practice

J. LOBO ANTUNES

Department of Neurosurgery, University of Lisbon, Lisbon, Portugal

Contents

Abstract

It has become more and more apparent that some aspects of current medical practice can no longer be kept solely within the private preserve of the profession. Medical error is now treated in an open fashion because it is clear that frank debate over its incidence, causes and mechanisms are crucial to effective prevention. This has always been one of our worst kept secrets. Equally conflicts of interest [1] assume particular relevance in an occupation whose foundation values demand a robust ethical identity. This is the topic of this essay.

Keywords: Ethics; conflicts of interest, medical professionalism.

The ethical paradox

Medical professionalism has some unique characteristics, which need to be preserved. In simple terms, it means the protection by competent people, specially qualified professionals, of vulnerable people and/or values, which, in our case, are our patients and the delivery of health care in all our areas of intervention [2–4]. This is our social contract, which implies professional autonomy and the correlative right and duty of self-regulation. This requires that we place the interests of the ones we care for above our own and, furthermore, to define and maintain patterns, of competence and integrity and play the role of social partners, with an independent voice based on knowledge and experience. All this has to be anchored in the absolute confidence on a peculiar fiduciary relationship between doctor and patient.

Although it is always claimed that doctors should place the interest of patients above all others, the truth is that this value is often jeopardized by the social, economical and cultural realities of our time and, as noted by Bloche [5], by the ubiquity of clinical work which serves mainly non-clinical goals. In fact, doctors have gotten increasingly involved in a complex web of relationships with other partners, and certainly a neurosurgeon working for an insurance company or a sports club, or acting as an expert in a judicial dispute, is playing a role quite distinct from the traditional medical act. The unequivocal one to one relationship between a doctor and his patient is nowadays just one of the multiple facets of medicine, albeit the noblest and of the longest tradition. But it is pure hypocrisy to claim that it dominates all of the other professional duties of a physician.

In this regard, it is no longer possible to ignore the deep moral paradox that has afflicted us since the time of our father Hippocrates, as noted by Jonsen [6]. This paradox emerges from the perpetual conflict between two basic moral principles: altruism and self-interest, which in its more extreme form is just plain egoism. As pointed out by Jonsen, many social and economic questions in healthcare delivery stem from this same paradox, and the fair balance between these two opposing values constitutes one of the most pungent challenges to our profession. On one side, self-interest promotes values that guarantee self-satisfaction, progression in the academic or professional career, public recognition, financial comfort, in sum, happiness or its illusion.... On the other hand, altruism demands the promotion of these same values, but in favour of others and, if needed, with sacrifice of our own. It is certainly naïve to believe that it is possible to create a health care system without taking into account this reality.

In simple terms, it may be said that doctors have their types of self-interests. The first one is easy to quantify and readily appreciated by lay people, and is the financial interest. The second may be called "academic" and includes the contributions to scientific progress, the recognition by peers, competition for the financing of research, the broadening of the referral basis of patients, attention by the media and, why not saying it simply, the wish to become famous.

The third type is more difficult to define, but its goal is to keep a certain comfort, by not taking on the difficult or risky cases, that could perhaps threaten professional or social reputation.

The sensibility of the public has always been particularly touched by news that doctors are given all sorts of gifts (money, luxury trips) in exchange for prescribing drugs or using certain tools, marketed by the companies that reward them so magnanimously. One should be reminded that in fact the primary aim of such gifts is to engrave in the mind of the receiver the identity of the donor and to create openly or subliminally, the obligation to reattribute [7]. The sociologists also point out that, in our case, gifts create the expectancy of reciprocity which may increase the health costs, affect the objectivity of the clinical decision, and bite the moral core of the profession, inevitably creating the appearance of a conflict of interest. It is important then, to deal openly with this issue.

The conflicts of interest

A conflict of interest arises whenever an individual or an institution has a primary duty and simultaneously a secondary one, that may overwhelm the other, or is sufficiently tempting to create the possibility or the appearance that this may occur [8]. In other words, a conflict of interest may occur in situations in which a primary duty (such as the patients well being or the validity of a research project) is unduly influenced by a secondary interest (such as a financial gain). It is important to emphasise that a conflict of interest is an occurrence, not a kind of systematic behaviour [9].

On the other hand, it is not necessarily a manifestation of wrong doing from a clinical or scientific perspective, as it remains, quite often, just an unjustified suspicion.

It is of interest to note that most of the literature on this topic is being published in the USA and the United Kingdom, but more and more countries are increasingly aware of its relevance, and its socioeconomic repercussions that go well beyond the medical profession. What Relman [10] aptly called the medical-industrial complex is one of most striking realities of our modern economics, and the industry is playing an increasing role industry in the financing and sponsorship of academic research. But perhaps the most decisive factor is that we are now living in an open society, and lawyers, economists, politicians, consumer-advocate groups, and all sorts of lay people are anxious to get into the game and to play a role in areas that were, until now, the province of a tremendously powerful corporation: the doctors.

Financial conflicts

Financial conflicts of interest are certainly the ones that have deserved a closer scrutiny. Besides the fees received for their medical acts, doctors are now being paid by the industry for lectures presenting new drugs or products, or as legal or workman's compensation experts. In these circumstances, conflicts of interest may occur.

It is also clear that physicians are increasingly investing in companies that sell products or drugs in whose investigation or trial, they are involved. As an example, in a paper [11] comparing the effectiveness of different coronary stents, seven of the twelve authors had received consulting or speaking fees from the manufacturers, and three of them owned stock of the company. Although in this case there was a clear disclosure, it is possible that, as noticed by Katz [12], doctors may somehow lose some of their moral authority to speak on health matters as the result of their financial interests.

It should be said, that this is not a question that regards exclusively the medical profession [13, 14]. The journal "Science and Engineering Ethics" of April 2001 reported that only 0.5% of 61134 papers published in 1997 in 181 peer-reviewed journals, contained a disclosure of conflict of interest of the authors.

Perhaps the most ancient economic conflict relates to professional fees. George Bernard Shaw whom, it is well known, was not particularly fond of doctors, wrote in the famous preface of "Doctor's Dilemma": "it is simply unscientific to allege or believe that doctors do not under existing circumstances, perform unnecessary operations and manufacture and prolong illnesses." This accusation is vague and difficult to substantiate, but there is evidence in the North American literature that the system of "fee for service" increases the number of unnecessary procedures. Moreover, in the "managed-care" systems in which doctors receive incentives to reduce the number of procedures or consultations with other specialities, incentives constitute forms of pressure that may affect the quality of the services rendered [15, 16].

Another delicate situation is the so called "self-referral" in which the patients are requested to obtain tests or therapeutic services in facilities owned by the referring physician. An American study demonstrates that the owners of these techniques ordered 54% more MRI, and 28% CTI scans [17]. Equally problematic is the situation that has risen in systems of "managed care" in which the patients are obligated to use contractualized services which may not have an acceptable quality level.

It is increasingly clear, that the technological and scientific growth of modern medicine has made it a very attractive business inviting doctors to take advantage of potential investment opportunities.

Intellectual conflicts

Intellectual conflicts of interest constitute a fascinating question. As noted by Marshall [18] scientists are human beings, thus subject to whims and passions, and tend to surround their own research with a mystic aura. The case of Symon LeVay, a homosexual neurobiologist who published a much publicized paper on gender differences in the size of one of the hypothamic nuclei between the brain of homosexuals (similar to the female brain) and heterosexuals, is often quoted as exemplary. This observation, which was not confirmed by other researchers, might have been tainted by the strong wish to find a biological support for homosexuality.

A strong adversary stance against the risks of tobacco, alcohol or certain drugs may likewise determine the design of the research methodology or the way the results are reported. An ideological bias enforced by repressive political systems was responsible for the infamous research by Nazi doctors which led to death penalties imposed to seven physicians during the Nuremberg trials. The imposition of the absurd genetic theories of Lyssenko or the abject use of psychiatry to eliminate the foes of the regime, in the former Soviet Union, also illustrate the perversity of these types of conflicts. Recently, it is being questioned the complicity of researchers associated with the prestigious "Kaiser Wilhelm Institute" in Germany, who were involved in studies on racial differences, using material collected from victims of concentration camps [19].

Other forms of intellectual conflict were pointed out by Horrobin [8]. For instance, an ideological stance against capitalism or the pharmaceutical industry may oppose any form of financing by it. A philosophical bias may again determine scientific agendas and policies. For some, nutritional factors or a medicine of life-styles is crucial for health maintenance, while others deny the importance of their role.

Finally, Horrobin cites as the most important cause of intellectual conflict the passionate defence of a certain theoretical model and imagines a scientist writing as a conclusion of a paper: "I am delighted by these results since they justify the 25 years I have spent following this line of research".

Conflicts in surgery

There are two types of conflict that are peculiar to surgical specialities. One is related to the surgeon–inventor of instruments, devices or prosthesis [20]. In this situation, the author is both interested not only in demonstrating the safety and efficacy of its product, but also in its promotion, from which he expects to receive dividends. It should be noted that, in this situation, neither efficacy nor safety can usually be demonstrated by randomized controlled trials. Furthermore, in the evaluation of new products, the surgeon may tend to exclude patients whose condition and hence prospect of unsatisfactory results may affect the reputation of the product under scrutiny. It is also likely that the surgeon-inventor will try his product in his/her own patients which may cause a certain psychological coercion. Equally, if he/she does not test the device on his/her own patients, other surgeons would ask why not.

The second type of surgical conflict is more subtle and relates to what Foster [7] calls "funkionslust", a concept based on the behaviourist theories of Konrad Lorenz, which describes the pleasure and pride in performing certain functions well, which may be the reward for many years perfecting a certain technique. But in surgery this may bring conflicts: the preference for a more complex procedure when a simpler one would do the job, reluctance to send the patient to another specialist, or the resistance to learn a new technique. The primary interest of the patient may be relegated in favour of more personal, albeit understandable human foibles.

We believe that a point of major concern relates to the increasing role neurosurgeons play in promoting industry driven medical devices. This is particularly blatant in the field of spine surgery, with the use of prosthetic material which has not been subjected to a rigorous critical evaluation not only of its therapeutic usefulness, but also in a cost-efficacy perspective. The conflict of interest in these areas are now being subjected to increased scrutiny by health authorities, particularly in the USA". I think this addresses all the points raised.

It is unquestionable that much of the progress in our field is due to innovation and technological developments and contributions from physicians in these areas are invaluable. It is therefore an undeniable professional duty, with correlative ethical implications, for surgeons to participate in the critical evaluation of new technologies and this includes, by necessity, cost-benefit analysis. We shouldn't forget that we are our patients' best advocates and should strive for putting the new technologies at their service. However, the tremendous increase in health care costs demands from us to be concerned with our patients, the patients of our colleagues and even the future patients, and therefore, we should play a decisive role as independent partners in the definition of health care policies. It should be reminded that recent concerns about the threats to medical professionalism demand that we should fight to maintain its foundational values such as altruism, compassion, integrity, truth and competence, and these should not collide with management goals.

Conflicts in academic duties

The academic physician often faces the challenging dilemma of how to balance equitably the time spent in academic, clinical, teaching and managerial activities. Each one of them seeks to claim precedence, their relevance and relative weight varies according to the circumstances, and each one being subject to different and increasingly demanding forms of evaluation. At present, more and more time is asked of clinical and academic leaders to spend on administrative duties, in part due to increasing scrutiny on the use of finite resources and legal constraints.

As educators, doctors have to deal with the inevitable tension between the duty to care for their patients and the training of future specialists. Foster [7] has rehearsed the question of how and when to decide that a resident is ready to operate on his or her first patient and how is he or she chosen. Are we aware of this conflict of interest when we delegate this responsibility to our junior colleagues? There is, however, clear evidence of the high quality of the services rendered by teaching hospitals and that, with adequate supervision, there is no difference between the results obtained by the trainees or their tutors. But it is crucial that the patient himself understands that he is fulfilling an important social duty, as he constitutes, a vital teaching tool, provided that the quality of care is guaranteed. Bernstein [21] has emphasized that open recognition of the potential ethical tension inherent in the teaching of surgical technique is the first and most important step in solving the intrinsic conflict generated.

The relationship with industry

Most of the literature on conflicts of interest in clinical practice pertains to relationships with industry particularly with the pharmaceutical industry [22–26].

In countries like the USA and the United Kingdom, the funding of biomedical research by industry has grown remarkably. In the USA the industry paid 32% in 1980, and 62% in 2000, of the expenses of clinical trials. The influence of the industry goes well beyond this aspect. Shamasunder and Bero [27] have called attention to the relationships between the pharmaceutical industry and the tobacco companies and how the latter have tried to soften up the marketing of programs for giving up smoking.

In biomedicine, it is the private sector and not academic medicine that develops most of the diagnostic techniques and products used in the treatment and prevention of illnesses, and is also responsible for their marketing. In the most industrialized countries, the universities are deeply involved in investing in "start-up" companies and support research by their members. Many neurosurgeons involved in the research and development of products, have financial ties with the companies that promote them.

Two factors have contributed to the recent interest in the topic of conflicts of interest in these areas. Firstly, was the news of the death of a patient who was participating as a volunteer in a phase I gene therapy trial in which the researcher and the hospital had financial interests [28].

Secondly there has been the suspicion of bias in the reporting of the results of therapeutical trials when the authors have financial ties with the manufacturing companies. The study of Stelfox *et al.* [29] on calcium antagonists is frequently cited and purportedly demonstrates a positive bias when the authors were associated with the manufacturer. Davidson [30] showed that the report of positive results with new drugs increases if the study is financed by the producer. Finally, and there are many more examples, Friedberg *et al.* [31] showed that studies of the pharmo-economics of oncological drugs supported by the industry reported 5% of unfavourable results in contrast to 38% by non financed studies.

This is certainly a complex and confused issue. Some have pointed out that the methodology of these sort of trials may be designed to favour positive results. This may be achieved by selecting patient groups with a lower rate of co morbidities, or less severe forms of disease [32] called the attention to the fact that in efficacy studies of anti-inflammatory non-steroidal drugs, only 21% of the target population were younger than 65 years of age [33]. It should be noticed, however, that for a drug to reach a phase III, trial it has to go through a strict process of evaluation, and therefore the industry anticipates a probability of success that justifies the investment made. On the other hand, some have suggested that the new drugs are tested against sub optimal doses of other medications already approved and, some studies may include multiple surrogate endpoints, but only the ones which shed a more favourable light on the "new" drug are published.

Montagner *et al.* [34] quote a study that demonstrates that there is no qualitative difference in the methodology of studies funded by the industry and the ones which are not so funded, but others found the first type more reliable. It is possible that the preponderance of positive results in funded trials is due to a tighter pre-selection of the drugs that are pursued to further advanced stages of clinical evaluation.

It is useful to consider the different interests that come into play in biomedical research. From the standpoint of the public, what really matters is that research that is paid for indirectly by the consumer is geared towards the search to independent truth. It matters that those discoveries with potential therapeutic benefit be transferred as soon as possible, after careful, well designed studies, to clinical practice. Finally, it is essential that participation in clinical trials be safe, supported by informed consent, with rapid access to the results, and with an adequate follow-up. The patients or volunteers should also be informed about all possible side-effects that may influence their decision to participate.

This is an area that has deserved a lot of attention because of the death of some volunteers [28, 35]. These cases have raised a number of very important issues concerning both the researchers individually, and the institutional review boards, such as the excessive haste in obtaining results, the incomplete search for possible toxicity of the products tried, the potential vulnerability of employees or medical students to the pressure to serve as volunteers, and the influence of payments received [34]. The need to change the rules of functioning of the review boards and the use of external boards, have been advocated particularly for multicentre studies.

Finally, it has to be guaranteed that the researcher is not subjected to any kind of external pressure that may affect the selection of the subjects or the publication of results. As mentioned by Bodenheimer [25] many research contracts submitted by the industry have unacceptable publication clauses that have to be renegotiated.

The primary interest of researcher is simply stated the publication in first rate journals of the result of their work. Clearly, this sort of recognition is indisputably a professional asset and may contribute to progression up the academic ladder and strengthens the ties with the industry, with increasing participation in new projects and consequent financial reward.

The interests of the industry are equally simple to enunciate and are the approval and commercialization of new products. Publication of results without peer review is not worth much but publication of results in a first rate journal is very important for the marketing of a new product [25].

It is understandable that there is an inevitable tension between health care delivery and the investigation of new drugs or techniques. The clinician involved in this kind of research is interested in gathering patients for the study, the speedy conclusion of the project and the publication of results. But he has to safeguard the medical component of his task, in a context that may create what has been called "therapeutic misunderstanding" [36]. In fact, "patient-volunteers" may believe that the experimental procedures or drug in trial are prescribed for an anticipated real benefit, even when this is explicitly denied in the consent form. In fact, although the possibility of benefit may be implicit in any therapeutic trial, this is not usually its primary goal. Freedman [37] has indicated the attention that some phase I studies of oncological drugs called studies of efficacy and safety, are designed objectively to determine the maximum tolerated dose, and to call them efficacy studies is misleading.

It is, however, important to consider that an inappropriate "clinical bias" may undermine the scientific validity of the study, by bypassing the randomization process or the "blind" evaluation of the results. Miller at al. [26] have suggested monitoring by a non-participating physician, who may act as a patient's advocate and verify the ethical competence of the researchers.

The relationships between industry and the universities have been raised in numerous debates [38–43], particularly in the American literature, and some have even asked rhetorically if academic medicine is "not for sale". As pointed out by Marciall Angell [44], the ties between clinical researchers and industry assume multiple forms such as grants, consulting fees, dividends, the agreement to borrow the name for articles written by request, the promotion of products in seminars and congresses, etc. The generosity of the industry, in Angell's critical view, knows no limits, has nefarious consequences, and may create in the young physician the mistaken impression that for every problem there is a pill and somebody from the company to push it.

There is a remarkable variety of policies in dealing with the conflicts of interest in various medical schools and research institutes [35] and, given the diversity of the regulations of different journals and financing agencies, the present rules may no longer be adequate to preserve scientific integrity.

It is not my purpose to discuss this matter in further detail, and although this may seem primarily an "American" problem, the truth is that globalization of medical research makes this a question that should be dealt with openly in any country involved in this type of research. It is known that nowadays about 60% of trials of new drugs in the USA are conducted by private organizations, the "Contract Research Organizations", that contract directly the physicians involved, many of them without hospital affiliations [25, 40, 45]. Since some hospitals or clinics are not particularly suitable or used to this kind of work the so-called "Site Management Organizations", which are independent business enterprises, may help to do the job. Furthermore, there are now private ethical review committees, which also may raise puzzling ethical questions, as it is reasonable to assume that committees with more benevolent criteria may be preferred to the ones with more stringent criteria.

Another concern is mentioned in the literature and relates to the academic output of doctors that are subsidized by industry. A study by Blumenthal *et al.* [46] indicates that there is no difference between them and the non-paid doctors. There are, however, two differences. The "industry physicians" are more productive from the commercial standpoint, and more reserved in communicating their results to their own colleagues. There is therefore, a legitimate fear that the emphasis on commercially rewarding research may have negative repercussions on basic science which is without immediate foreseeable applications.

Conflicts over communication

Publication of the results of industrially financed research is now a matter of grave concern, particularly since it has become apparent that there is a strong resistance to the publication of negative results, by delaying the reporting of unfavourable outcomes. Furthermore, there is evidence that the access of the researchers to the results may be restricted, and there is an occasional practice of hiring "ghost-writers", who did not participate in the investigation to write of the manuscript. On the other hand, historically there has not always been a well defined policy of disclosure of conflict of interest of the authors, the reviewers of the manuscripts, and even of the authors of review articles [47]. However this situation is rapidly changing. The editors of some of the most prestigious international medical journals [48] (such as Lancet, JAMA,

New England Journal of Medicine) have proposed new guidelines to correct a situation that was challenging the credibility of scientific communication in clinical medicine. In fact, an interesting study by Chaudhry *et al.* [49] analyzing whether the disclosure of conflict of interest affected the evaluation by the readers of the reliability of the results, seems to confirm that trust was a diminished when the authors were financed by the industry, in the case of this article, a fictious company.

The journals that have approved such guidelines now demand a clear statement on the personal and financial ties with industry. Moreover, they call the attention for the need for research contracts to guarantee that there should be no limitation of access to the data, and no interference with their analysis, and with the preparation and publication of the manuscript.

It is therefore necessary to describe in detail the role of the sponsor in the collection, analysis, interpretation and publication of the data. It is the role of the editors to assure that there is no conflict of interest involving the reviewers and the editors themselves should abstain from participating in decisions in which they may have a vested interest, personally, professionally or financially.

In such a complex area, the academy must play a leading role, starting with the safety and well being of the participants in clinical trials [50]. It should be the guardian of such fundamental values as the freedom to publish, the objectivity and integrity of the data, and the regulation of economic incentives, which should contemplate both senior and junior scientists. This is underscored in the recommendations of the Task Force of the American Association of Medical Colleges in 2003 [51, 52], that emphasize the importance of distinguishing the strictly scientific aspects of any research project from investment and technological transfer policies.

Conclusions

As I pointed out at the beginning, one of the fundamental aspects that characterize professionalism is the duty to self-regulate. This is carried on by legal and ethical codes, as well as by the intervention of a number of professional regulatory bodies. Ethical codes have to preserve the basic foundation of professional values but the changes in social, economic, political and cultural conditions, as well as the new ethical challenges that the scientific and technological progress are continuously raising, demand the clarification of some rules and even the definition of new ones.

This occurred, for instance, in regard to such questions as medical advertising, relationships with industry and, sooner or later, to complex maters such as "enhancement" technologies, (like searching for better memory, more intelligence, longer life span or engineering desired traits, thus creating the so called "design-babies") therapeutic cloning or even euthanasia.

Professional regulation has extended also to domains such as certification and recertification of competence, accreditation of services and hospitals in matters of teaching and training. Societal scrutiny of medical activity is increasingly vigilant. This is performed informally by the "media" for which the "bad deeds" of doctors are always news and formally by various organizations public or private, including insurance companies and other third party payers.

They are particularly attentive to areas such as professional competence, which were, until quite recently, the exclusive domain of physicians' organizations, but also to the management of resources and the overview of potential conflicts of interest.

The mechanisms of regulation of professionalism have become more demanding and sophisticated, with proliferation of statutes, regulations and guidelines. The statements of the editors of medical journals mentioned before, or the recommendation of the task-force of the Association of American Medical Colleges to regulate the financial conflicts of interest of researchers and institutions clearly illustrate this point [51, 52]. Even research institutions such as the Howard Hughes Medical Institute [53] have found it necessary to define their own code which, in the latter case, limits to 5% the amount of stock owned by scientists in the companies with which they collaborate. They are also concerned about preserving the scientific autonomy including the right to publish their results, and establishing a maximum limit of 90 days to obtain a patent, if required.

The American College of Physicians and the American Society of Internal Medicine have also drafted guidelines concerning the ethical aspects of the relationships between industry and the clinical practice [54]. The fact that they felt it necessary to address such questions as the new modalities of "e-commerce" illustrates the tremendous revolution in this field.

Many of the control mechanisms should be supported by prophylactic rules that have to be included in ethical codes. The disclosure of conflicts of interest should be open and this is certainly better to the profession that the persistent suspicion of illegitimate gains [54, 55] that undermines its credibility and prestige. It is also important to accept the fact that ethical scrutiny is no longer the exclusive duty of the physician, and he should favour a plural and multidisciplinary intervention. This may contribute to finding the right equilibrium between the role to guarantee the safety and protection of patients and volunteers and the aim to pursuing the scientific inquiry whilst abiding by the rules of methodological rigor. The review boards should therefore include scientists, informed lay people, and patients' representatives, who may actually not be totally immune to pressures or dangerous liaisons [56]. This is the only way to achieve what Hannah Arendt called the art of representative thinking. In any circumstance, as Henry Beecher [57] wrote in a celebrated article published in 1966 on the ethics of clinical investigation, "the most reliable safeguard (is) provided by the presence of an intelligent, informed, conscientious, compassionate, responsible investigator".

References

1. Hazard GC Jr (1996) Conflicts of interest in the classic professions. In: Spece Jr RG, Shim DS, Buchanan AE (eds) Conflicts of interest in clinical practice and research. Oxford University Press, pp 85–104
2. Medical professionalism in the new millennium: a physicians' charter. Lancet 359: 520–522, 2002
3. Rothman DJ (2000) Medical professionalism – focusing on the real issues. N Engl J Med 342: 1284–1286
4. Swick HM (2000) Toward a normative definition of medical professionalism. Acad Med 75: 612–616
5. Bloche MG (1999) Clinical loyalties and the social purposes of medicine. JAMA 281: 268–274
6. Jonsen A (1983) Watching the doctor. N Engl Med 308: 1531–1532
7. Foster RS Jr (2003) Conflicts of interest: recognition, disclosure, and management. J Am Coll Surg 196: 505–517
8. Horrobin DF (1999) Non-financial conflicts of interest are more serious than financial conflicts. BMJ 318: 466
9. Cohen JJ (2001) Trust us to make a difference: ensuring public confidence in the integrity of clinical research. Acad Med 76: 209–214
10. Relman AS (1980) The new medical-industrial complex. N Engl J Med 303: 963–970
11. Moses JW, Leon MB, Popma JJ *et al.* (2003) Sirolimus-eluting stents versus standard stents in patients with stenosis in a native coronary artery. N Engl J Med 349: 1315–1323
12. Katz J (1996) Informed consent to medical entrepreneurialism. In: Spece RG Jr, Shim DS, Buchanan AE (eds) Conflicts of interest in clinical practice and research. Oxford University Press
13. Can you believe what you read? Nature 416: 360–363, 2002
14. Holden C (2001) Few authors disclose conflicts, survey finds. Science 292: 829
15. Armour BS, Pitts MM, Maclean T *et al.* (2001) The effect of explicit financial incentives on physician behavior. Arch Intern Med 161: 1261–1266
16. Grumbach K, Osmond D, Uranizan K *et al.* (1998) Primary care physicians' experience of financial incentives in managed – care systems. N Engl J Med 339: 1516–1521
17. Mitchell JM (1996) Physician joint ventures and self-referral: an empirical perspective. In: Spece RG Jr, Shim DS, Buchanan AE (eds) Conflicts of interest in clinical practice and research. Oxford University Press
18. Marshall E (1992) When does intellectual passion become conflict of interest? Science 257: 620–622
19. Koenig R (2000) Reopening the darkest chapter in German science. Science 288: 1576–1577
20. Elks ML (1995) Conflict of interest and the physician-researcher. J Lab Clin Med 126: 19–23
21. Bernstein M (2003) Surgical teaching: how should neurosurgeons handle the conflict of duty to today's patients with the duty to tomorrows? Br J Neurosurg 17: 121–123
22. Agnew B (2000) Financial conflicts of interest get more scrutiny in clinical trials. Science 289: 66–67

23. Alpert JS, Furman S, Smaha L (2002) Conflicts of interest. Science, money and health. Arch Intern Med 162: 635–637
24. Bekelman JE, Li Y, Gross CP (2003) Scope and impact of financial conflicts of interest in biomedical research. A systematic review. JAMA 289: 454–465
25. Bodenheimer T (2000) Uneasy alliance. Clinical investigators and the pharmaceutical industry. N Engl J Med 342: 1539–1544
26. Miller FG, Rosenstein DL, De Renzo EG (1998) Professional integrity in clinical research. JAMA 286: 1449–1454
27. Shamasunder B, Bero L (2002) Financial ties and conflicts of interest between pharmaceutical and tobacco companies. JAMA 288: 738–744
28. Lewinsky NG (2002) Nonfinancial conflicts of interest in research. N Eng J Med 347: 759–761
29. Stelfox HT, Chua G, O'Rourke K *et al.* (2000) Conflict of interest in the debate over calcium-channel antagonists. N Engl J Med 342: 1539–1544
30. Davidson RA (1986) Source of funding and outcome of clinical trials. J Gen Intern Med 1: 155–158
31. Friedberg M, Saffran B, Stinson TJ *et al.* (1999) Evaluation of conflict of interest in economic analyses of new drugs in oncology. JAMA 282: 1453–1457
32. Rochon PA, Berger PB, Gordon M (1996) The evolution of clinical trials: inclusion and representation CMAJ 159: 1373–1374
33. Rochon PA, Gurwitz JH, Simons RW *et al.* (1994) A study of manufacturer – supported trials of nonsteroidal anti-inflammatory drugs in the treatment of arthritis. Arch Intern Med 154: 157–163
34. Montagner JSG, O'Shaughnessy MV, Shetchter MT (2001) Industry sponsored clinical research: a double edged sword. Lancet 358: 1893–1895
35. Lo B, Wolf LE (2000) Berkeley? Conflict-of-interest policies for investigators in clinical trials. N Eng J Med 343: 1616–1620
36. Appelbaum PS, Roth LH, Lidz CW *et al.* (1987) False hopes and best data: consent to research and the therapeutic misconception. Hastings Cent Rep 17: 20–24
37. Freedman B (1996) The ethical analysis of clinical trials: new lessons for and from cancer research. In: Vanderpool HY (ed) The ethics of research involving human subjects. Frederick, MD. University Publishing Group
38. Cho MK, Shohara R, Schissel A *et al.* (2000) Policies on faculty conflicts of interest at US Universities. JAMA 284: 2203–2208
39. Gross CP, Gupta AR, Krumholz HM (2003) Disclosure of financial competing interests in randomised controlled trial: cross sectional review. BMJ 326: 526–527
40. Johns MME, Barnes M, Florencio PS (2003) Restoring balance to industry – academia relationships in an era of institutional financial conflicts of interest. Promoting research while maintaining trust. JAMA 289: 741–746
41. Korn D (2002) Industry, academy, investigator: managing the relationships. Acad Med 77: 1089–1095
42. Martin JB, Kasper DL (2000) In whose best interest? Breaching the academic – industry wall. N Engl J Med 343: 1646–1649
43. Schulmann KA, Seils DM, Timbie JW *et al.* (2002) A national survey of provisions in clinical-trial agreements between medical schools and industry sponsors. N Engl J Med 347: 1335–1341

44. Angell M (2000) Is academic medicine for sale? N Engl J Med 342: 1516–1518
45. Morin K, Ratansky H, Riddick FA Jr *et al.* (2002) Managing conflicts of interest in the conduct of clinical trials. JAMA 287: 78–84
46. Blumenthal D, Campbell EG, Causino N *et al.* (1996) Participation of life science faculty in research relationships with industry. N Engl J Med 335: 1734–1739
47. Angell M (2000) Disclosure of authors' conflicts of interest: a follow-up. N Engl J Med 342: 586–587
48. Davidoff F, De Angelis CD, Drazen JM *et al.* (2001) Sponsorship, authorship and accountability. Lancet 358: 854–856
49. Chaudhry S, Schroter S, Smith R *et al.* (2002) Does declaration of competing interests affect readers' perceptions? A randomised trial. BMJ 325: 1391–1392
50. Steinbrook R (2002) Improving protection for research subjects. N Engl J Med 346: 1425–1430
51. AAMC Task Force on financial conflicts of interest in clinical research. Protecting subjects, preserving trust, promoting progress I: policy and guidelines for the oversight of individual financial interests in human subject's research. Acad Med 78: 225–236, 2003
52. AAMC Task Force on financial conflicts of interest in clinical research. Protecting subjects, preserving trust, promoting progress II: principles and recommendations for oversight of an institution's financial interests in human subjects research. Acad Med 78: 237–245, 2003
53. Cech TR, Leonard JS (2001) Conflicts of interest – moving beyond disclosure. Science 291: 989
54. Coyle SL *et al.* (2002) Physician – industry relations. Part 1: individual physicians. Ann Intern Med 136: 396–402
55. De Angelis CD, Fontanarosa PB, Flanagin A (2001) Reporting financial conflicts of interest and relationships between investigators and research sponsors. JAMA 286: 89–91
56. Little M (1999) Research, ethics and conflicts of interest. J Med Ethics 25: 259–262
57. Beecher HK (1966) Ethics and clinical research. N Eng J Med 274: 1354–1360

Offprint from
Advances and Technical Standards in Neurosurgery, Vol. 32
Edited by J.D. Pickard

Neurosurgical treatment of perineal neuralgias

R. ROBERT[1], J. J. LABAT[2], T. RIANT[1], M. KHALFALLAH[3], and O. HAMEL[1]

[1] Service de Neurotraumatologie, Nantes, France
[2] Service d'Urologie, Nantes, France
[3] Service de Neurochirurgie, Centre Hospitalier de la côte Basque, Bayonne, France

With 9 Figures

Contents

Abstract

Perineal pain is the basis of presentation to different specialities. This pain is still rather unknown and leads the different teams to inappropriate treatments which may fail.

For more than twenty years, we have seen these patients in a multidisciplinary consultation. Our anatomical works have provided a detailed knowledge of the nervous supply of the perineum which allowed us to propose the description of an entrapment syndrome of the pudendal nerve. Other disturbances of different origins were highlighted helping colleagues to a better analysis of this enigmatic painful syndrome.

Cadaveric studies have been done to guide treatments by blocks and surgery if necessary according to well defined criteria.

A randomized prospective study validated the surgery. The retrospective study concluded that two thirds of the patients improved after treatment. New anatomical concepts are leading us to enlarge the field of this type of surgery, with the hope of improving the success rate.

Keywords: Perineal pain; pudendal neuralgias; Alcock's tunnel syndrome; pudendal nerve surgery; blocks of the pudendal nerve.

Introduction

Perineal neuralgias are usually misunderstood and lead patients to medical nomadism and misdiagnosis.

Very often specialised medical teams relate such pain to the pathology of one organ, more often pelvic than perineal. The treatment is then guided by this target organ and leads to surgical techniques (hysterectomy, prostatectomy...) which fail and leave a disappointed patient. Radiological data is verified to be normal and then we may think that the pain arises from a truncal palsy. The fact is that the pain is situated in the sensory territory of the pudendal nerve and that it occurs when in the seated position. We undertook an anatomical study to define possible sources of entrapment along the course of the nerve by positioning cadavers in the seated position. Subsequently a neurophysiological approach led us to consider that in many cases prolonged distal motor latency was usually found just like in carpal tunnel syndrome. Treatment is based on nerve blocks guided by CT scan and surgery by a transgluteal approach. We consider that perineal neuralgia is not commonly a pudendal nerve palsy, and is, an entrapment syndrome in the deep spaces of the buttock.

We will exclude all pain with a local explanation (dermatological infections, tumours and so on).

Anatomy, pathology and nosology

Pelvi-perineal pains (PPP) are not rare. It is estimated that up to 3.8% of women aged between 15 and 73 years old suffer from PPP which is more than migraine (2.1%), identical to asthma, and a little less than lumbar pain (4.1%). 15% of gynaecological consultations are for vulvodynia. Pelvic pain is excluded from this study. The pelvis and the perineal spaces are separated from each other by the levator ani muscle. Local disorders such as tumour, dermatological lesions, haemorrhoid, etc. must be recognized and treated. This chapter considers only perineal neuropathic pain of which three different groups must be distinguished:

Neuropathic somatic perineal pain

The perineum is supplied by somatic nerves which are divided into two groups

- sacral origin: pudendal and inferior cluneal nerves
- thoraco-lumbar origin: ilio-hypogastric, ilio-inguinal, genito-femoral and obturator nerves.

Neuropathic visceral pain

This is mediated by the sympathetic system and constitutes most pelvic pain as the sympathetic system infiltrates all the viscera of this area (interstial cystitis, vulvar vestibulitis, levator ani syndrome, orchialgias ...). Urethralgias are typical perineal visceral pain and may be the equivalent of interstial cystitis. Their presentation is quite different from somatic pain. Nevertheless, sympathetic dysfunction can be noted even when only the pudendal nerve is damaged, as this nerve includes sympathetic fibers.

Myofascial pain

This consists of myofascial syndromes which may be components of fibromyalgia. On the other hand, "single" muscular contractures may lead to pathological disorders. Piriformis or internal obturator muscles syndromes lead to a gluteal pain with an ischiatic component in the inferior limb. They can be encountered with a true pudendal palsy.

Pudendal nerve entrapment

Clinical features [34]

The population is mostly in the 50–70-year old age group, with 60% being females. This incidence may be the result of pregnancy which causes a pulling effect which leads to a kind of fragility of the nerves.

The standard clinical presentation is an adult patient with uni- or bilateral pain in the anal, uro-genital or both areas of the perineum, exacerbated in the seated position [15, 23]. It's a neuropathic pain [7]. Pain is located in the territory of the pudendal nerve. We must be careful and distinguish a scrotal pain (pudendal nerve) from a testicular pain (thoraco-lumbar pathology).

Mostly the onset is insidious, but a lot of patients believe that the starting point of the pain is from a pelvi-perineal surgery, forgetting the fact that this surgery was first done to relieve pain. Anyway, surgery of the hip joint with traction of the leg may induce pudendal nerve compression [11, 32]. Gynaecological surgery with hysterectomy by a trans perineal approach may be responsible for pain as the surgeons hang the vagina with wires around the sacrospinal ligament and may then entrap the nerve in the suture [1, 29, 35].

Sitting on the toilet is not painful. Pain is absent in the early morning and increases during the day, and leads to a complete avoidance of the seated position. Cycling is a classic factor which leads to pain [2]. Driving too. A fall can also be advocated. Standing or lying makes the pain decrease or vanish at the beginning of the symptoms. It is usually a burning pain without any dysfunction of the sphincters and perineal function. Associated signs may lead to a wrong diagnosis: sciatica may be noted, which is incomplete most of time, reaching only the popliteal fossa. The muscular component explains such radiation. Pollakiuria may be noted as well as dysuria, but they are just functional syndromes referred to the pain. Sexual disturbances are not frequent although such activities are avoided because of pain. Constipation is more frequent and leads to perineal efforts which damage the nerve.

Neurological examination is normal (no sensory impairment, no motor weakness, positive reflexes). Intra rectal manipulation reproduces a pain mostly at the ischiatic spine level and in Alcock's canal.

Intractable chronic pain has significant emotional consequences and a psychological component is an integral part of the pain process. After surgery performed on an organ that brings no benefit, patients are in a state of distress being unable to enjoy their lives (no cinema, no restaurant, difficulties for driving cars and bikes or motorbikes, no desire for sex because of the pain).

To summarize:

- it is a neuropathic pain (burning pain) with sometimes allodynia, corresponding to the territory of the pudendal nerve;
- pain increases or only exists in the seated position.

Anatomical datas

We thought from the beginning of our studies that this perineal pain was due to a pudendal nerve pathology. The fact that the seated position would lead to pain led us to believe that an entrapment syndrome might exist [15, 23, 25].

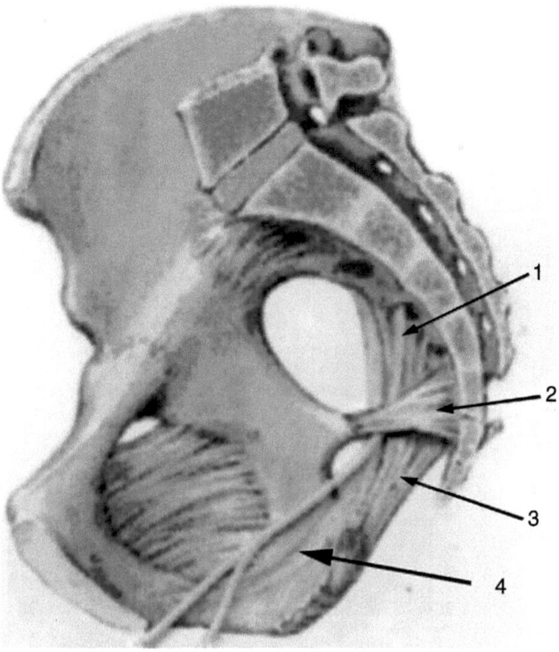

Fig. 1. Medial view of a right hemipelvis showing the course of the pudendal nerve. *1* Pudendal nerve, *2* sacrospinous ligament, *3* sacrotuberal ligament, *4* falciform process

The pudendal nerve (Fig. 1) arises mostly from the S3 root, sometimes from S2 and S4. Its course starts in the presacral area, then it goes laterally to penetrate the greater ischial aperture under the piriformis muscle medial to the ischiatic nerve. In the gluteal region, it crosses behind the distal insertion of the sacro-spinal ligament, then goes medially to enter the pudendal tunnel in the inner aspect of the ischial tuberosity. In its perineal course, the nerve is in the infra-levatori space, and is situated within the internal obturator muscle fascia (Alcock's canal) (Fig. 2). Its branches perforate this fascia to reach their target zones (Fig. 3). The motor branches supply the external striated sphincters of the anus, the urethra and the erector muscles. The sensory fibres supply the skin of the anal region, the intermediate perineum, the penis or the clitoris, the scrotum or the labia.

According to our work on cadavers, three potential entrapment zones can be described:

- In the gluteal region, between the sacro-tuberal and the sacro-spinous ligaments which cross each other;
- At the entry to Alcock's canal by the falciform process of the sacro-tuberal ligament;
- In the pudendal canal, among the splitting of the internal obturator fascia.

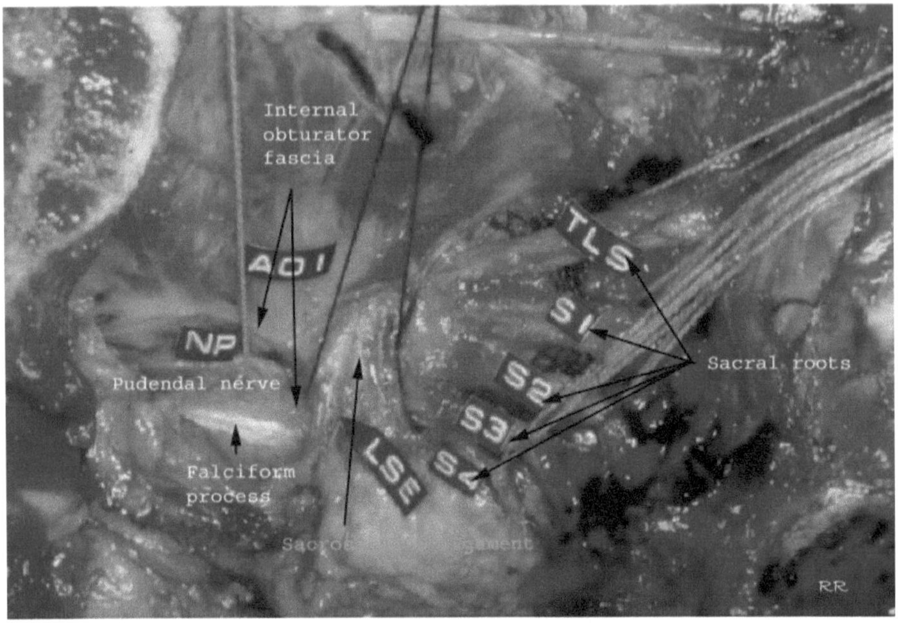

Fig. 2. Medial view of a right hemipelvis. The pudendal nerve starts from mainly the third sacral root in the presacral area, then enters the gluteal region around the sacrospinous ligament, and then goes through the pudendal tunnel in the fascia of the internal obturator muscle which has been resected here

In the seated position on cadavers we can see the ascension of the ischiorectal fat tissue which leads to compression of the nerve trunk at the 3 levels mentioned above (Fig. 4).

Neurophysiological data

An objective test was required to confirm a compression component. According to evaluation of other well known entrapment syndromes such as carpal tunnel syndrome, we have devised a distal motor latency (DML) test by stimulating with a finger electrode in the rectum, and recording the responses in the erector muscles. This DML must be less than 5 milliseconds [3].

Radiological data

Tumoral pathology must be excluded in the pelvi-perineal area by an MRI or at least a CT scan. Sometimes, calcification of the sacro-spinal ligament or benign osteogenic tumor of the ischiopubic branch can be noted and may induce a compression of the nerve.

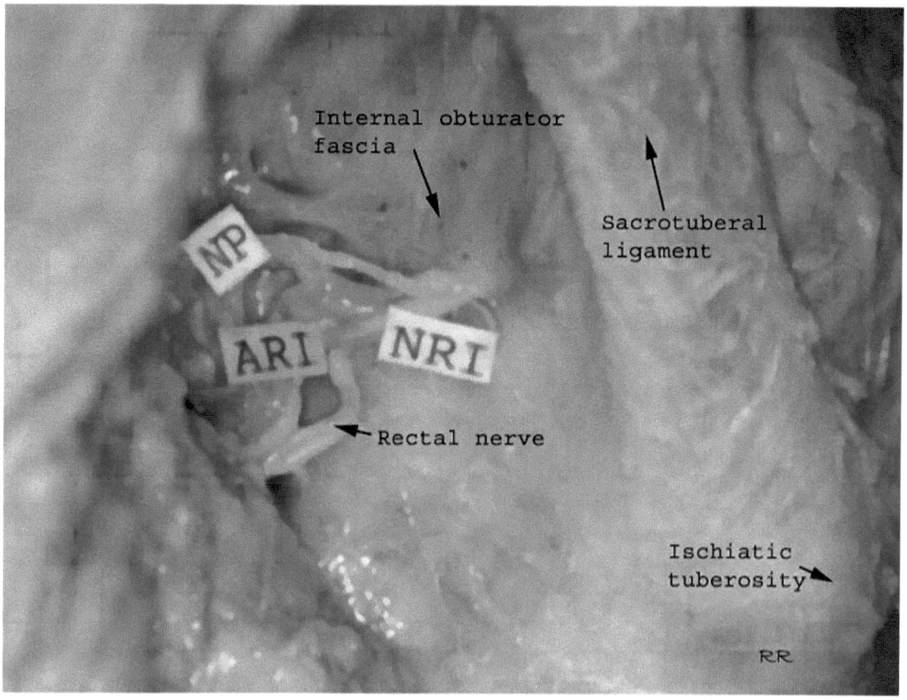

Fig. 3. Posterior view of the right side of the entry of the pudendal nerve in the pudendal (Alcock's) tunnel. The proximal branches of the nerve perforate the fascia of the internal obturator muscle to reach the anal region

Treatment

Medical therapy

Medical treatments based on anti-convulsivant and anti-depressant medications for neuropathic pain are insufficient, but can bring mild relief.

Blocks

Such techniques are both diagnostic and therapeutic.

Those techniques must be performed under very standardised conditions [6, 13]. A CT scanner must be used with injection of local anaesthetic and steroids. The patient is in a prone position in the CT scanner. The needle is inserted under local anaesthesia toward the ischiatic spine and displaced in the inner part of it. Paraesthesias may occur which signifies the good position of the injection. Contrast product is then injected, followed by local anaesthetic and steroids. For a block in the internal obturator fascia, the same conditions are required. The needle must be parallel to the muscle, in the inner part of it.

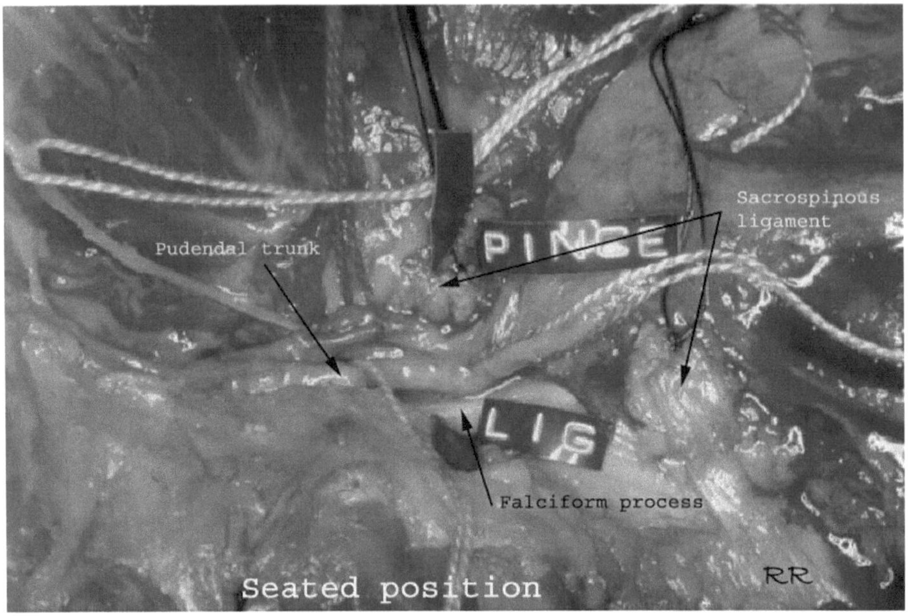

Fig. 4. Medial view of a right hemipelvis. The cadaver is in a seated position. The fat of the ischiorectal fossa lifts and may entrap the nerve in the internal obturator muscle fascia, and in the claw between the sacrotuberal and the sacrospinous ligaments. The falciform process if tall may also damage the nerve

Just after the blocks, the patient is kept in a seated position for half an hour. Then a Visual Analogic Scale (VAS) is established to appreciate the analgesic effect of the local peritruncular block which is an important diagnostic test. The efficacy of the steroid will be judged two or three weeks later. This treatment can be sufficient and done two or three times. Only patients with a positive diagnostic test and no long term side effect of the steroids should be offered surgery.

Surgical procedure

This has been described previously in the literature [23]. We started using a perineal approach in 1986. The problems encountered were deep incision through the firm fat tissue in the ischio-rectal space; problems with hemostasis of huge and numerous veins; difficulties in reaching the main point of entrapment, i.e. the claw between the sacro-tuberal and the sacro-spinal ligaments. There were significant risks of sepsis. Moreover, patients felt pain when sitting on their perineal scar for some days following surgery. Hence, we decided to use a transgluteal approach which has been adopted with good results by other

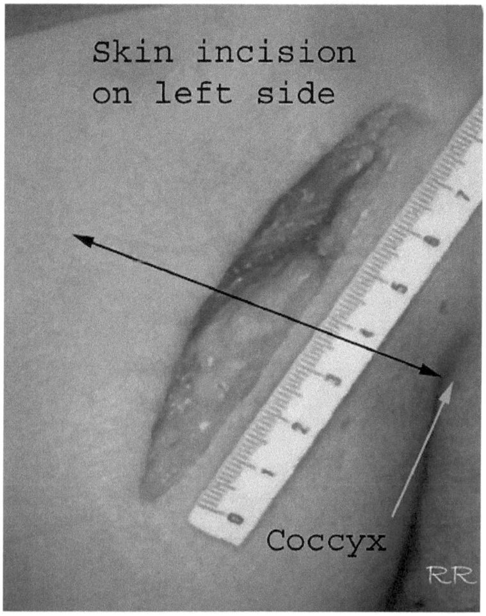

Fig. 5. Skin incision on the left side according to the obliquity of the gluteus maximus muscle fibres

teams [4, 22, 28]. Recently, a transperineal approach has been analyzed nevertheless [5].

Our transgluteal approach [25] allows all possible entrapments that we have detailed to be corrected easily in a single incision. Under general anesthesia, the patient is placed in the so called genu-pectoral position. In this position that we have only been using for a couple of months, the exploration is easier deep in Alcock's canal, better than in the "classical" single lying position. A gluteal incision of about 7 cm in length is made uni or bilaterally on both sides of a transversal line from the top of the coccyx, oriented obliquely according to the direction of the gluteus maximus fibres which are dissected and disinserted from the sacro-tuberal ligament (Fig. 5). The narrow section of this structure is resected transversely with the scissors (Figs. 6 and 7). We must remember that the nerve can go through a layer of the sacro-tuberal ligament and could be severed when cutting it. It is situated at the exact level of the ischiatic spine. The pudendal neurovascular bundle is then visible and released from the dorsal surface of the sacro-spinous ligament. A simple retractor holding medially the ischio-rectal fossa fat is sufficient to open Alcock's canal and to follow the distal branches of the nerve (Fig. 8). If the fascia of the internal obturator muscle is thickened or the falciform process is obstructing, these can be incised. The sacro-spinous ligament is cut and the nerve can be transposed frontally to the ischial spine (Fig. 9).

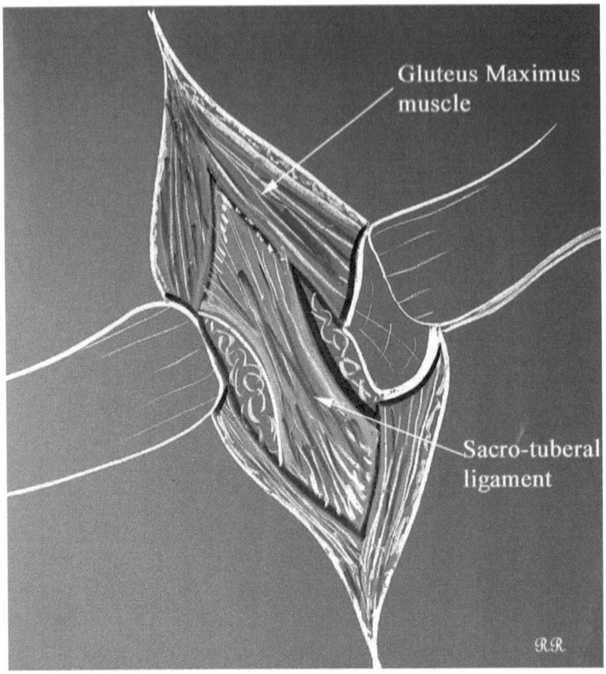

Fig. 6. Surgical approach on the right side of the superficial layers. After the skin incision, the fibers of the gluteus maximus muscle are divided and resected from the posterior aspect of the sacrotuberal ligament

One may then assess the diameter of the nerve and its potential variations [22, 25], its shape (flattened or not), its inflammatory appearance, peritruncular fibrosis and satellite veins dilatations, vasculo-nervous conflict, abnormalities of the nerve course (such as trans sacro-spinous or trans sacro-tuberal pathways) [26] and the shape of the ischiatic spine [4]. The combination of normal anatomical conditions and a normal nerve is a bad prognostic factor of course [26]. The closure is done in two planes. Drainage is usually unnecessary. A 3–5 days hospital stay is required. The duration of this procedure is 20–30 minutes for one side. The sacrifice of the two ligaments has no morbid consequences for the sacro-iliac joint in normal cases. If patients are complaining of a true sacro-iliac instability prior to surgery, we can preserve the sacrotuberal ligament and only cut the sacrospinous one. The approach is then done a little more medially than the standard technique. The nerve is reached in the inner and ventral part of the sacro-tuberal ligament.

Sitting is allowed the day after surgery according to the neuropathic pain. The wound is above the pressure area. All the different pathological considerations during surgery must be clearly noted in a report.

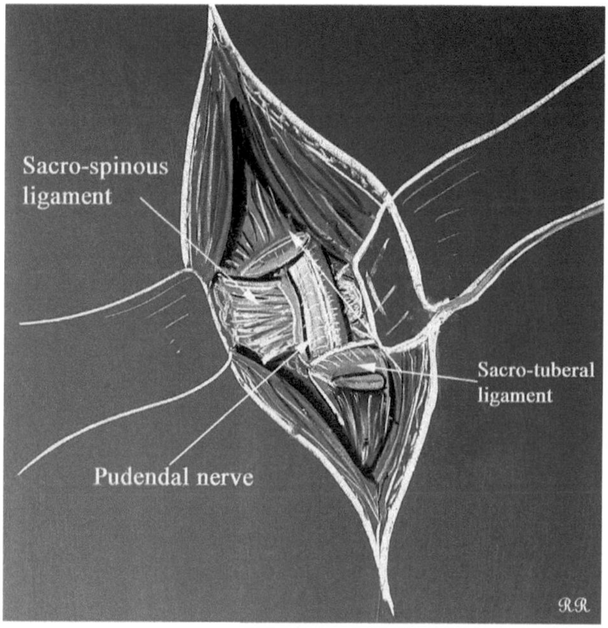

Fig. 7. Surgical approach; the sacrotuberal ligament is cut and resected. The pudendal nerve and vessels appear behind to sacrospinous ligament

Results

We have analyzed our results both in a prospective randomised study and retrospectively.

Randomized prospective controlled trial [27]

Method

Study inclusion criteria: patients eligible for inclusion had chronic perineal pain for at least one year's duration. The pain, uni or bilateral, was exacerbated in the seated position. Patients had to be between the ages of 18 and 70 and had pain intensity of at least 70 on 100 according to the VAS score. We also used a behavioural scale and the Hamilton depression rating scale (minimum score at 3 for the first and 9 or below for the latter).

A positive diagnostic response to an anesthetic block of the pudendal nerve was required and also the persistence of perineal pain in spite of at least two steroid blocks. Every patient had a normal pelvi-perineal CT scan, avoiding all the tumour pathology which could lead to pain.

The study design was a sequential, randomized controlled trial without blinding. Patients were assigned randomly to one of the two treatment groups: surgery or control. The only difference in the treatment between the two

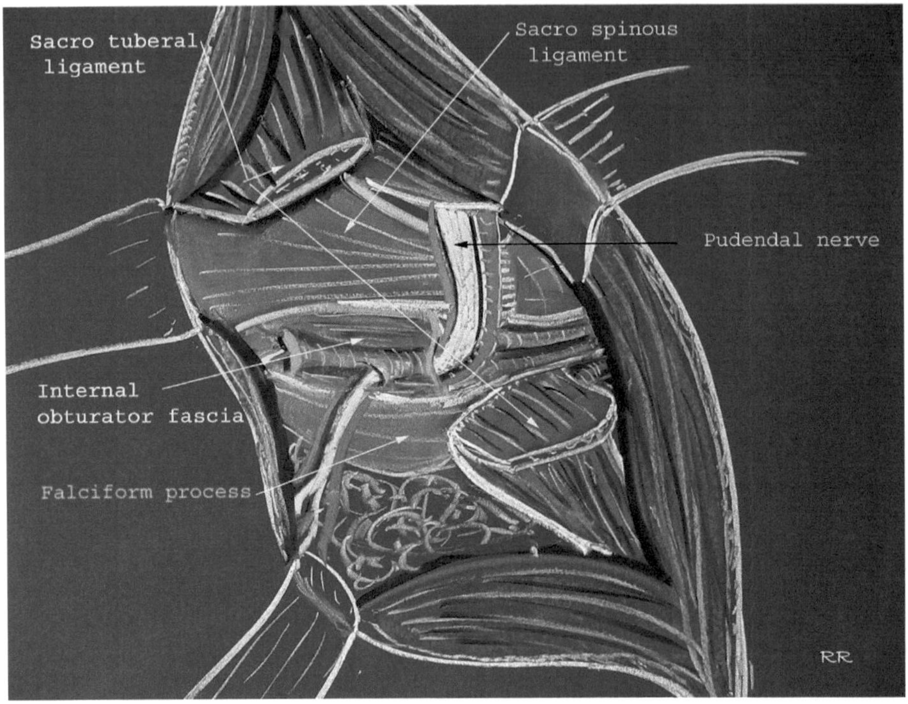

Fig. 8. A deep spreader is used to open the inner part of the ichiatic region. The pudendal canal appears; the pudendal nerve enters the tunnel in an undoubling of the internal obturator muscle fascia. The anal branch perforates this layer to reach the anal area

groups is related to the fact that only the patients of the first group were operated on.

Outcome measures: the primary endpoint of the study was the proportion of patients judged to have improved three months following surgery or after 3 months of medical treatment. Treatment was considered effective if the pain score had decreased by at least 30 on the VAS and less than 3 on the behaviour scale. We followed up both groups 1 year after the inclusion and the surgical group was assessed again 4 years later to find out whether improvement was maintained.

Results

Thirty-five patients were eligible for the study among 181 patients seen in a multidisciplinary clinic over a two years period. Three patients refused and the other 32 were recruited, 16 to each of the study groups. At 3 months, 50% of the surgery group were improved versus 6% of the control group. At 12 months by analysis to treat protocol, 71% in the surgical group and 13% of the control group had a successful outcome. The surgical procedure is there-

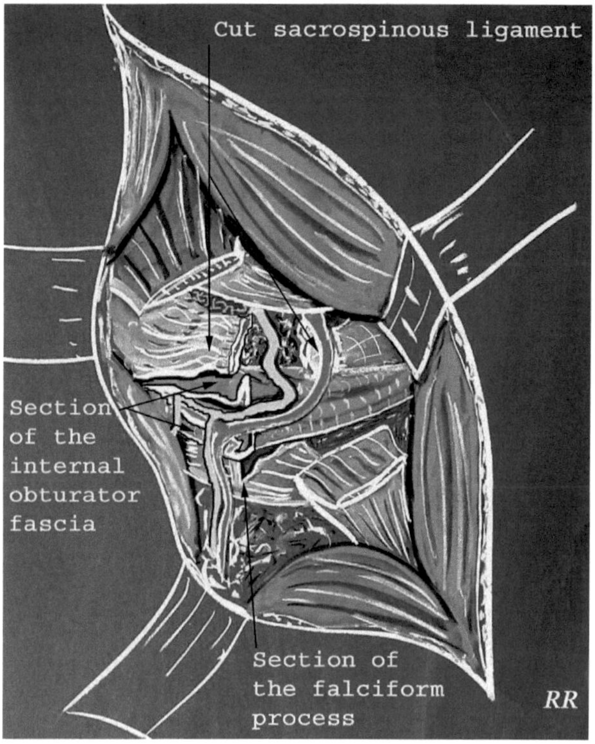

Fig. 9. The fascia of the internal obturator muscle is opened, the falciform process and the sacrospinous ligament are cut. The nerve is then transposed ventrally to the ischiatic spine. The nerve is then free all along its course

fore validated and can be reasonably proposed for perineal pain patients, according to the clinical signs mentioned above. The efficacy of the surgery confirms the etiology of these postural perineal pain syndromes previously considered as reflecting pathology within the pelvic visceras idiopathic or psychogenic.

Failure analysis: diagnostic error is always possible of course but long lasting or tight compression preoperatively could account for irreversible nerve fiber damage initiating chronic neuropathic pain. With this aim in view, the earlier people are operated on, the better the result will be. Incomplete release of the nerve by the transgluteal approach should be avoided. Recently we have positioned the patient in a genu-pectoral installation which allows a better view of the distal part of the nerve trunk.

Retrospective study

From January 1994 to December 2000, 500 patients were operated on by a single surgeon. Only 158 patients were selected, i.e. 248 nerves. The fact is that most of them came from abroad or far from Nantes.

Pain

Preop VAS was 77% which reflects very intense pain. Patients improved if the VAS decreased by 28 or more. Excellent results were considered if VAS decreased to 52 or more, no improvement for 1 mm or the same as before.

Age

Most of the patients were between 40 and 75 years old. The mean was 56. Not improved patients were 5 years older than improved ones. After 70, the success rate decreased significantly.

Sex

57% were females, 43% males. The better results in the men was not statistically significant.

Side

51% of patients had bilateral pain; 49% unilateral (51% left side, 49% right side). No difference was noted between each side. People with a unilateral pathology had a better result.

Characteristic of pain

The above mentioned clinical presentation is of course a good guide for the diagnosis. This pain is typically located in the perineal area, consisting of a burning feeling, increased with seated position. In fact, numerous patients have pain irradiation to the thigh, the abdominal wall, the pubis, complaints about sensation of a foreign body in the rectum or vagina, have pain even when standing or at night when lying. The results are the same even if the clinical presentation is atypical.

Time for evaluation

We must wait at least one year after surgery to evaluate the pain on the VAS score. Patients are informed that the definitive result will not be appreciated sooner, in spite of some early improvements.

Time for surgery since the beginning of pain

66% of patients suffering for less than 6 years improved versus 40% after 7 years duration of pain. This is an important point. Diagnosis must be made much earlier if we want to improve the results.

Neurophysiological data

The distal motor latency is, in our experience, the best test to confirm that the pudendal nerve is entrapped. Normal score is less than 5 milliseconds. When the score is more than 9 milliseconds, results are poor.

Blocks

They constitute a therapeutic weapon and a diagnostic test.

When the preoperative anaesthetic block at the level of the ischiatic spine is negative, only 17% of patients improve. If the block is positive and a per operating conflict is found, 65.5% of patients improve. If no conflict is found at this level, only 50% improve. Among them, 50% had a conflict at the level of Alcock's canal.

59% of patients with a positive diagnostic block at Alcock's canal improved. Among them, 91% had also a conflict at the level of the ischiatic spine and a positive diagnosis test at this level.

The steroid preop blocks seem to persist longer in improved patients.

Origin of pain

67% of post traumatic pain improved which is a little better than spontaneous neuralgias.

Peri-operative findings

They are very important to consider. Normal anatomy leads to a bad result as mentioned above. To summarize, the best condition is to find a flattened nerve with a conflict at the level of the ischiatic spine only. 74% of these patients improve. If the entrapment is noted in Alcock's canal, only 50% improve. If the entrapment is at the two levels, the success rate is 60%.

Results

Finally, fewer than two third of patients improve after the surgery, nearly one third stay in the same condition, 1% feel worse than before.

Complications of the surgery

We never encountered any hypoesthesia nor motor complication after surgery. There was less than 1% of hematomas and sepsis. Less than 1% of the patients felt worse after surgery. Most of them estimated their pain at 100 on the VAS prior to surgery.

Comments

The results of this retrospective study pointed out some failures for nerves entrapped in Alcock's canal. To obtain a good distal decompression we defined a new preoperative position i.e. in genu pectoral. It allows us to enter deeply into the canal and to cut the fascia of the internal obturator muscle under visual control. With the same aim, we have started to cut the nerve to this muscle to obtain a definitive amyotrophy reducing the pressure in the tunnel. We will publish our results later.

The prospective randomized study validated the surgery. It must be clearly keep in mind that before our clinical work, the patients were considered as psychiatric. Blocks and surgery have transformed the life of patients from a terrible social condition in two third of cases.

These results could be considered rather poor, but are consistent with results obtained in the surgery of the spinal lumbar disc for example. If we consider that the blocks definitively improve about 50% of patients and that among them 65% improve after surgery, only 17% of the patients we treat failed to improve.

Other diagnoses

Symptomatic pain provoked by acute dermatological infections of the perineum are easy to diagnose and leads to symptomatic treatment.

Pain persisting at night suggests a tumour to be excluded radiologically. Other neuropathic pains must be explored and analysed in their context. Surgery requiring trans abdominal or pelvic wall approaches may cut sensory nerves such as the ilio-hypogastric, ilio-inguinal or genito-femoral trunks [8, 16, 21, 30]. They invade partly the supplying area of the pudendal nerve. The patient's story is clear enough and a trigger zone must be sought (Tinel's sign) leading to the diagnosis of a post traumatic neuroma.

The possibility of radicular pain arising from orthopaedic problems at the thoraco-lumbar area must be considered and can be treated by physiotherapy and specific blocks [18].

Testicular [9] and urethral [36] pains must be carefully analysed. Their nervous supply arises from the autonomic system which is situated at the thoraco-lumbar junction. Specific blocks may be helpful.

Vestibulodynias (vulvar pain) are very special [12]. Women suffer from an allodynia which is the main sign and any local contact is unbearable.

Bladder pain is frequently encountered during our consultations. The pain increases during the filling up of the bladder and stops after the micturition.

Proctalgia fugax is a paroxysual pain in the anal region during the night, awaking the patients, leading even to syncope and resolves within half an hour. Its origin is unknown.

Some patients may complain about a sciatic pain without back ache which can be the main pain or in association with a perineal pain. Different presentations occur: a sciatic pain may reach only the posterior aspect of the buttock and of the thigh. A compression of the posterior cutaneous nerve of the thigh can be provoked. The entrapment is caused by the piriformis muscle [10, 33] which can damage both the posterior cutaneous muscle of the thigh and the pudendal nerve. A sciatica which reaches, without any lumbar pain, the inferior limb until the foot may be due to a compression of the anterior part of the ischiatic trunk and/or the pudendal nerve by the internal obturator muscle [19]. A deep gluteal syndrome has been described when the two muscles are involved [17]. Physiotherapy focussed on the stretching of these muscles, specific blocks, and even surgery may help.

A pain situated laterally to the anal region when sitting could be explained by a compression of the inferior clunial nerve. Patients with this pathology complain of pain when sitting on a hard seat. Pudendal pain arises when seating on a soft seat most of the time.

The obturator neuralgia is different, being located away from the perineum and reaching the superior and medial aspect of the thigh. Walking or stepping on one foot is then painful. Herniations must be evoked [20]. A real entrapment syndrome has been established [31]. We have one case of such a pain after surgery for urethral incontinence (unpublished observation).

Coccydynias start in the coccygeal area, back from the anal region, occur when sitting and when standing up and then become very acute. People therefore sit in a bending position avoiding the compression of the coccyx. A radiological instability may be demonstrated by dynamic X-rays in sitting and standing position. Clinically, intra rectal pressure brings on the pain when moving the coccyx. The instability, if found is between the coccygial vertebre. Blocks may be positive. Surgery is rarely required.

Herpetic infection especially in women may later induce chronic pain which is not influenced by any position and persists during the night.

Chronic prostatitis [14] is a fashionable syndrome but, unfortunately, the bacteriological proof is rare. Very often a true pudendal pain may be called prostatitis.

Sacral root pains are quite different. They are mostly accompanied by lumbar pain, and reflexes are absent. Anesthesia is noted and mild motor disturbances are frequent.

Conclusion

Perineal pain constitutes a difficult diagnostic problem. Nevertheless, patients may describe a typical history of burning pain in the territory of the pudendal nerve when sitting. An entrapment syndrome of the pudendal nerve must be diagnosed and complementary investigations must be done to be sure that there is no other explanation for the pain.

Neurophysiological tests are performed, searching for an increase of the distal motor latency. Blocks are proposed under CT scan control which are at the same time a diagnostic test and a therapeutic weapon. Surgery is then performed if the pain is still present. The transgluteal approach allows the release of all compressive factors. Nearly two thirds of patients improve after surgery. Long duration of the illness, advanced age of the patients, are predictive factors, and must be reduced by an earlier diagnosis.

References

1. Alevizon SJ, Finan MA (1996) Sacrospinous colpopexy: management of postoperative pudendal nerve entrapment. Obstet Gynecol 88: 713–715
2. Amarenco G, Lanoe Y, Perrigot M, Goudal H (1987) Un nouveau syndrome canalaire, la compression du nerf pudendal dans la canal d'Alcock ou paralysie périnéale du cycliste. Presse Med 16: 399
3. Amarenco G, Ismael SS, Bayle B, Denys P, Kerdraon J (2001) Electrophysiological analysis of pudendal neuropathy following traction. Muscle Nerve 24: 116–119
4. Antolak SJJ, Hough DM, Pawlina W, Spinner RJ (2002) Anatomical basis of chronic pelvic pain syndrome: the ischial spine and pudendal nerve entrapment. Med Hypotheses 59: 349–353
5. Bautrant E, de Bisschop E, Vaini-Elies V *et al.* (2003) La prise en charge moderne des névralgies pudendales. A partir d'une sériede 212 patientes et 104 interventions de décompression. J Gynecol Obstet Biol Reprod (Paris) 32: 705–712
6. Bensignor-Le Henaff M, Labat JJ, Robert R, Lajat Y, Papon M (1991) Douleur périnéale et souffrance des nerfs honteux internes. Agressologie 32: 277–279
7. Bouhassira D, Attal N, Alchaar H *et al.* (2005) Comparison of pain syndromes associated with nervous or somatic lesions and development of a new neuropathic pain diagnostic questionnaire (DN4). Pain 114: 29–36
8. Chevallier JM, Wind P, Lassau JP (1996) La blessure des nerfs inguino-fémoraux dans le traitement de hernie. Un danger anatomique des techniques traditionnelles et laparoscopies. Ann Chir 50: 767–775
9. Costabile RA, Hahn M, McLeod DG (1991) Chronic orchialgia in the pain prone patient: the clinical perspective. J Urol 146: 1571–1574
10. Fishman LM, Schaefer MP (2003) The piriformis syndrome is underdiagnosed. Muscle Nerve 28: 646–649
11. France MP, Aurori BF (1992) Pudendal nerve palsy following fracture table traction. Clin Orthop 276: 272–276
12. Friedrich EGJ (1987) Vulvar vestibulitis syndrome. J Reprod Med 32: 110–114
13. Hough DM, Wittenberg KH, Pawlina W *et al.* (2003) Chronic perineal pain caused by pudendal nerve entrapment: anatomy and CT-guided perineural injection technique. AJR Am J Roentgenol 181: 561–567
14. Krieger JN, Ross SO, Riley DE (2002) Chronic prostatitis: epidemiology and role of infection. Urology 60: 8
15. Labat JJ, Robert R, Bensignor M, Buzelin JM (1990) Les névralgies du nerf pudendal (honteux interne). Considérations anatomo-cliniques et perspectives thérapeutiques. J Urol (Paris) 96: 239–244
16. Liszka TG, Dellon AL, Manson PN (1994) Iliohypogastric nerve entrapment following abdominoplasty. Plast Reconstr Surg 93: 181–184

17. McCrory P (2001) The "piriformis syndrome" myth or reality? Br J Sports Med 35: 209–210
18. Maigne R (1981) Le syndrome de la jonction dorso-lombaire. Douleur lombaire basse, douleur pseudo-viscérale, pseudo douleur de hanche et pseudo douleur pubienne. Sem Hop 57: 545–554
19. Meknas K, Christensen A, Johansen O (2003) The internal obturator muscle may cause sciatic pain. Pain 104: 375–380
20. Mondelli M, Giannini F, Guazzi G, Corbelli P (2002) Obturator neuropathy due to obturator hernia. Muscle Nerve 26: 291–292
21. Perry CP (2003) Peripheral neuropathies and pelvic pain: diagnosis and management. Clin Obstet Gynecol 46: 789–796
22. Ramsden CE, McDaniel MC, Harmon RL, Renney KM, Faure A (2003) Pudendal nerve entrapment as source of intractable perineal pain. Am J Phys Med Rehabil 82: 479–484
23. Robert R, Labat JJ, Lehur PA *et al.* (1989) Réflexions cliniques, neurophysiologiques et thérapeutiques à partir de données anatomiques sur le nerf pudendal (honteux interne) lors de certaines algies périnéales. Chirurgie 115: 515–520
24. Robert R, Brunet C, Faure A *et al.* (1993) La chirurgie du nerf pudendal lors de certaines algies périnéales: évolution et résultats. Chirurgie 119: 535–539
25. Robert R, Prat-Pradal D, Labat JJ *et al.* (1998) Anatomic basis of chronic perineal pain: role of the pudendal nerve. Surg Radiol Anat 20: 93
26. Robert R, Bensignor M, Labat JJ *et al.* (2004) Le neurochirurgien face aux algies périnéales: guide pratique. Neurochirurgie 50: 533–539
27. Robert R, Labat JJ, Bensignor M *et al.* (2005) Decompression and transposition of the pudendal nerve in pudendal neuralgia: a randomized controlled trial and long-term evaluation. Eur Urol 47: 403–408
28. Roche B, Dembe JC, Mavrocordatos P, Rap JR, Cahana A (2004) Approche anatomo-chirurgicale des névralgies du nerf pudendal. Le courrier de l'algologie 3: 109–112
29. Sagsoz N, Ersoy M, Kamaci M, Tekdemir I (2002) Anatomical landmarks regarding sacrospinous colpopexy operations performed for vaginal vault prolapse. Eur J Obstet Gynecol Reprod Biol 101: 74–78
30. Sippo WC, Burghardt A, Gomez AC (1987) Nerve entrapment after Pfannenstiel incision. Am J Obstet Gynecol 157: 420–421
31. Sorenson EJ, Chen JJ, Daube JR (2002) Obturator neuropathy: causes and outcome. Muscle Nerve 25: 605–607
32. Soulie M, Vazzoler N, Seguin P, Chiron P, Plante P (2002) Conséquences urologiques du traumatisme du nerf pudendal sur table orthopédique: mise au point et conseils pratiques. Prog Urol 12: 504–509
33. Stewart JD (2003) The piriformis syndrome is overdiagnosed. Muscle Nerve 28: 644–646
34. Turner ML, Marinoff SC (1991) Pudendal neuralgia. Am J Obstet Gynecol 165: 1233–1236
35. Verdeja AM, Elkins TE, Odoi A, Gasser R, Lamoutte C (1995) Transvaginal sacrospinous colpopexy: anatomic land marks to be aware of to minimize complications. Am J Obstet Gynecol 173: 1468–1469.la
36. Wesselmann U, Burnett AL, Heinberg LJ (1997) The urogenital and rectal pain syndromes. Pain 73: 269–294

Technical standards

Offprint from
Advances and Technical Standards in Neurosurgery, Vol. 32
Edited by J.D. Pickard

Spinal cord stimulation for ischemic heart disease and peripheral vascular disease

J. DE VRIES[1], M. J. L. DE JONGSTE[1], G. SPINCEMAILLE[2], and M. J. STAAL[3]

[1] Department of Cardiology, Thoraxcenter, University Medical Center Groningen, The Netherlands
[2] Department of Neurosurgery, University Medical Center Maastricht, The Netherlands
[3] Department of Neurosurgery, University Medical Center Groningen, The Netherlands

With 7 Figures

Contents

Abstract

Ischemic disease (ID) is now an important indication for electrical neuromodulation (NM), particularly in chronic pain conditions. NM is defined as a therapeutic modality that aims to restore functions of the nervous system or modulate neural structures involved in the dysfunction of organ systems. One of the NM methods used is chronic electrical stimulation of the spinal cord (spinal cord stimulation: SCS).

SCS in ID, as applied to ischemic heart disease (IHD) and peripheral vascular disease (PVD), started in Europe in the 1970s and 1980s, respectively. Patients with ID are eligible for SCS when they experience disabling pain, resulting from ischaemia. This pain should be considered therapeutically refractory to standard treatment intended to decrease metabolic demand or following revascularization procedures.

Several studies have demonstrated the beneficial effect of SCS on IHD and PVD by improving the quality of life of this group of severely disabled patients, without adversely influencing mortality and morbidity. SCS used as additional treatment for IHD reduces angina pectoris (AP) in its frequency and intensity, increases exercise capacity, and does not seem to mask the warning signs of a myocardial infarction.

Besides the analgesic effect, different studies have demonstrated an anti-ischemic effect, as expressed by different cardiac indices such as exercise duration, ambulatory ECG recording, coronary flow measurements, and PET scans. SCS can be considered as an alternative to open heart bypass grafting (CABG) for patients at high risk from surgical procedures. Moreover, SCS appears to be more efficacious than transcutaneous electrical nerve stimulation (TENS).

The SCS implantation technique is relatively simple: implanting an epidural electrode under local anesthesia (supervised by the anesthesist) with the tip at T1, covering the painful area with paraesthesia by external stimulation (pulse width 210, rate 85 Hz), and connecting this electrode to a subcutaneously implanted pulse generator.

In PVD the pain may manifest itself at rest or during walking (claudication), disabling the patiënt severely. Most of the patients suffer from atherosclerotic critical limb ischemia. All patients should be therapeutically refractory (medication and revascularization) to become eligible for SCS. Ulcers on the extremities should be minimal.

In PVD the same implantation technique is used as in IHD except that the tip of the electrode is positioned at T10-11. In PVD the majority of the patients show significant reduction in pain and more than half of the patients show improvement of circulatory indices, as shown by Doppler, thermography, and oximetry studies. Limb salvage studies show variable results depending on the stage of the trophic changes. The underlying mechanisms of action of SCS in PVD require further elucidation.

Keywords: Neuromodulation; spinal cord stimulation; ischaemic heart disease; peripheral vascular disease; pain.

Preface

Neuromodulation (NM) is defined as the recruitment of nerves through electrical stimulation as a therapeutic approach for patients with chronic non-fatal anomalies varying from neuropathic and ischemic pain to movement and psychiatric disorders. One of the therapeutic options is chronic electrical stimulation of neural structures, including peripheral nerves (PNS: peripheral nerve stimulation), the spinal cord (SCS: spinal cord stimulation) and part(s) of the brain (DBS: deep brain stimulation). Although the use of electrical current might be associated with empirical and medically obscure treatments, the value of chronic electrical stimulation of neural structures has been demonstrated on a long term base over the last 40 years. It sometimes shows dramatic, instant and long-lasting effects on pain, improvement of circulatory insufficiency or movement and psychiatric anomalies. It produces convincing improvement in quality of life and social rehabilitation.

Multidisciplinarity is the key word in NM. NM is applied by a variety of medical specialists: e.g. vascular surgeons, cardiologists, anaesthesiologists, rehabilitation specialists, neurologists, and neurosurgeons, supported by dedicated paramedical personnel. The clinical application and the background research require the ability to think and work together in an interdisciplinary way. This makes NM such an attractive, challenging and often a very rewarding concept. Nevertheless it is remarkable how little representatives of the various medical disciplines are engaged in NM despite its high level of efficacy in otherwise therapeutically refractory chronic anomalies. How is it that it is relatively unknown that "untreatable" angina pectoris or chronic back and/or leg pain ("failed back surgery syndromes") is suitable for NM treatment? And why are so few neurosurgeons interested in NM? We sincerely hope that this monograph will draw the attention of the neurosurgical reader to two severe ischemic diseases: ischemic heart and peripheral vascular diseases (PVD). Both anomalies are very suitable targets for NM treatment with SCS. These patients have very little to loose (except their legs in cases of PVD). NM offers real possibilities for substantial pain relief and improvement of quality of life.

Part I: Spinal cord stimulation for ischemic heart disease

Introduction: Background and definition

Increased knowledge of the pathophysiology of ischemic heart disease has generated improved diagnostic opportunities, which in turn has promoted the development of a large armamentarium of therapies for this illness. However, to date ischemic heart disease is still one of the most substantial plagues, concerning morbidity and mortality, in the Western World [54]. In addition to the reduction in mortality from cardiovascular disease during the last three decades, the quality of life of patients suffering from ischemic heart disease has been improved. This can be attributed to improved primary prevention measures, such as lifestyle changes and treatment of risk factors for heart diseases, advances in pharmacotherapeutical and surgical treatment strategies. Subsequently, more patients survive their heart disease for longer periods of time, albeit ultimately without options for further treatment [72]. So, in general, notwithstanding the therapeutic merits usually supplying appropriate symptom relief in the majority of patients [83], in an increasing number of patients with ischemic cardiovascular disease the major goal of control of pain is not met [60]. These patients, with an unmet medical need, have severe disabling chest pain, occurring during minimal exercise or even at rest. They are suffering from chronic pain that is therapeutically refractory to standard therapies. The term "chronic stable refractory cardiovascular pain" has been designated to patients with severe pain, resulting from (coronary) artery disease that is uncontrollable by both pharmacological (aspirins, β-blocking agents, calcium-channel blockers, long-acting nitrates etc.) and revascularization procedures (percutaneous coronary interventions [PCI] and coronary artery bypass surgery [CABG]) [37]. However, the severity of pain is to the judgement of the patients. Therefore, the European Study Group on the treatment of refractory angina pectoris has recently redefined the cardiac disorder as: "a chronic condition characterized by the presence of angina, caused by coronary insufficiency in the presence of coronary artery disease, which cannot be adequately controlled by a combination of medical therapy, angioplasty, and coronary artery bypass surgery. The presence of myocardial ischemia should be clinically established to be the cause of symptoms" [46].

Patients enduring this condition are usually characterized by a long history of artery disease, have often been treated with revascularization procedure(s) previously, are in their sixties, predominantly male and, have on the average a slightly reduced left ventricular ejection fraction. Furthermore, as a result of an acute worsening of their disease, these patients frequently need hospital admissions [55]. Therefore, the search for and evaluation of adjunct therapies has to be encouraged in order to identify novel strategies which are capable of reducing the burden of ischemic pain and subsequently improve the quality of life, without adversely influencing the prognosis, of these often severely disabled patients.

For these patients suffering from chronic debilitating ischemic pain, refractory to conventional therapies such as pharmacological approaches and revascularization procedures, adjunct therapies have become available. One of the most promising of these additional therapies appears to be electrical neuromodulation, albeit that the accumulating body of clinical and experimental data is still not very dramatic, mainly related to the lack of studies with a large sample size. However, electrical neuromodulation has become accepted as an additional therapy for refractory angina pectoris in the ACC/AHA guidelines, since 2002 [28].

It is our purpose to discuss the literature on electrical neuromodulation for ischemic cardiovascular disease and provide practical strategies.

History of neuromodulation for ischemic heart disease

Since 1967 modulation of the nervous system has been performed to obtain a reduction in pain in ischemic cardiovascular disease [9]. Starting with transthoracic [58], or endoscopic [40, 78] denervation of specific parts of the sympathic nerve such as the stellate ganglion [79], gradually medical attention has become re-focussed on modulation of nerves. This may be performed by means of vagal stimulation [82], by creating a temporary sympathetic block through injections with local anesthetics into the stellate ganglion [14], or through application of electrical current on different sites (nerves, spine, skin, subcutis) of the body (i.e. 'electrical neuromodulation'). The latter is either executed by spinal cord stimulation (SCS) or by transcutaneous electrical nerve stimulation (TENS). Among the available adjunct therapies SCS may be considered as one of the most effective and safe adjuvant treatments for patients with ischemic cardiovascular pain resistant to conventional strategies [23, 52].

The first report on antianginal effect of SCS on the dorsal aspect of the spinal cord in patients with chronic refractory angina pectoris was published by Murphy and Giles, in 1987 [53]. They observed a reduction in both the frequency and severity of angina attacks in conjunction with a reduction in sublingual intake of nitrogen tablets. In contrast with the favorable results, the therapy initially met with great skepticism [45]. Since the nineties many authors have advocated SCS as an effective additional approach for patients chronically disabled by their angina [2, 7, 18, 19, 23, 28, 29, 31, 37, 45, 46, 48, 53, 55, 63, 69, 77, 83]. To date, in selected patients, SCS may even be considered as an alternative to bypass surgery [48]. However, in view of the partially understood mechanism of action, it is substantive to demonstrate the safety of SCS in patients suffering from chronic refractory angina pectoris, resulting from unmanageable coronary artery disease. Therefore, recent research has been performed to determine whether the observed electro-analgesic effect of SCS is accompanied by an antiischemic effect.

Effects of SCS

The analgesic effect

Both observational and randomized studies on SCS have demonstrated beneficial effects, expressed in a reduction in severity of angina complaints and the number of short acting nitrate tablets, and perceived quality of life [77], in conjunction with an improvement in exercise capacity [19, 31, 48]. In approximately 80% of patients the beneficial effects of SCS last for at least one year [2, 19, 31, 37, 48, 55] and in nearly 60% of these patients improvement in exercise capacity and quality of life has been reported for up to 5 years [7]. There has been concern with regard to the safety of spinal cord stimulation as it might deprive the patient of an important angina 'warning' signal. The fear of a potential increase in myocardial events does not seem to be justified [2, 7, 48, 55, 57]. Rather than abolishing anginal pain, SCS enhances the angina threshold. As a consequence patients report an increase in exercise capacity and a reduction in the severity, without a complete elimination, of symptoms of angina on intact pain perception during acute myocardial infarction [2, 7, 38, 57]. This is congruent with the absence of an adverse effect on mortality as demonstrated in prospective and retrospective studies on SCS for refractory angina pectoris [48, 69]. In addition, SCS was not able to suppress the conduction of cardiac pain signals to the cerebrum during cardiac distress [32].

The antiischemic effect

In addition to analgesic achievements, SCS employs antiischemic effects. Both, open and randomized studies have demonstrated that the reduction in anginal pain during SCS enables the patient to prolong the exercise without aggravating myocardial ischemia. Furthermore, the antiischemic effects of SCS have been demonstrated by a reduction in ST-T segment depression on ECG recordings during exercise stress testing [19, 31, 48, 63] and ambulatory ECG monitoring [18, 31]. One study showed an increased tolerance to atrial pacing and delayed onset of anginal complaints during SCS [47]. All patients ultimately experienced angina pectoris. In addition, Chauhan *et al.* [13] demonstrated an increase in coronary flow velocity, using Doppler flow catheters following 5 min of transcutaneous electrical neuromodulation. The rise in the anginal threshold is likely to be related to a redistribution of coronary blood flow from myocardial regions with a normal perfusion in favor of regions with impaired myocardial perfusion [30]. Therefore, the reduction in ischemia appears to be related to homogenization of myocardial blood flow, most likely this phenomenon is resulting from improved collateral flow. Since collateral flow is individually determined, this might very well be the explanation why in some patients ischemia is improved instantaneously and in others it may take up to a year [20]. In spite of the above, many concerns remain among physicians regarding the potential risk on an increase in myocardial ischemia through SCS, when spinal cord stimulation is indeed depriving the patient of the anginal 'warning' signal. Because SCS elevates the anginal threshold and patients are subsequently reporting a reduction, and not a complete elimination of anginal attacks during SCS, this concern is obviously not rational.

Moreover, evidence is growing that electrical neuromodulation prevents and reduces ventricular arrhythmia's [34, 84].

In conclusion, since SCS appears to employ an antiischemic effect, without increasing mortality [48, 69] and without concealing the anginal warning signal during an acute myocardial infarction [27, 31, 32, 38, 57], or increasing serious arrhythmia's, neuromodulation is considered a safe therapy for patients invalidated by chronic therapeutically refractory angina pectoris.

Mechanisms of action of spinal cord stimulation

At the level of the central nervous system

In 1965, Melzack and Wall published the 'gate-control theory' [51]. The model was based on the theory that stimulation of myelinated relatively fast conducting A-fibers modulate the processing of "pain" signals in the non-myelinated slower conducting C-fibers in the dorsal horn. Following ischemia, which is the consequence of a divergence between myocardial oxygen supply and demand, primary nociceptive nerve endings containing capsaicin (vanilloid receptor 1 or VR_1) receptors are stimulated in the heart or around the peripheral arteries [59].

It has been postulated that electrical neuromodulation can effectively remodel neural pathways [43], and subsequently re-scales the neural hierarchy in cardiac control [4]. At the most peripheral level, the intra-cardiac neurons (ICN) are considered as the final common integrator of the nervous system in the heart [5]. Preliminary data of animal experiments showed that SCS modulates, in a consistent pattern, the firing rate of ICN. Furthermore, during ischemic challenges, it was demonstrated that SCS stabilizes the activity of ICN [25]. In higher brain centers, both angina pectoris and neuromodulation have been found to affect areas involved in cardiovascular control [32, 62].

In addition to these putative actions at different levels in the central nervous system (CNS), a variety of neurotransmitters and vasoactive compounds, like GABA, adenosine, bradykinin, K^+, lactate, endorphins etc, are thought to link shifts in the activity in CNS' centers to control cardiovascular state.

At the cardiac level

In both open and randomized studies it has repeatedly been demonstrated that the reduction in anginal pain during spinal cord stimulation enables the patients to prolong their exercise. In this respect it was found that SCS was not able to suppress conduction to the cerebrum of a cardiac pain signal, acting as an alarm signal of cardiac distress [32]. Initially, the antiischemic effect of SCS was subscribed to modulation of the autonomic nervous system, more specifically, to the sympathetic branch. However, clinical data does not support this hypothesis, since no change in heart rate variability, or in (nor)-epinephrine metabolism has been found during spinal cord stimulation [19, 31, 33, 56].

The rise in the anginal threshold, causing the delayed onset of angina, may be related to a redistribution in coronary blood flow from normal perfused (non-ischemic) to impaired perfused (ischemic) myocardial regions, causing a homogenization of myocardial perfusion [30]. Subsequently, the moment of critical balance between myocardial oxygen supply and demand is deferred. Whether or not this suggested redistribution in coronary blood flow results from recruitment of collaterals [39] or that other mechanisms are involved such as angiogenesis [71] or preconditioning [49] is a matter of further research.

The increased anginal threshold was emphasized by a study in which patients with refractory angina and a SCS were randomized to control or stressed by right atrial pacing until ischemic threshold [45]. During SCS the anginal threshold was higher, perhaps secondary to the antiischemic effect, albeit that all patients ultimately reported angina. In a letter to the editor it was claimed that the results could be alternatively explained by preconditioning [49]. Preconditioning and collateral recruitment are likely to play an important role in determining the ischemic threshold in patients with refractory angina pectoris. Furthermore, preconditioning can be induced by either pharmacological or ischemic stimuli. Electrically induced preconditioning may interact with both pathways. With regard to pharmacological preconditioning adenosine and opoids are found to influence the G protein-coupled receptors which, on their turn up-regulate protein kinase C, that is thought to phosphorylate the ATP-sensitive K channel, playing a key role in preconditioning. Since adenosine has vasodilatory effects and is involved in pain transmission adenosine may couple the involved neural and cardiac interactions. Moreover, SCS may blunt the effect of dipyridamole, an adenosine re-uptake inhibitor [30].

Finally, the intake of caffeine, which influences the adenosine handling via xanthine metabolism, has been demonstrated to impair the effects of neuromodulation [50].

Patients selection

Patients who are referred to our hospital and fulfil the inclusion criteria (see Table 1) are considered for SCS. A team consisting of an anesthesiologist, a cardiologist, a neurosurgeon, a nurse practitioner and a psychologist make the final decision, whether to implant a SCS. For a beneficial outcome it is essential

Table 1. *Inclusion and exclusion criteria SCS for IHD*

Inclusion criteria
1. Severe chest pain (NYHA classes III–IV or VAS score >7)
2. Optimal tolerated pharmacological therapy
3. Significant coronary artery disease (i.e. >1 stenosis of 75%)
4. Not eligible for Percutaneous Transluminal Intervention or Coronary Artery Bypass Surgery
5. No prognostic benefit from surgical revascularization (according to guidelines)
6. Patient considered intellectually capable to manage the SCS device
7. No acute coronary syndrome during last 3 months

Exclusion criteria
1. Myocardial infarction within the last 3 months
2. Uncontrolled disease such as hypertension or diabetes mellitus
3. Personality disorders or psychological instability
4. Pregnancy
5. Implantable cardioverter defibrillator (ICD) and pacemaker dependency
6. (Local) infections
7. Insurmountable spinal anatomy
8. Contraindication to withheld anti-platelet agents or coumarins
9. Addictive behavior

to perform cardiac, neuro-logical/-surgical and psychological examination, provide essential information (brochure with "frequently posed questions", device information) and train the patients to let them adequately manage the device, making use of a rehabilitation program. In this respect TENS application before implanting a SCS is not used for screening, but merely for getting the patients used to the paresthesias. Clinically we sometimes have to deal with patients who are upset when confronted with a device that has to be implanted. Some patients therefore insist to remain on TENS therapy. Others later proceed to SCS, mainly for reasons of an ortho-ergic reaction, which is rather frequently observed when TENS, or occasionally other external stimulating devices, are applied onto the chest [66].

In and exclusion criteria are mentioned in Table 1.

Implantation technique

The implantation device (Fig. 1) consists of a lead, eventually an extension cable and a pulse generator, all parts to be implanted internally. An external patients programmer is used after the operation to program the pulse generator through the skin. The key to the success of SCS is an accurate placement of the stimulation lead in the dorsal epidural space. The procedure is performed under local anesthesia, with the patient in prone position.

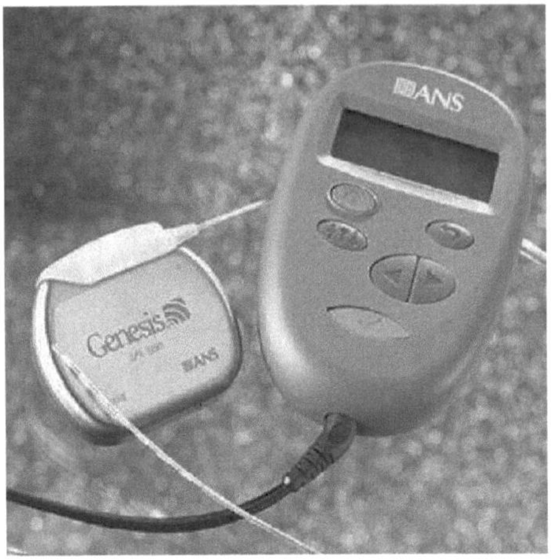

Fig. 1. Complete SCS system: electrode, pulse generator and patient programmer

However in IHD the presence and the vigilance of an anesthesiologist is mandatory: most of these patients have a high cardiac risk even for a "local anaesthesia" operation, specifically when aspirin is withheld. Haemodynamic monitoring is essential. To increase the patients comfort additional i.v. analgesics and/or anesthetics can be used, all to be given in close interdisciplinary communication. The patient is in a prone and comfortable position. Fluoroscopy is used to verify the position of the lead. Peri-operative antibiotics are administered (1 gr cephazoline). After infiltration of the soft tissue with a local anaesthetic at the level of T4–5, an incision is made up to the spinous processus and the epidural is punctured with a Touhy needle. The lead is introduced through this needle into the dorsal epidural space.It is connected to an external stimulator to elicite paraesthesia that have to be felt by the patient within the area of pain.

When the tip of the electrode is correctly positioned, usually at the T1 level (see Figs. 2 and 3) the lead is anchored and (eventually via an extension cable) connected to a pulse generator, generally placed in a subcutaneous pocket

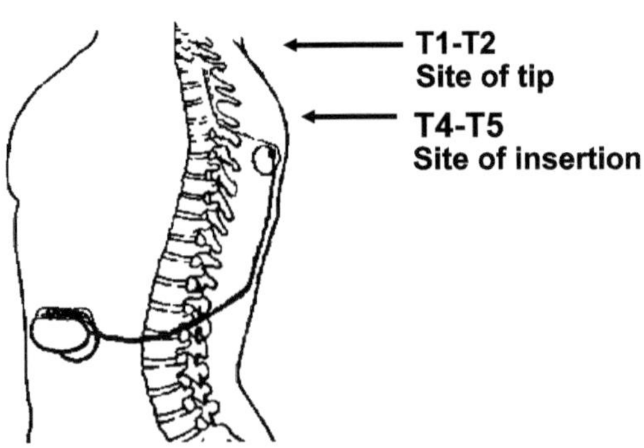

Fig. 2. Diagram of implanted SCS system

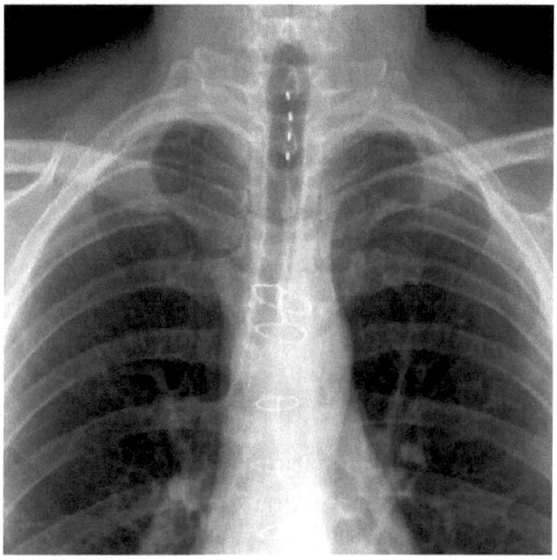

Fig. 3. Epidural quapripolar SCS electrode placed at T1

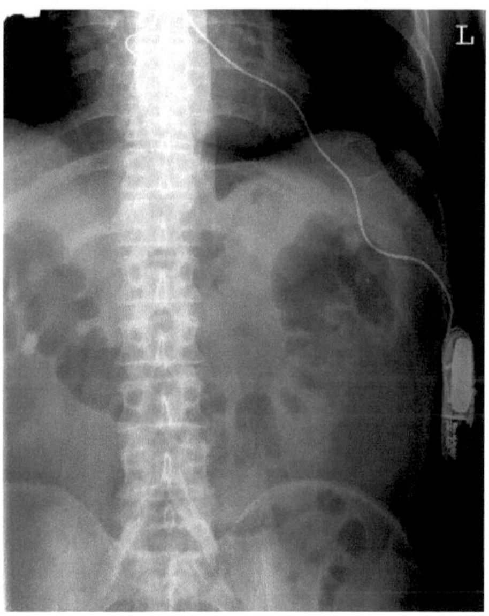

Fig. 4. Pulse generator in the lateral abdominal wall

in the lateral abdominal wall (see Fig. 4). The stimulator can be activated (or deactivated) by the patient, by using a patient programmer.

Cost-effectiveness

Several studies have consistently showed that SCS is cost-effective following a variable period (16 months–3 years) after the initial costs for the system have been made. After 2-year follow-up of 104 randomized patients participating in the ESBY study (electrical stimulation versus coronary artery bypass surgery in severe angina pectoris) hospital care costs, morbidity and causes of death after spinal cord stimulation (SCS) and coronary artery bypass grafting (CABG) were assessed. SCS was less expensive than CABG ($p<0.01$) and the patients had fewer hospitalization days related to the primary intervention ($p<0.0001$) and fewer hospitalization days due to cardiac events ($p<0.05$). The groups did not differ with regard to causes of death. No serious complications were observed related to the SCS treatment [66]. In a retrospective study Wei and colleagues showed that 16 months after the implantation of the device, SCS was already cost-effective compared to a control group with respect to the prevention of, among others hospitalizations [3]. Taylor *et al.* performed a systematic review and identified and evaluated 14 studies of the cost effectiveness of spinal cord stimulation (SCS) for the treatment of chronic pain [68]. They demonstrated that the initial costs of the SCS are offset by a reduction in post-implant healthcare resource demand and costs. The need for acute admissions for chest pain in patients with refractory angina pectoris was, in retrospect, analyzed in 19 consecutive patients implanted for SCS by Murray *et al.* [55]. Annual admission rate after revascularization was 0.97/patient/year and 0.27 after SCS ($p=0.02$). The average time the patients were in the hospital after revascularization was 8.3 days per year versus 2.5 days per year after SCS ($p=0.04$). The authors concluded that SCS was effective in preventing hospital admissions in patients with refractory angina, without masking serious ischemic symptoms or leading to (silent) myocardial infarction.

Conclusions

SCS is an effective and safe additional therapy that improves the quality of life of patients who are severely disabled by their angina complaints. In addition, SCS improves exercise tolerance in conjunction with antiischemic properties and does not mask angina pectoris during a myocardial infarction. The mechanisms of action are multi-factorial and are thought to take place at different levels in the heart and the brain.

Suggestions for further reading

Electrical Stimulation and the Relief of Pain. (2003) In: Simpson BA (ed), Pain research and clinical management, vol 15. Elsevier, Amsterdam

Operative Neuromodulation vol 1: Functional neuroprosthetic surgery. An introduction. (2006) In: Sakas D, Simpson B, Krames E (eds) Acta Neurochin Suppl 47 (7)

Part II: Spinal cord stimulation for peripheral vascular disease

Introduction: Background and history

Peripheral vascular disease (PVD) and spinal cord stimulation (SCS) have a long history in common. Cook was the first to notice that spinal cord stimulation in patients with a neurological disease such as multiple sclerosis and spinal cord lesions, resulted in autonomic changes. He assumed that a regional increase in blood flow might be the underlying mechanism. Three years later he published a small study of nine patients, with varying degrees of limb ischemia resulting from failure of sympathectomy or bypass procedures. He observed a striking pain relief, while infarcted tissue was not restored but healing of wounds was promoted after SCS. He concluded: "It is indeed probable that persistent spinal cord stimulation will avert the need for amputation in some patients. It certainly can be considered as another alternative before progression to amputation after failure of all other known therapeutic modalities" [16]. Dooley observed the same phenomenon of increased blood flow in patients stimulated for central nervous system disorders such as multiple sclerosis, olivopontocerebellar atrophy, amyotrophic lateral sclerosis and Friedreich's ataxia [21]. Trying to elucidate the phenomenon he used transcutaneous electrical stimulation in a patient with a cervical radiculitis. Electrodes were placed over the right side of the cervical spine. A one-channel impedance plethysmograph was connected to the right finger. Electrostimulation during 2½ minutes resulted in a fall in impedance that was interpreted as equivalent to a 154% increase in blood flow to the finger. He concluded: "Electrostimulation over the posterior spinal roots and the spinal cord, although not new, has not been used extensively for the treatment of patients with arterial disease. Electrostimulation of the nervous system is not designed to replace standard therapeutic measures of treatment of patients with vascular disease, but to supplement them."

In the second half of the eighties and the beginning of the nineties, epidural SCS was seen as a possible alternative treatment for patients with peripheral arterial occlusive disease (PAOD) who were no longer eligible for vascular reconstruction. Spinal cord stimulation seemed to be useful whatever the origin of pain. Relieving pain would result in improved mobilization of the patient, which in turn would enhance blood flow and heal ulcers. If this was indeed the case, then the need for amputation would decrease.

Over a period of 10–15 years, case reports and series of patients have been published demonstrating that SCS was a very effective pain treatment. As inclusion criteria were frequently ill-defined, many reports contained a highly inhomogeneous group of patients (atherosclerosis, vasospastic diseases, like Raynaud's and Buerger's disease, and others) sometimes at different stages of the disease. As pain treatment was the first objective of SCS, many reported an excellent result of pain relief following SCS. Due to the success with pain relief and the fact that patients without pain could walk again, the next step towards possible limb salvage was obvious. The belief that an amputation could be avoided in at least in 40–50% of the patients, motivated an increasing number of physicians to use the technique.

The positive sentiment towards the therapy was further driven by the publication of Augustinsson, who stated that indeed almost all patients (90%) conservatively treated were amputated, while in the case of SCS this was only 34% [6]. Some reports mentioned a near normalization of the blood flow in larger vessels as seen by a normalization of Doppler ankle pressure or even Doppler waves. Although one might expect some criticism on these data, reports of a significant increase in microcirculatory parameters sustained the effect of SCS. Due to a growing evidence, but considering the different way these results were reported, vascular surgeons produced a European Consensus document in order to at least harmonize the patient population under treatment.

If SCS could avoid limb amputation in a substantial proportion of the patients with critical limb ischemia, this would be an important gain for patients in whom the mortality rate was already 45–75% within 5 years [8, 22].

Mechanisms of action

Tallis suggested three possible mechanisms whereby SCS could influence blood flow [67].

1. Conventional pain relief might reverse the sympathetic vasoconstriction that occurs in response to pain. The observation that adequate pain relief correlates with improved capillary flow would be in accordance with this.
2. SCS induces an electrical sympathetic paralysis (with or without concomitant stimulation of cholinergic vasodilators).
3. The antidromic stimulation of dorsal root afferents causing sustained vasodilatation has been demonstrated both in man and animals.

Ghajar found that depending on the level of stimulation, there was an increase in capillary blood flow and skin temperature if the stimulation electrode was placed below the vertebral level T10 or preferably at T12 [27].

In his thesis, Linderoth [44] formulated the following general conclusions on the possible action of SCS:

1. In man dorsal column stimulation (DCS) induces increased CSF levels of substance P (SP), presumably of spinal origin.
2. Spinal microdialysis is suitable for studies of SP-release in the dorsal horn in response to noxious electrical stimulation of a peripheral nerve.

3. In response to peripheral noxious stimuli SP is released both in the ipsi- and contralateral dorsal horn of the spinal cord.
4. In the cat DCS induces release of both serotonin and SP in the dorsal horn of the spinal cord as measured with microdialysis.
5. The activation of SP release by DCS probably requires the involvement of supraspinal mechanisms. SP released in the dorsal horn by noxious stimulation and that released by DCS presumably originate from separate neuronal pools, possibly with different functional properties.
6. The alleviation of ischemic and other types of pain by DCS may involve at least partly different mechanisms.
7. The vasodilatation hypothetically underlying the suppression of the ischemic pain is not dependent on intact connections with the supraspinal centres or on antidromic activation of primary afferent fibres, whether of large or small diameter.
8. The vasodilatory effects of DCS involve spinal and segmental mechanisms and require intact transmission through the ventral roots and sympathetic paravertebral ganglia via postganglionic noradrenergic neurones.
9. DCS exerts its influence in the peripheral vascular bed predominantly via transitory suppression of sympathetic vasoconstrictor control.

Some of the biochemical aspects of pain have been described in greater detail in many review articles. In his thesis, Cui gives an extensive description of the history of SCS and the pathophysiological and biochemical background of neuropathic pain [17]. If spontaneous pain due to a hyperexcitatory state of primary or secondary order neurones, SCS seems to be able to inhibit the excitatory status. Recent publications on the pathophysiological processes involved in the generation of different types of pain indicate that tremendous progress has been made in unravelling the biochemical processes involved. The rapid evolution in genetic manipulation also provides the opportunity in pain research to "turn genes on and off", producing specific alterations in animals and thus facilitating the study of specific characteristics of receptors and the related neurotransmitters.

Patients selection

The second European consensus document on chronic critical leg ischaemia defines critical limb ischaemia (CLI) in non-diabetic patients as the presence of rest pain or tissue necrosis (ulceration or gangrene; Fig. 5) with an ankle systolic pressure of 50 mm Hg or less, or a toe pressure of 30 mm Hg or less [64]. Normal oxidative processes of cells need an oxygen supply. When blood flow to a tissue drops below the level needed for normal metabolic function, anaerobic metabolism temporarily tries to compensate. This phenomenon is known as ischaemia. It becomes critical when blood flow drops to a level

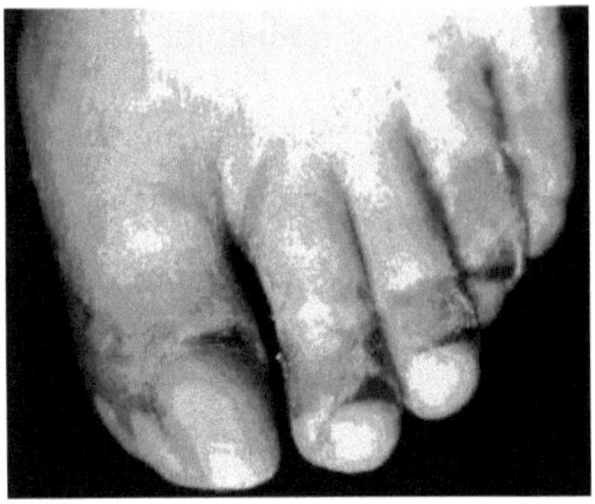

Fig. 5. Ischemic ulcers of the foot

where cell survival is in danger. Cell death results in tissue necrosis. The best known symptom in the early stages of tissue necrosis, is intermittent pain (vascular claudication).

CLI as defined is equivalent to Fontaine stages III and IV plus the blood pressure criteria. None of the criteria of the European consensus have been evaluated for its prognostic value in predicting outcome of the threatened limb. Jacobs and Thompson both found in their series that 50% of the patients classified as severely ischaemic fulfilled the criteria of the consensus document [35, 70]. The other 50% had an ankle systolic pressure greater than 50 mm Hg and an outcome similar to those with an ankle systolic pressure less than 50 mm Hg. It is, however, agreed that patients with ulcers greater than 3 cm^2 have a much lower limb salvage rate [10, 67]. Wolfe and Wyatt [80] presented an overview of the different definitions of CLI. Their suggestion to look for high- and low-risk patients is a step in the right direction. However, they do not mention the microcirculatory measurements. Carter [12] and Bunt and Holloway [11], proposed modified haemodynamic definitions for critical and subcritical ischaemia, which include measurements of pressures and indices of microcirculation.

The debate which might lead to a better classification of patients with CLI belongs to the vascular surgeons. An important part of the discussion will certainly be the value of microcirculatory measurements.

There are different ways to assess blood flow and there is no consensus on the best prognostic indicator. In a leading article [36] Jacobs and Jorning stated: "systolic ankle/arm pressure measurements at rest and after treadmill exercise are generally accepted as the best non-invasive method to document arterial obstruction of lower extremities. It should be emphasised, however, that in patients with Fontaine stages III and IV not only is the macrocirculation inadequate but, especially in patients with ulcerations and gangrene, the microcirculation is also threatened. Tissue oxygen pressure measurement,

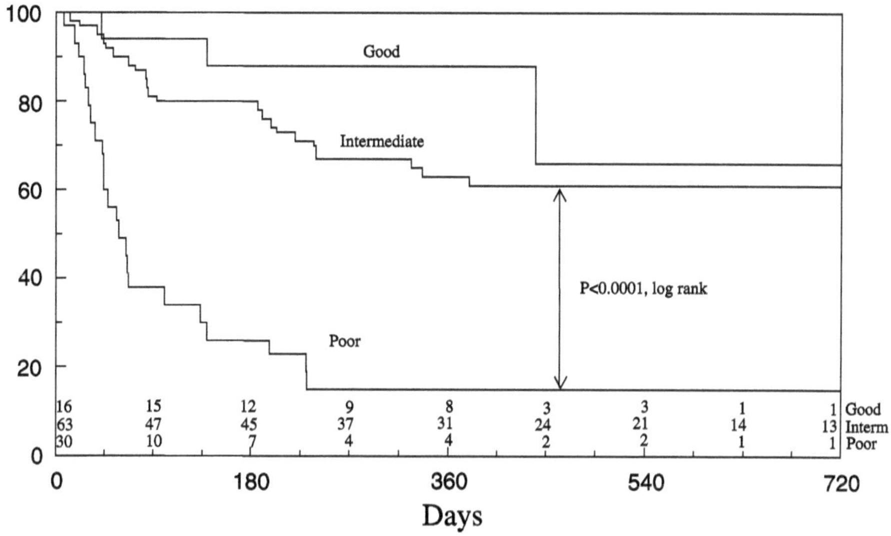

Fig. 6. Cumulative limb survival in the three microcirculatory categories. A dotted line indicates a standard error >10%. The numbers per category indicate the number of patients at risk. Good = $TcpO_2$ >30 mm Hg, Intermediate = $TcpO_2$ between 10 and 30 mm Hg, Poor = $TcpO_2$ <10 mm Hg [76, 77]

laser Doppler flowmetry and isotope clearance techniques can be performed to study cutaneous blood flow. Intravital skin capillary microscopy is a direct and non-invasive method of studying the morphological pattern of skin microcirculation and allows the measurement of red blood cell velocity in the skin capillaries, which specifically reflects nutritional blood flow". This means that further studies are needed to find out which method has the best prognostic value and can discriminate responders (limb salvage) from non-responders. Ubbink suggests that a combination of toe blood pressure and transcutaneous oxygen tension (TcpO2), using cut-off values of 38 mm Hg for toe blood pressure and 35 mm Hg for TcpO2 in the supine position, has a better prognostic value [75, 76] (Fig. 6). Gersbach uses the difference between sitting and supine TcpO2 as a better predictor of outcome [26]. Fiume reported that pain relief was obtained only in patients who showed an improved TcpO2 during trial stimulation [24], an observation also made by Jacobs [36].

Petrakis suggested that a trial period of two weeks should be considered before final implantation, because those who show a significant increase in TcpO2 in that period have a better outcome [61]. The criteria of the second European consensus document concern patients with 'chronic' CLI. This means a constant pain persisting for at least more than 2 weeks as used in the Dutch trial [41]. Kumar included only those patients treated conservatively for 6 months; this represents a different population [42]. With regard to limb survival of patients with CLI, it is obvious that the first two to three months after the diagnosis of CLI are very important because a large number of patients undergo amputation within this period. Recently, in a consensus document on the definition of CLI, some recommendations have been proposed both for the definition and for the trials on CLI. It is clear from this document that there is no real consensus on inclusion criteria and investigation of patients at risk of an amputation within months of diagnosis of CLI [15].

Patients selected for SCS are surgically non reconstructable and must have a critical limb ischemia, not evolving dramatically in a couple of days or weeks to a situation urging a minor or major amputation. In general they belong to the clinical grading of Fontaine III and IV. This means that patient has pain at rest and/or skin lesions in the region of the foot which may not exceed 3 cm^2.

In addition macrovascular criteria were added as Doppler ankle systolic pressure $\leq$50 mm Hg or a ankle/brachial index $\leq$35%. More recently microvascular criteria completed selection criteria adding transcutaneous pO2 (TpO2). Values between 10 and 30 mm Hg were accepted as compatible with CLI. General accepted selection criteria are found in Table 2.

Table 3 shows characteristics of patients included in the Dutch trial [41] for standard or SCS treatment. It also shows the high rate of other concomitant ischemic diseases.

Table 2. *Inclusion and exclusion criteria SCS for PVD*

Inclusion criteria

1. Persisting pain at rest for at least 2 weeks,
2. And/or skin lesions (ulcerations or gangrene) in the region of the feet or toes, which surface may not exceed 3 cm^2.
3. Doppler ankle systolic pressure $\leq$50 mm Hg or ankle/brachial pressure index $\leq$35%. For patients with diabetes mellitus and incompressible ankle arteries, absence of arterial ankle pulsations on physical examination.
4. Patient's written informed consent.

Exclusion criteria

1. Vascular disorders other than atherosclerotic disease.
2. No rest pain (e.g., only intermittent claudication) and no gangrene or ulceration.
3. Ulcerations deeper than the fascia or gangrene with a diameter larger than 3 cm^2.
4. Intractable existing infection of the ulceration o gangrene area
5. Neoplastic or concomitant disease restricting life expectancy to less than a year.
6. Presence of a cardiac pacemaker
7. Inadequate patient compliance due to psychological or social incompetence.

Table 3. *Characteristics of patients ($n = 120$) included in a Dutch randomized trial (Klomp et al.* [41])

Characteristics	*Standard* % (n)	*SCS* % (n)
Female	38% (23)	45% (27)
Age (mean + SD)	72 ± 10.6	73 ± 9.8
Diabetes	38% (23)	37% (22)
Contralat.leg		
– symptomatic	48% (29)	32% (19)
– amputated	12% (7)	15% (9)
Smoking		
– not for >1year	27% (16)	37% (22)
– still smoking	44% (26)	30% (18)
CVA/TIA	27% (16)	22% (13)
Myocardial infarction	37% (22)	38% (23)
Angina pectoris	25% (15)	20% (12)
Ulcerations/gangrene	68% (41)	63% (38)
Gangrene		
– dry	38% (23)	40% (24)
– wet	8% (5)	13% (8)
Previous vascular surgery		
– none	18% (11)	25% (15)
– 1 or 2	48% (29)	42% (25)
– >3	33% (20)	32% (19)
Sympathectomy (randomized leg)	32% (19)	35% (21)
Ankle pressure (mean + SD)	41.6 ± 21.8	35.2 ± 24.8
Ankle-brachial index (mean + SD)	0.28 ± 0.1	0.23 ± 0.1
$TcpO_2$ (mm Hg)	10	10

Clinical studies/level of evidence

Spincemaille *et al.* [65] published a systematic review on patients with CLI and SCS. Characteristics of patients treated for PAOD (Peripheral Arterial Obstructive Disease) were very similar in non-randomised studies and randomised controlled studies (RCTs). In the randomised studies standard treatment resulted in a limb salvage of 40–50% after two years follow-up. More specific treatments, such as prostaglandins or spinal cord stimulation (SCS) had slightly higher limb salvage ranging from 55 to 65%. The transcutaneous oxygen pressure ($TcpO_2$) was the parameter most frequently used to evaluate skin microcirculation. Limb survival of patients with an intermediate $TcpO_2$ value was 76% for SCS treatment compared to 52% in the conservative treated patients ($p = 0.08$). A limb salvage of 88% was found in patients treated with SCS if the difference between the supine and sitting $TcpO_2$ baseline values ($\Delta TcpO_2$) was ≥ 15 mm Hg. A rise in $TcpO_2$ after trial stimulation of at least 15% resulted in a limb salvage of 77% at 18 months ($p < 0.01$).

A recent systematic review and meta-analysis of the available controlled trials was done by Ubbink *et al.* [73]. He reported: "main endpoints were limb salvage, pain relief and clinical situation. Eighteen reports were found of which 5 RCTs. Nine studies were used for the analysis. The 12 month survival appeared significantly greater in the SCS group (risk difference (RD) −0.13, 95% CI −0.04 to −0.22)) Significant pain relief occurred in both treatment groups, but patients who received SCS required significantly less analgesia and reached Fontaine stage II more often than those who did not have SCS (RD 0.33 (95% CI 0.19–0.47)) This article however does not stress the importance of the initial $TcpO_2$. Further selection on the basis narrows the targeted population but clearly select the patients who will benefit from SCS. Amann *et al.* [1] reported at 12 months follow up a cumulative limb survival of patients treated with SCS which was significantly better than the control group. Their selection criteria were a baseline forefoot $TcpO_2$ of <30 mm Hg and both sufficient pain relief and paresthesia coverage (>75%) after test stimulation for 72 h. This kind of selection was already discussed and proposed in two other articles mentioned in this paragraph. $TcpO_2$ seems the best promising way of selecting patients for SCS treatment.

Implantation technique

In most cases, local anaesthesia is used to position the lead in the epidural space. General anaesthesia makes a correct placement of the electrode nearly impossible, because patients cannot provide information on the exact area where paraesthesia are felt. An epidural or a good regional block with complementary sedation even makes it possible to perform a laminectomy. These paraesthesia are phantom sensations created by SCS which activates the dorsal column neurones. When treating patients with critical limb ischemia, it is essential to obtain/produce paraesthesia in the painful region of the limb, but the same is true for several other chronic pain conditions. The site of puncture of the epidural space with a Touhy needle is two or three levels below the area where the tip of the lead will finally be positioned (T10). The best technique is an oblique (45° to the surface) and paramedian route in order to avoid sharp angles of the lead when perforating the ligamentum flavum of the epidural space (Fig. 7). The lead is always positioned medially or slightly lateral to the midline in the dorsal part of the epidural space. Fluoroscopic control during the procedure is mandatory. Positioning of the lead in the epidural canal is the most important part of the procedure. One should be careful to avoid migration of the lead during the subsequent stage of the procedure. Fixation of the lead at the level of the superficial fascial layer is

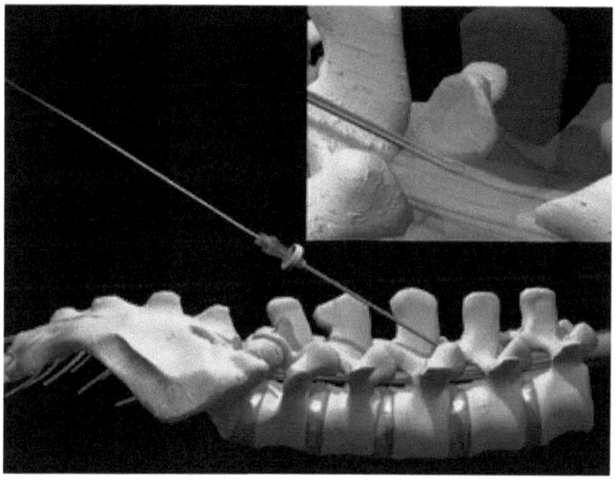

Fig. 7. Diagram showing insertion of epidural lead

necessary. The lead is connected to an extension cable, which in turn is connected to the pulse generator. The whole system is implanted subcutaneously in the same way as a pacemaker. The patient obtains an external programmer which allows the generator to be switched on and off. Another feature is the possibility of changing amplitude, pulse width and pulse rate; usually only the option of changing amplitude is activated. The physician can, however, fully control and programme the pulse generator using a remote external programmer.

Cost effectiveness

In the Dutch randomized study a cost calculation was performed [41]. At that time costs were calculated in Dutch guilders which are equivalent to 0.5€. The study was performed almost 10 years ago. Most of the costs derived from staying in hospital and in rehabilitation facilities. These costs were similar for both groups: mean *f*25957 and *f*14870 per patient in the spinal-cord-stimulation group vs *f*27153 and *f*16465 in the standard group. The mean cost for operative procedures per patient was *f*18428 in the stimulator group and *f*918 in the standard group. The cost of implanting the stimulator was *f*15900. Costs for professional care at home and in homes for the elderly, were similar. Outpatient cost, medications, medical supplies, and non-medical costs were a small part of the cost. Total cost at 2 years was *f*80439 per patient in the spinal-cord stimulator group, *f*17376 (28%) higher than in the standard group ($p = 0.009$). Adjusted for mortality, the mean cost per patient was *f*69066 in the stimulator group and *f*52407 in the standard group, $p = 0.002$.

Ubbink calculated the costs for SCS in case of CLI in his review article [73] and stated: "pooled data but not the individual RCTs revealed a significant beneficial effect in terms of limb salvage, at the cost of a significantly higher number of correctable complications and apparently higher costs. The finding that eight patients need to be treated to save one more leg, together with the higher cost of SCS treatment (about 8000€ for 2 years), suggests that about 64000€ extra needs to be spent to achieve this end. This should be weighted against any improvement in quality adjusted life years and the eventual cost of a major amputation, itself accompanied by ongoing high costs and high mortality rate".

Both studies give about the same differences in costs for both treatments. However regarding a better selection procedure the superiority of SCS must be easier to prove.

Conclusions

It seems from the available literature that SCS in CLI with a good selection algorithm is able to select those patients able to respond to SCS thereby reducing the number of amputations under SCS treatment. This group of patients with chronic CLI has a 50% survival of 5 years. So if amputation can be avoided and quality of life is enhanced, the short life expectancy for these patients is considerably ameliorated. The best recent reference is the Cochrane report of Ubbink giving all information on the effectiveness of SCS in PVD [74].

Suggestions for further reading

Electrical stimulation and the relief of pain. (2003) In: Simpson BA (ed), Pain research and clinical management, vol 15. Elsevier, Amsterdam.

Operative neuromodulation vol 1 (2006) In: Sakas D, Simpson B, Krames E (eds), Functional neuroprosthetic surgery. An introduction. Acta Neurochir Suppl 97/1

For more practical information

http://www.ans-medical.com/
http://www.medtronic.com/neuro/paintherapies/pain_treatment_ladder/neurostimulation/neuro_neurostimulation.html
http://www.neuromodulation.com/

References

1. Amann W, Berg P, Gersbach P, Gamain J, Raphael J, Ubbink DT (2003) Spinal cord stimulation in the treatment of non-reconstructable stable critical leg ischaemia: results of the European peripheral vascular disease outcome study. Eur J Vasc Endovasc Surg 26: 280–286
2. Andersen C, Hole P, Oxhoj H (1994) Does pain relief with spinal cord stimulation for angina conceal myocardial infarction? Br Heart J 71: 419–421
3. Andréll P, Ekre O, Eliasson T, Blomstrand C, Börjesson M, Nilsson M, Mannheimer C (2003) Cost-effectiveness of spinal cord stimulation versus coronary artery bypass grafting in patients with severe angina pectoris – long-term results from the ESBY Study. Cardiology 99: 20–24

4. Armour JA (2004) Cardiac neuronal hierarchy in health and disease. Am J Physiol Regul Integr Comp Physiol 287: R262–R271
5. Armour JA (1999) Myocardial ischaemia and the cardiac nervous system. Cardiovasc Res 41: 41–54
6. Augustinsson LE, Carlsson A, Holm J, Jivegard L (1985) Epidural electrical stimulation in severe limb ischemia. Evidences of pain relief, increased blood flow and a possible limb-saving effect. Ann Surg 202: 104–111
7. Bagger JP, Jensen BS, Johannsen G (1998) Long-term outcome of spinal electgrical stimulation in patients with refractory chest pain. Clin Cardiol 21: 286–288
8. Bertele V, Roncaglioni MC, Pangrazzi J, Terzian E, Tognoni (1999) Clinical outcome and its predictors in 1560 patients with critical leg ischaemia. Eur J Vas Endovasc Surg 18: 401–410
9. Braunwald E, Epstein SE, Glick G, Wechsler AS, Braunwald NS (1967) Relief of angina pectoris by electrical stimulation of the carotid-sinus nerves. New Engl J Med 277(24): 1278–1283
10. Broseta J, Barbera J, de Vera JA, Barcia-Salorio JL, March G, Gonzalez-Darder J, Rovaina F, Joanes V (1986) Spinal cord stimulation in peripheral arterial disease. A cooperative study. J Neurosurg 64: 71–80
11. Bunt TJ, Holloway GA (1996) $TcpO_2$ as an accurate predictor of therapy in limb salvage. Ann Vasc Surg 10: 224–227
12. Carter SA (1997) The challenge and importance of defining critical limb ischemia. Vasc Med 2: 126–131
13. Chauhan A, Mullins PA, Thuraisingham SI, Taylor G, Petch MC, Schofield PM (1994) Effect of transcutaneous electrical nerve stimulation on coronary blood flow. Circulation 89: 694–670
14. Chester M (2000) Long-term benefits of stellate ganglion block in severe chronic refractory angina. Pain 87: 103–105
15. Chronic critical limb ischaemia (2000) In: Management of peripheral arterial disease (PAD). Transatlantic inter-society consensus (TASC). Section D. Eur J Vasc Endovasc Surg 19 (Suppl A): S144–S243
16. Cook AW, Oygar A, Baggenstos P, Pacheco S, Kleriga E (1976) Vascular disease of extremities: electrical stimulation of spinal cord and posterior roots. NY State J Med 76: 366–378
17. Cui JC (1999) Spinal cord stimulation in neuropathy. Experimental studies of neurochemistry and behaviour. Thesis, Stockholm
18. DeJongste MJL, Haaksma J, Hautvast RW, Hillege HL, Meyler JW, Staal MJ, Sanderson JE, Lie KI (1994) Effects of spinal cord stimulatiom on daily life myocardial ischemia in patients with severe coronary artery disease. A prospective ambulatory ECG study. Br Heart J 71: 413–418
19. DeJongste MJL, Hautvast RWM, Hillege H, Lie KI (1994) Efficacy of spinal cord stimulation as an adjuvant therapy for intractable angina pectoris: a prospective randomized clinical study. J Am Coll Cardiol 23: 1592–1597
20. Diedrichs H, Zobel C, Theissen P *et al.* (2005) Symptomatic relief precedes improvement of myocardial blood flow in patients under spinal cord stimulation. Curr Control Trials Cardiovasc Med 6(7): 1–7
21. Dooley D, Kasprak M (1976) Modifications of blood flow to the extremities by electrical stimulation of the nervous system. Soth Med J 69: 1309–1311

22. Dormandy JA, Thomas PRS (1988) What is the natural history of a critical ischaemic patient with and without his leg? In: Greenhalgh RM, Jamieson CW, Nicolaides AN (eds) Limb salvage and amputation for vascular disease. Saunders, Philadelphia, pp 11–26
23. Fallen EL (1999) Evidence-based cardiovascular medicine, 3.20
24. Fiume D, Palombi M, Sciassa V, Tamorri M (1989) Spinal cord stimulation (SCS) in peripheral vascular disease. Pace 12: 698–704
25. Foreman RD, Linderoth B, Ardell JL, Barron KW, Chandler MJ, Hull SS Jr, TerHorst GJ, DeJongste MJ, Armour JA (2000) Modulation of intrinsic cardiac neurons by spinal cord stimulation: implications for its therapeutic use in angina pectoris. Cardiovasc Res 47: 367–375
26. Gersbach P, Hasdemir MG, Stevens RD, Nachbur B, Mahler F (1997) Discriminative microcirculatory screening of patients with refractory limb ischaemia for dorsal column stimulation. Eur J Vasc Endovasc Surg 13: 464–471
27. Ghajar AW, Miles JB (1998) The differential effect of the level of spinal cord stimulation on patients with advanced peripheral vascular disease in the lower limbs. Br J Neurosurg 12: 402–408
28. Gibbons RJ, Abrams J, Chatterjee K (2003) ACC/AHA 2002 guideline update for the management of patients with chronic stable angina – summary article: a report of the American College of Cardiology/American Heart Association Task Force on Practice Guidelines (Committee on the Management of Patients With Chronic Stable Angina). Circulation 107(1): 149–158
29. Gonzalez-Darder JM, Canela P, Gonzalez-Martinez V (1991) High cervical spinal cord stimulation for unstable angina pectoris. Stereotact Funct Neurosurg 56: 20–27
30. Hautvast RW, Blanksma PK, DeJongste MJ, Pruim J, van der Wall EE, Vaalburg W, Lie KI (1996) Effect of spinal cord stimulation on myocardial blood flow assessed by positron emission tomography in patients with refractory angina pectoris. Am J Cardiol 77: 462–467
31. Hautvast RW, DeJongste MJ, Staal MJ, van Gilst WH, Lie KI (1998) Spinal cord stimulation in chronic intractable angina pectoris: a randomized, controlled efficacy study. Am Heart J 136: 1114–1120
32. Hautvast RW, ter Horst GJ, DeJong BM, DeJongste MJ, Blanksma PK, Paans AM, Korf J (1997) Relative changes in regional cerebral blood flow during spinal cord stimulation in patients with refractory angina pectoris. Eur J Neurosci 9: 1178–1183
33. Hautvast RWM, Brouwer J, DeJongste MJL, Lie KI (1998) Effects of spinal cord stimulation on heart rate variability and myocardial ischemia in patients with chronic intractable angina pectoris. A prospective ambulatory electrocardiographic study. Clin Cardiol 21: 33–39
34. Issa ZF, Zhou X, Ujhelyi MR, Rosenberger J, Bhakta D, Groh WJ, Miller JM, Zipes DP (2005) Thoracic spinal cord stimulation reduces the risk of ischemic ventricular arrhythmias in a postinfarction heart failure canine model. Circulation 111(24): 3217–3220
35. Jacobs MJ, Jörning PJG, Beckers RCY, Ubbink DT, van Kleef M, Slaaf DW, Reneman RS (1990) Foot salvage and improvement of microvascular blood flow as a result of epidural spinal cord electrical stimulation. J Vasc Surg 12: 354–360
36. Jacobs MJHM, Jorning PJGIs (1998) Epidural spinal cord stimulation indicated in patients with severe lower limb ischaemia?. Eur J Vasc Surg 2: 207–208
37. Jessurun GAJ, Meeder JG, DeJongste MJL (1997) Defining the problem of intractable angina. Pain Rev 4: 89–99
38. Jessurun GAJ, TenVaarwerk IAM, DeJongste MJL *et al.* (1997) Sequalae of spinal cord stimulation for refractory angina pectoris. Reliability and safety profile of long-term clinical application. Cor Artery Dis 8: 33–37

39. Jessurun GAJ, Tio RA, DeJongste MJL, Hautvast RWM, Den Heijer P, Crijns HJGM (1998) Coronary blood flow dynamics during transcutaneous electrical nerve stimulation for stable angina pectoris associated with severe narrowing of one major coronary artery. Am J Cardiol 82: 921–926
40. Khogali SS, Miller M, Rajesh PB, Murray RG, Beattie JM (1999) Video assisted thorascopic sympathectomy for severe intractable angina. Eur J Cardiothorac Surg 16 (Suppl I): S95–S98
41. Klomp HM, Spincemaille GH, Steyerberg EW, Habbema JD, van Urk H (1999) Efficacy of spinal cord stimulation in critical limb ischemia. Lancet 353: 1040–1044
42. Kumar K, Toth C, Nath RK, Verma AK, Burgess JJ (1997) Improvement of limb circulation in peripheral vascular disease using epidural spinal cord stimulation: a prospective study. J Neurosurg 86: 662–669
43. Latherop DA, Spooner PM (2001) On the neural connection. J Cardiovasc Electrophysiol 12: 841–844
44. Linderoth B (1992) dorsal column stimulation and pain. Experimental studies of putative neurochemical and neurophysiological mechanisms. Thesis, Stockholm
45. Mannheimer C, Augustinsson LE, Carlsson CA (1988) Epidural spinal electrical stimulation in severe angina pectoris. Br Heart J 59: 56–61
46. Mannheimer C, Camici P, Chester MR, Collins A, DeJongste M, Eliasson T, Follath F, Hellemans I, Herlitz J, Luscher T, Pasic M, Thelle D (2002) The problem of chronic refractory angina; report from the ESC Joint Study Group on the Treatment of Refractory Angina. Eur Heart J 23: 355–370 (Review)
47. Mannheimer C, Eliasson T, Andersson B *et al.* (1993) Effects of spinal cord stimulation in angina pectoris induced by pacing and possible mechanisms of action. Br Med J 307: 477–480
48. Mannheimer C, Eliasson T, Augustinsson L-E *et al.* (1998) Electrical stimulation versus coronary artery bypass surgery in severe angina pectoris. Circulation 97: 1157–1163
49. Marber M, Walker D, Yellon D (1993) Spinal cord stimulation or ischemic preconditioning? Br Med J 307: 737
50. Marchand S, Li J, Charest J (1995) Effects of caffeine on analgesia from transcutaneous electrical stimulation. N Eng J Med 333: 325–326
51. Melzack R, Wall PD (1965) Pain mechanisms: a new theory. Science 150: 971–979
52. Mulcahy D, Knight C, Stables R, Fox K (1994) Lasers, burns, cuts, tingles and pumps: a consideration of alternative treatments for intractable angina. Br Heart J 71: 406–408
53. Murphy DF, Giles KE (1987) Dorsal column stimulation for pain relief from intractable angina pectoris. Pain 28: 365–368
54. Murray CJ, Lopez AD (1997) Mortality by cause for eight regions of the world: Global Burden of Disease Study. Lancet 349: 1296
55. Murray S, Carson KG, Ewings PD, Collins PD, James MA (1999) Spinal Cord Stimulation significantly decreases the need for acute hospital admission for chest pain in patients with refractory angina pectoris. Heart 82: 89–92
56. Norsell H, Eliasson T, Mannheimer C, Augustinsson LA, Bergh CH, Andersson Waagstein F, Friberg P (1997) Effects of pacing-induced myocardial stress and spinal cord stimulation on whole body and cardiac norepinephrine spillover. Eur Heart J 18: 1890–1896
57. Oosterga M, DeJongste MJL (2000) Neurostimulation in patients with intractable angina pectoris. Acta Chir Austriaca 32: 58–60

58. Palumbo LT, Lulu DJ (1966) Anterior transthoracic upper dorsal sympathectomy; current resuls. Arch Surg 92: 247–257 Maseri A. Chapter 4: The Coronary Circulation. In: Ischemic Heart Disease. Maseri A (ed). Churchill Livingston, New York 1995, p 71
59. Pan HL, Chen SR, Sensing tissue ischemia (2004) Another new function for capsaicin receptors? Circulation 110: 1832–1837
60. Parmley WW (1997) Optimal treatment of stable angina. Cardiology 88 (Suppl 3): 27–31 (Review)
61. Petrakis IE, Sciacca V (1999) Epidural spinal cord stimulation in diabetic critical lower limb ischemia. J Diabetes Complications 13: 293–299
62. Rosen SD, Paulescu E, Frith CD, Frackowiak RS, Davies GJ, Jones T, Camici PG (1994) Central nervous pathways mediating angina pectoris. Lancet 344: 147–150
63. Sanderson JE, Brooksby P, Waterhouse D, Palmer RBG, Neuhauser K (1992) Epidural spinal electrical stimulation for severe angina. A study of effects on symptoms, exercise tolerance and degree of ischemia. Eur Heart J 13: 628–633
64. Second European consensus document on chronic critical leg ischemia (1992) European Working Group on critical leg ischemia. Eur J Vasc Surg (Suppl A): 1–32
65. Spincemaille G, de Vet H, Ubbink Th, Jacobs M (2001) The results of spinal cord stimulation in critical limb ischaemia. Eur J Vas Endovasc 20: 99–105
66. Strobos MA, Coenraads PJ, De Jongste MJ, Ubels FL (2001) Dermatitis caused by radiofrequency electromagnetic radiation. Contact Dermatitis 44(5): 309
67. Tallis R, Jacobs M, Miles J (1992) Spinal cord stimulation in peripheral vascular disease (Editorial). Br J Neurosurg 6: 101–105
68. Taylor R, Taylor RJ, Van Buyten JP, Buchser E, North R, Bayliss S (2004) The cost effectiveness of spinal cord stimulation in the treatment of pain: a systematic review of the literature. J Pain Symptom Manage 27: 370–337
69. Ten Vaarwerk IA, Jessurun GA, DeJongste MJ, Anderson C, Mannheimer C, Eliasson T, Tadema W, Staal MJ (1999) Clinical outcome of patients treated with spinal cord stimulation for therapeutically refractory angina pectoris. The working Group on Neurocardiology. Heart 82: 82–88
70. Thompson MM, Sayers RD, Varty K, Reid A, London NJM, Bell PRF (1993) Chronic critical leg ischaemia must be redefined. Eur J Vasc Surg 7: 420–426
71. Tio RA, Tan ES, Jessurun GA *et al.* (2004) PET for evaluation of differential myocardial perfusion dynamics after VEGF gene therapy and laser therapy in end-stage coronary artery disease. J Nucl Med 45: 1437–1443
72. Tunstall-Pedoe H, Kuulasmaa K, Mahonen M *et al.* (1999) Contribution of trends in survival and coronary-event rates to changes in coronary heart disease mortality: 10-year results from 37 WHO MONICA project populations. Monitoring trends and determinants in cardiovascular disease. Lancet 353: 1547
73. Ubbink DT, Vermeulen H, Spincemaille G, Gersbach P, Amann W (2004) Systematic review and meta-analysis of controlled trials assessing spinal cord stimulation for inoperable critical leg ischaemia. Br J Surg 91: 948–955
74. Ubbink DT, Vermeulen H (2005) Spinal cord stimulation for non-reconstructable chronic critical leg ischaemia. Cochrane Database Syst Rev 20(3): CD 0004001
75. Ubbink DT, Spincemaille GHHM, Prins MH, Reneman RS, Jacobs MJ (1999) Microcirculatory investigations to determine the effect of spinal cord stimulation for critical leg ischemia: the Dutch multicenter randomized controlled trial. J Vasc Surg 30: 236–244

76. Ubbink DT, Spincemaille GH, Reneman RS, Jacobs MJ (1999) Prediction of imminent amputation in patients with non-reconstructible leg ischemia by means of microcirculatory investigations. J Vasc Surg 30: 114–121
77. Vulnink NCC, Overgaauw DM, Jessurun GAJ, TenVaarwerk IAM, Kropmans TJB, VanderSchans CP, Middel B, Staal MJ, DeJongste MJL (1999) The effects of spinal cord stimulation on quality of life in patients with therapeutically refractory angina pectoris. Neuromodulaton 2(1): 29–36
78. Wettervik C, Claes G, Drott C, Emanuelsson H, Lomsky M, Radberg G, Tygesen H (1995) Endoscopic transthoracic sympathectomy for severe angina. Lancet 345: 97–98
79. Wiener L, Cox JW (1966) Am J Med Sci 252: 289–295
80. Wolfe JHN, Wyatt MG (1997) Critical and subcritical ischaemia. Eur J Vasc Endovasc Surg 37: 587–582
81. Yu W, Maru F, Edner M, Hellstrom K, Kahan T, Persson H (2004) Spinal cord stimulation for refractory angina pectoris: a retrospective analysis of efficacy and cost-benefit. Coron Artery Dis 15(1): 31–37
82. Zamotrinsky A, Afanasiev S, Karpov RS, Cherniavsky A (1997) Effects of electrostimulation of the vagus afferent endings in patients with coronary artery disease. Coron Artery Dis 8: 551–557
83. Zanger DR, Solomon AJ, Gersh BJ (2000) Contemporary management of angina: part II. Medical management of chronic stable angina. Am Fam Phys 61: 129–138
84. Zhou X, Vance FL, Sioms AL *et al.* (2000) Prevention of high incidence of neurally mediated ventricular arrhythmias by afferent nerve stimulation in dogs. Circulation 101(7): 819–824

Offprint from
Advances and Technical Standards in Neurosurgery, Vol. 32
Edited by J.D. Pickard

Surgical anatomy of the petrous apex and petroclival region

H.-D. FOURNIER[2], P. MERCIER[2], and P.-H. ROCHE[1]

[1] Departement de Neurochirurgie, Hôpital Ste Marguerite, Marseille, France
[2] Departement de Neurochirurgie, Laboratoire d'Anatomie, Faculté de Médecine, Angers, France

With 39 Figures

Contents

Abstract

Surgical exposure of the clivus, the ventral or lateral aspect of the brain stem, and all the intradural structures of the petroclival area remains difficult because of the presence of the petrous apex and peripetrous complex. However, a lateral skull base approach to the petroclival area is the most suitable approach if the lesion to be resected lies medial to the fifth nerve, in front of the acousticofacial bundles, extending towards the midline. The purpose of this study is to review the topographic anatomy of the petrous apex and peripetrous structures, with emphasis on the relationships important to the lateral approaches to the petroclival area. Such anatomical knowledge allows us to study the surgical technique, exposure, and pitfalls of the main lateral transpetrosal skull base approaches used to reach the petroclival area.

Keywords: Anatomy; petroclival tumors; petrous apex; transpetrosal approach; skull base.

Introduction (Fig. 1)

The petroclival region is a surgical entity rather than an anatomical one, recognized because of specific diseases, notably petroclival tumors. It is defined as including the upper clivus and the anterior third of the petrous pyramid in front of the internal acoustic meatus. The term petroclival tumor refers to a lesion originating or inserted in the upper two-thirds of the clivus or the petrous apex, medial to the trigeminal nerve. This definition distinguishes these tumors from lesions of the cerebellopontine angle or the posterior face of the petrous portion of the temporal bone, which originate or are inserted further back and which therefore do not entail the same surgical problems. Structures close to the clival dura mater are often involved by growing tumor masses in this region and in consequence, the cavernous sinus, the Meckel's cave, the sphenoidal sinus, the sellar region, the incisure of the tentorium, the porus and the ventral edge of the foramen magnum may be encroached

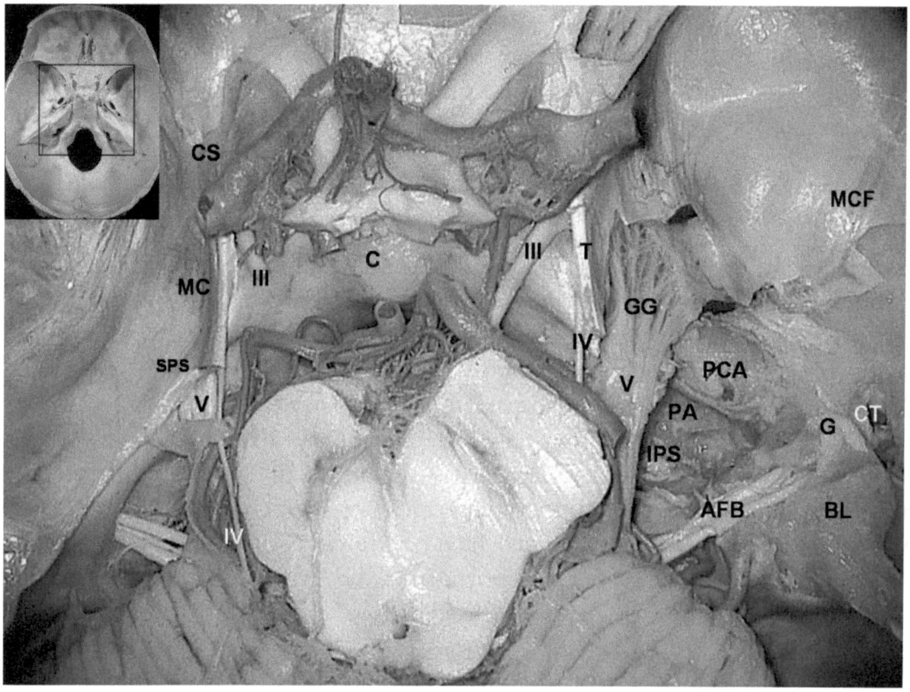

Fig. 1. Superior view of a cadaver skull base: the right middle cranial fossa has been drilled. See both petroclival areas. *CS* Cavernous sinus; *MC* Meckel's cave; *SPS* superior petrosal sinus; *C* clivus; *GG* gasserian ganglion; *T* tentorium; *PCA* petrous carotid artery; *PA* petrous apex; *IPS* inferior petrosal sinus; *MCF* middle cranial fossa; *AFB* acousticofacial bundles; *G* geniculate ganglion; *BL* bony labyrinth; *CT* cavum tympani; *III* 3rd cranial nerve; *IV* 4th cranial nerve; *V* 5th cranial nerve

upon and may need to be exposed. A lateral transpetrosal approach to this petroclival region is indicated when exposure is required beyond the lateral face of the cavernous carotid and, even more so, the petrous apex and the gasserian area. The main advantage of the lateral approach is that it creates considerably broader exposure than other approaches (e.g. a cisternal approach) at the same time as reducing cerebral retraction. Without any claim to solving all the problems of surgery of the skull base, such approaches bypass the potential pitfall represented in front by the septic craniofacial cavities and behind by the cerebellum and the brain stem itself. The problems boil down to those associated with the petrous and peripetrous barriers but these approaches probably constitute the shortest route to the clivus and the ventral surface of the brain stem.

Distinction can be made between two main types of lateral approach to the petroclival region and the ventral surface of the brain stem: antero-lateral approaches (in front of the cochlea) and posterolateral ones (which may or may not cover the labyrinthine mass). Almost every new description corresponds to a modification of an approach which is basically anterior or posterior and which constitutes one of the fundamental approaches already described.

Topographic anatomy

The petroclival region is a small cisternal space located in the most anterior part of the posterior cranial fossa (Fig. 2). It is defined by complex osteomeningeal edges but at the top, it opens onto the supratentorial sector, at the bottom onto the peribulbar area, and behind onto the area of the cerebellopontine angle. Various neurovascular structures pass through this space.

It is deeply located, below base of the brain and in front of the cerebellum. In front, it is blocked by the clivus and on the side, by the anterior third of the petrous pyramids and peripetrous elements. It is particularly difficult to expose the endocranial face of the clivus, the vertical aspect of the posterior face of the petrous portion of the temporal bone, the ventral surface of the brain stem, and all the intradural elements of the petroclival

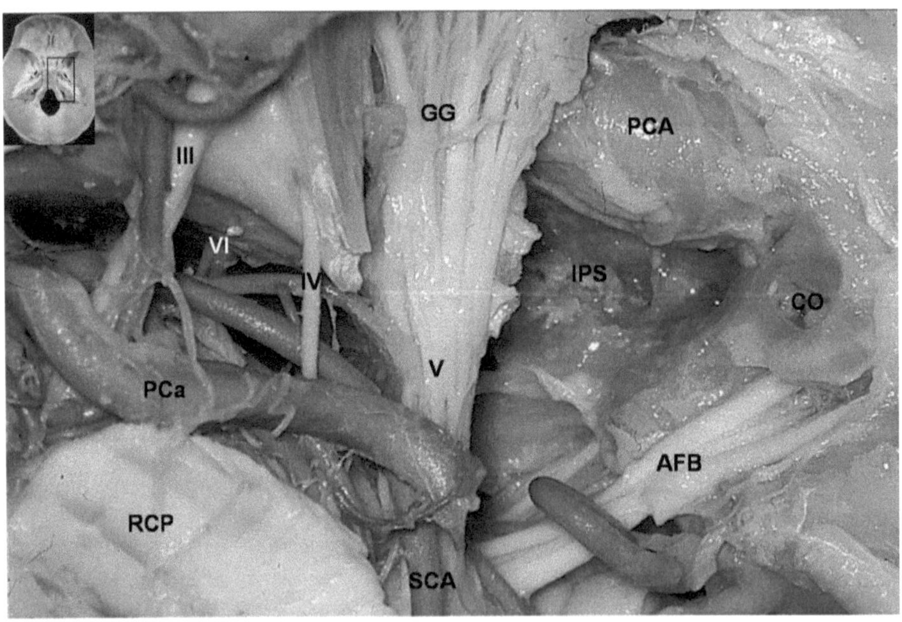

Fig. 2. Superior view of the right petroclival area: see the relationships between the petrous apex, the Vth nerve, and the petroclival area. *VI* 6th Cranial nerve; *PCa* posterior cerebral artery; *RCP* right cerebral peduncle; *SCA* superior cerebellar artery; *CO* cochlea; *GG* gasserian ganglion; *PCA* petrous carotid artery; *IPS* inferior petrosal sinus; *AFB* acousticofacial bundles

region, because of the presence of an "anatomical complex" comprising the following:

- The cavities of the petrous bone and what they contain (the middle ear, the bony labyrinth including the semicircular canals and the cochlea, the intrapetrous carotid in the carotid canal, and the facial nerve in the internal acoustic meatus and the fallopian canal).
- The dural sinuses (the superior and inferior petrosal sinuses)

To introduce the anatomical review of the surgical approaches, we will describe the complex of the petrous apex and its relationships with the main elements of the petrous pyramid. We will then focus on the region to which these approaches give access, namely the ventrolateral face of the brain stem and the cisternal petroclival region. We will also detail the cisternal configuration of the cranial nerves which are the elements that account for the morbidity associated with surgery in this region.

Petrous apex and its relationships within the petrous complex (Fig. 3)

The petrous apex or the apex of the petrous portion of the temporal bone comprises an upper surface which is part of the middle cranial fossa, and the anterior third of the posterior face of the petrous portion of the temporal bone which we are describing here. Triangular in shape with an anterior apex, both sides are clearly defined, at the top by the petrous ridge (which is the sulcus of the superior petrosal sinus [SPS]) and at the bottom by the petroclival suture (which itself forms a groove – that of the inferior petrosal sinus (IPS). Only the base of this triangle is an artificial boundary defined by a virtual line drawn vertically straight down from anterior edge of the porus acousticus. It should be specified here that the texture of the bone at the apex varies. As a rule, once the cortical is open, the bone is relatively soft, spongy and adipose – depending on the patient's age. However, in some cases, there is extensive pneumatization which helps when drilling. Moreover, it may be infiltrated by the tumor itself in which case it assumes the consistency of the tumor, be it a meningioma, a chordoma or an epidermoid cyst.

Superior aspect of the middle cranial fossa

This is formed by a forward concave face centered on the foramen spinosum, and a posterior convex face centered on the relief of the arcuate eminence. Continuous with the temporal scala, we will first address the tegmen tympani, a thin layer of bone which forms the roof of the tympanic cavity. Inside and behind the tegmen, there is the arcuate eminence, close to the petrous crest, where the external one-third and the internal two-thirds meet. This relief feature is an

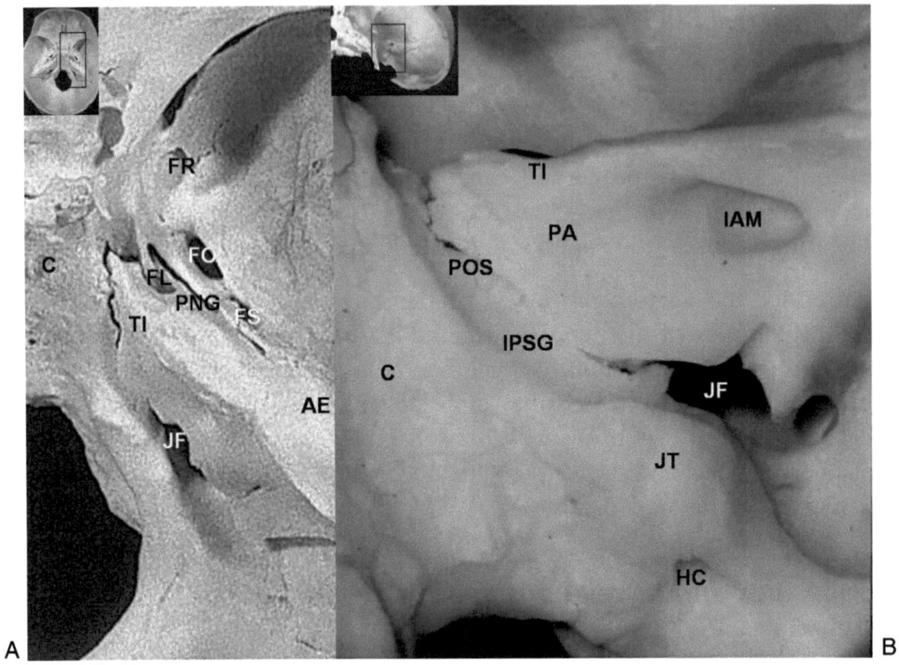

Fig. 3. Dry specimen of a right petrous bone: (A) Superior view, (B) lateral view. *C* Clivus; *FR* Foramen rotundum; *FO* foramen ovale; *FL* foramen lacerum; *TI* trigeminal incisura; *PNG* petrosal nerves groove; *FS* foramen spinosum; *JF* jugular foramen; *AE* arcuate eminence; *POS* petrooccipital suture; *PA* petrous apex; *IPSG* inferior petrosal sinus groove; *IAM* internal acoustic meatus; *JT* jugular tubercle; *HC* hypoglossal canal

important landmark since it can be used to locate the upper or anterior semicircular canal, the loop of which is found between 1 and 3.5 mm below the ventromedial face [31]. In front of the arcuate eminence, there is the meatal space which corresponds to the roof of the internal acoustic meatus. In front of the meatal space, there is a prominence out over the fossa or trigeminal pit on the petrous apex. Inside this relief is the foramen lacerum. This broad opening is oblique in front and inside and is located between the petrous apex and the dorsolateral wall of the sphenoidal sinus. Its lower half is filled with fibrocartilaginous tissue. It measures approximately one centimeter in length and is not completely traversed by the internal carotid [30]. The carotid only crosses the upper half of the foramen lacerum. It passes over and not across the lower half of the opening. The terminal part of the horizontal segment of the carotid canal opens at its upper half. The medial part of this foramen may or may not be covered in bone, exposing or hiding the horizontal segment of the intrapetrous carotid at the floor of the middle cranial fossa. Outside of the foramen lacerum, there is the sulcus of the greater petrosal nerve which comes from the hiatus of the canal for the lesser petrosal nerve which is located in front and inside the arcuate eminence. The lesser petrosal nerve, coming from the accessory hiatus, runs parallel to the former. The foramen ovale is anteromedial to the foramen spinosum. These two openings located in front of the carotid canal do not belong the petrous bone but their relationships need to be considered. The foramen spinosum is on average 4.7 mm (2.5 to 8) from the carotid canal [30]. A line joining the centers of these two foramina is parallel to the axis of the horizontal segment of the intrapetrous carotid, thus constituting an important landmark once this segment has been exposed via an extradural approach [43, 44].

Posterior aspect of the petrous pyramid

This vertical structure is defined behind by the impression of the sigmoid sinus and at the bottom by the very wide groove of the inferior petrosal sinus, deeply marking the petro-occipital suture. The internal acoustic meatus, opening behind via its porus, is located just below the petrous crest which provides a thick upper edge for this opening. The fundus of the internal acoustic meatus is divided into four parts by vertical and transverse crests [29, 33]. The antero-superior quadrant corresponds to the passage of the facial nerve, the antero-inferior one to the cochlear nerve, and the postero-superior and postero-inferior quadrants to the upper and lower vestibular nerves respectively. The endolymphatic fossa, located one centimeter behind the porus, gives passage to the endolymphatic sac, a blind bulge of the endolymphatic canal which is in contact with the dura mater and which has to be protected if hearing is to be preserved. The posterior face of the petrous portion of the temporal bone cannot be described without brief mention of the lateral mass of the occipital. In the prolongation of the sulcus of the inferior petrosal sinus, this structure represents the lower lip of the endocranial opening of the jugular foramen. The jugular tubercle projects out from the lateral mass over the hypoglossal canal which it separates from the jugular foramen. The endocranial opening of the jugular foramen is divided in two by the jugular spine of the temporal bone: laterally, the jugular indentation which gives passage to the gulf of the jugular vein, and medially, the pyramidal fossa which gives passage to the lower cranial nerves. The pyramidal fossa terminates the sulcus of the inferior petrosal sinus in front, and the jugular indentation represents the termination of the sulcus of the sigmoid sinus.

Intrapetrous cavities and their relationships

We will begin by describing these cavities on dry specimen in order to understand how they are organized in space and their various inter-relationships. Then, by means of views from above of dissections through the middle cranial fossa, we will describe the cavities in the context of the regional anatomy as a whole, treating them as inseparable from their contents.

Inner ear, carotid canal and fallopian canal on dry specimen dissection: installation (Fig. 4)

Most of the inner ear is constituted by the bony labyrinth. It comprises an anterior and a posterior segment. The former is formed by the cochlea and the latter includes the semicircular canals and the vestibule. It is about two centimeters in length and is located in the middle part of the greater axis of the pyramid. The labyrinth is particularly well described in Pellet and Cannoni [31] so we will only address those structures which are relevant to our dissections. The superior or anterior, horizontal or lateral and posterior semicircular canals form incomplete loops with a diameter of 7–8 millimeters, arranged in an orthogonal configuration with respect to one another. The upper semicircular canal forms a convex loop at the top determining the relief of the arcuate eminence, a loop more or less perpendicular to the petrous axis. The posterior semicircular canal is perpendicular to the former, in a vertical plane, close to the cortical of the posterior face of the pyramid. The horizontal or lateral semicircular canal forms a laterally convex loop in the horizontal plane. These canals are implanted on the vestibule and have a common branch for the upper and lower canals. These

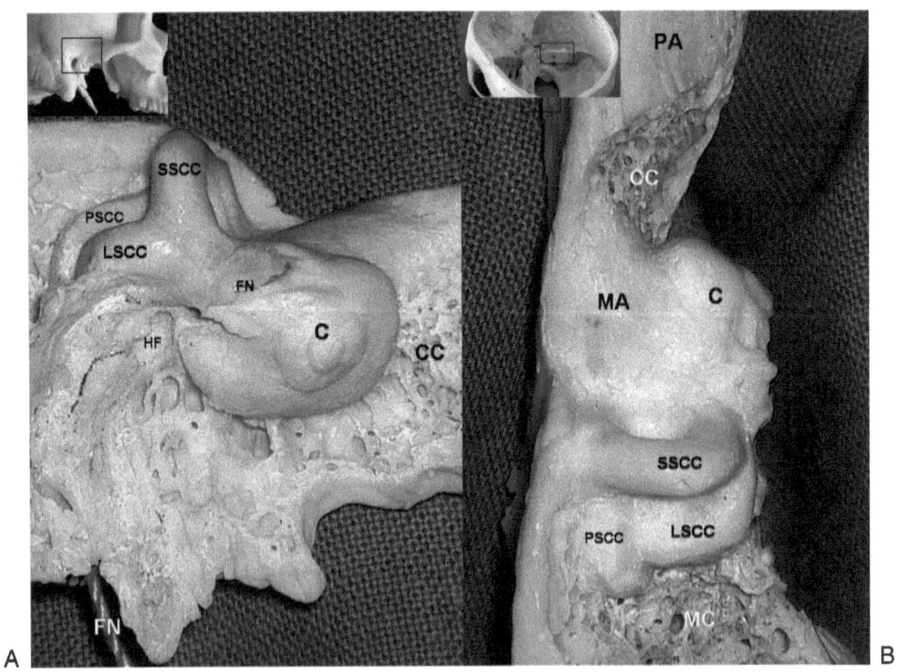

Fig. 4. Dry specimen of a right bony labyrinth: (A) Lateral view, (B) superior view. *SSCC* Superior semicircular canal; *PSCC* posterior semicircular canal; *LSCC* lateral semicircular canal; *FN* facial nerve; *HF* hemispheric fossa; *C* cochlea; *CC* carotid canal; *MA* meatal area; *PA* petrous apex; *MC* mastoidian cells

canals present ampullary dilatations. This dilatation is located on the anterior branch of the upper canal, on the lateral branch of the lateral canal, and on the posterior branch of the posterior canal. It is important to note two landmarks. The lateral branch of the lateral canal is in contact with the second portion of the facial nerve. The ampullary dilatations of the upper and lateral canals are in contact with the knee of the facial nerve. These relationships have to be borne in mind when drilling the labyrinthine mass to find the facial nerve. In our dissections, the vestibule is open. The hemispheric fossa bordered behind by the vestibular crest is exposed. Its wall separates it from the internal acoustic meatus.

The cochlea is joined to the cortical of the petrous apex. It is a tube rolled up on itself around a conical axis. We will look at relationships with the geniculate ganglion.

The carotid canal is located in front of the cochlea but in 33% of cases (as in this anatomical view), the knee and the vertical portion of the carotid canal are partly covered by the cochlea [30].

Intrapetrous cavities on fresh specimen dissections: description and relationships (Figs. 5–7)

Examination of the petrous portion of the temporal bone via the middle cranial fossa reveals its complex anatomy and makes it possible to define the important relationships between the intrapetrous carotid, the facial nerve, the porus, the cochlea, the geniculate ganglion, the petrosal nerves, the trigeminal ganglion, the middle ear, the eustachian tube, the tensor tympani muscle, and the middle meningeal artery.

Middle meningeal artery (Figs. 5 and 7). The first structure encountered on the floor of the middle cranial fossa, entering the skull via the foramen spinosum. It has a single trunk but in a few cases divides into two branches below the base of the skull, entering the cranium through two distinct openings [30]. If the middle meningeal artery arises from a persistent stapedial artery, a branch of the intrapetrous carotid, there will not be any foramen spinosum [23]. The petrosal artery arises from the middle meningeal artery, proximal to the foramen spinosum (58%) or distal to it (42%) [30]. It runs along with the greater petrosal nerve (or the lesser petrosal nerve in just 8% of cases) to supply the geniculate ganglion, the facial nerve and the middle ear (Fig. 5). There are also anastomotic ramifications with branches of the anterior and lower cerebellar arteries and branches of the stylomastoid artery (Fig. 7). These collaterals probably preclude peripheral facial paralysis if the petrosal artery is interrupted [24, 26].

The trigeminal ganglion (Figs. 1, 5, 6 and 8). Lying in the trigeminal fossa, the entry opening of which at the trigeminal incisure is located under the superior petrosal sinus (Figs. 1, 5 and 8). After resection of the sinus and opening of the

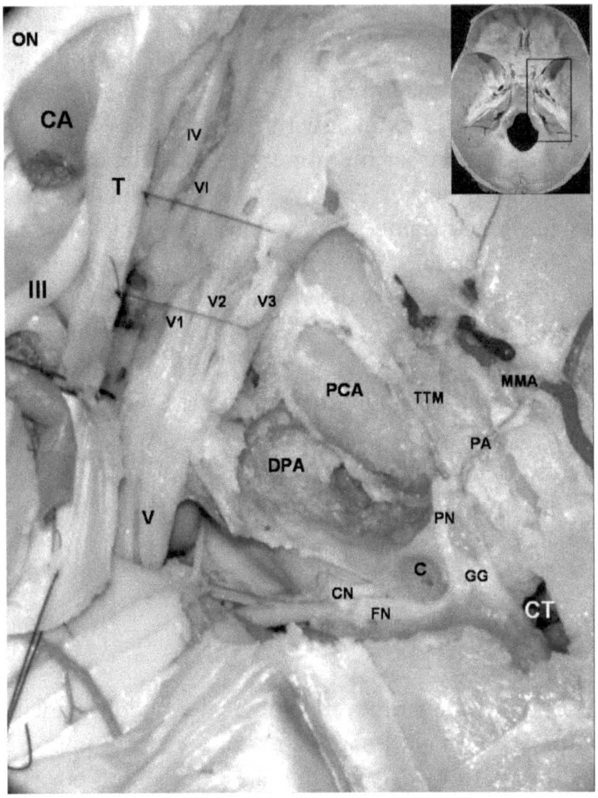

Fig. 5. Superior view of a right drilled middle cranial fossa: the third branch of the Vth nerve has been cut and displaced forwards to see the dural layer between the Vth nerve and the carotid artery. *ON* Optic nerve; *CA* carotid artery; *T* tentorium; *PCA* petrosal carotid artery; *DPA* drilled petrous apex: *TTM* tensor tympani muscle; *MMA* middle meningeal artery; *PA* petrosal artery; *PN* petrosal nerve; *C* cochlea; *CN* cochlear nerve; *FN* facial nerve; *GG* geniculate ganglion; *CT* cavum tympani; *IV* 4th cranial nerve; *VI* 6th cranial nerve; *V* 5th cranial nerve with first (*V1*) second (*V2*) and third (*V3*) divisions

dura mater covering the trigeminal ganglion and the origin of the dividing branches, it is seen that the infero-lateral angle of the ganglion is separated from the terminal portion of the horizontal carotid by only the dura mater (Fig. 6), as reported by Pait [29]. There is sometimes a thin bony sheet [30]. The supero-medial angle of the ganglion lies on the ascending portion of the intra-cavernous carotid. The ganglion usually lies on the ventral lip of the carotid canal (98% of cases according to Paullus) [30]. According to Pait, the carotid can be exposed laterally at the ganglion in 68% of cases [29].

Meckel's cave is a dural space occupying the middle fossa laterally to the cavernous sinus. It contains the trigeminal ganglion, the pars triangularis of the nerve and the origin of the branches of division that are wrapped in a cisternal

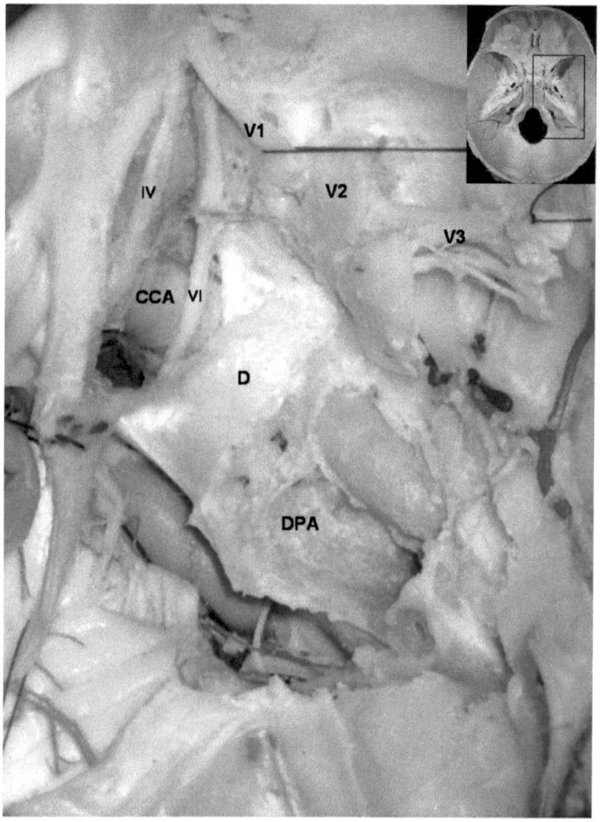

Fig. 6. Superior view of a right drilled middle cranial fossa: the Vth nerve has been removed. See the dura (*D*) and the cavernous sinus entrance. *CCA* Cavernous carotid artery; *D* dura; *V* 5th cranial nerve with first (*V1*) second (*V2*) and third (*V3*) divisions; *DPA* drilled petrous apex

space. This cistern is an extension of the cerebellopontine cistern. Communication between the posterior fossa and Meckel's cave is formed by a dural ring called the porus trigeminus through which pass the motor nerve and the sensory root of the nerve (Fig. 8) [42].

The facial nerve (intra-meatal and first portion) – petrosal nerves – the geniculate ganglion (Fig. 5). Using a diamond drill, the petrosal nerves, the geniculate ganglion, the facial nerve in the internal acoustic meatus together with its first portion are exposed, as well as the cochlear nerve and the upper vestibular nerve. The greater superficial petrosal nerve (GSPN) which is attached to the dura mater leaves the geniculate ganglion, emerges near the hiatus of the canal for the lesser petrosal nerve, and continues in an antero-medial direction towards the trigeminal ganglion. The proximal portion of the greater petrosal nerve is usually covered in bone. In 30% of cases [30], the

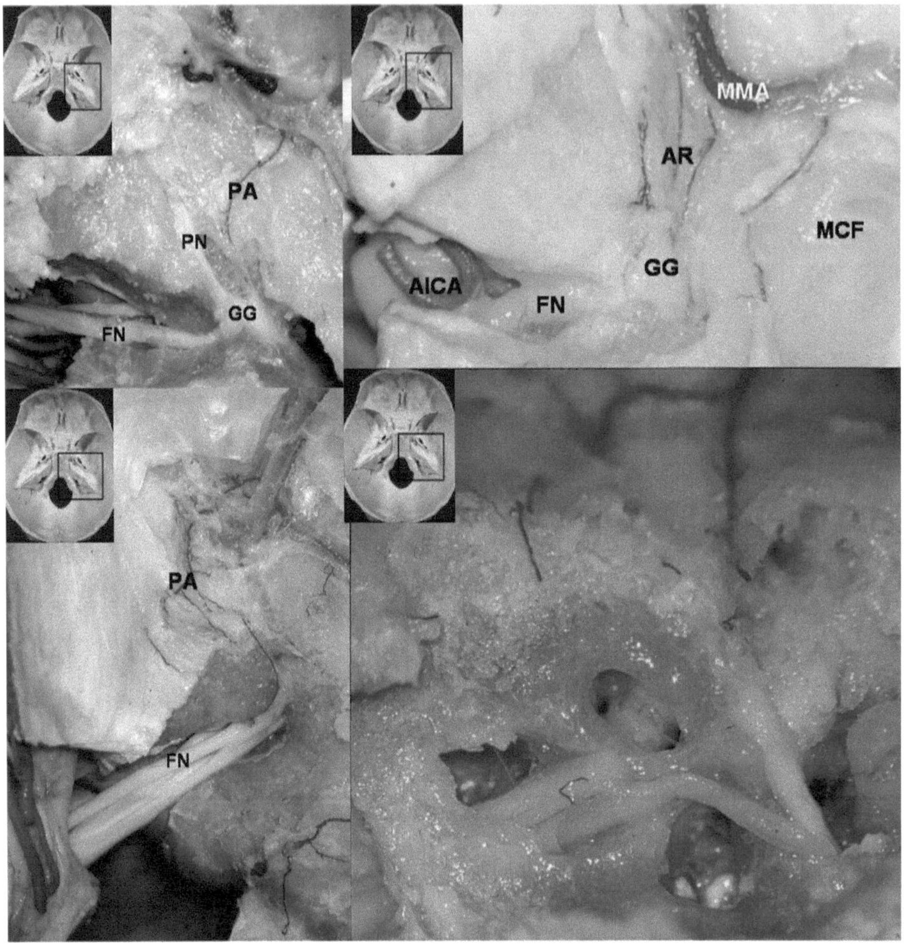

Fig. 7. Facial nerve vascular supply. Superior view of a right middle cranial fossa: *PA* petrosal artery; *PN* petrosal nerve; *FN* facial nerve; *GG* geniculate ganglion; *AICA* anterior inferior cerebellar artery; *AR* anastomotic ramifications; *MMA* middle meningeal artery

junction of this nerve with the geniculate ganglion is not covered. The average distance between the hiatus of the canal for the lesser petrosal nerve and the geniculate ganglion is 3.7 mm (range: 0.5–8 mm) [30]. The greater petrosal nerve runs parallel to the horizontal segment of the carotid, above its ventral edge in 66% of cases, and it can be located in front of it or above the anterior half of the canal [30]. The lesser petrosal nerve also arises from the geniculate ganglion and enters a sulcus located in front and outside of the canal for the tensor tympani muscle. The geniculate ganglion is postero-lateral (38%) posterior (26%) or lateral (16%) to the carotid knee [30], at an average distance of 6.5 mm (range: 3–13 mm). Usually covered with bone, the geniculate ganglion can be exposed

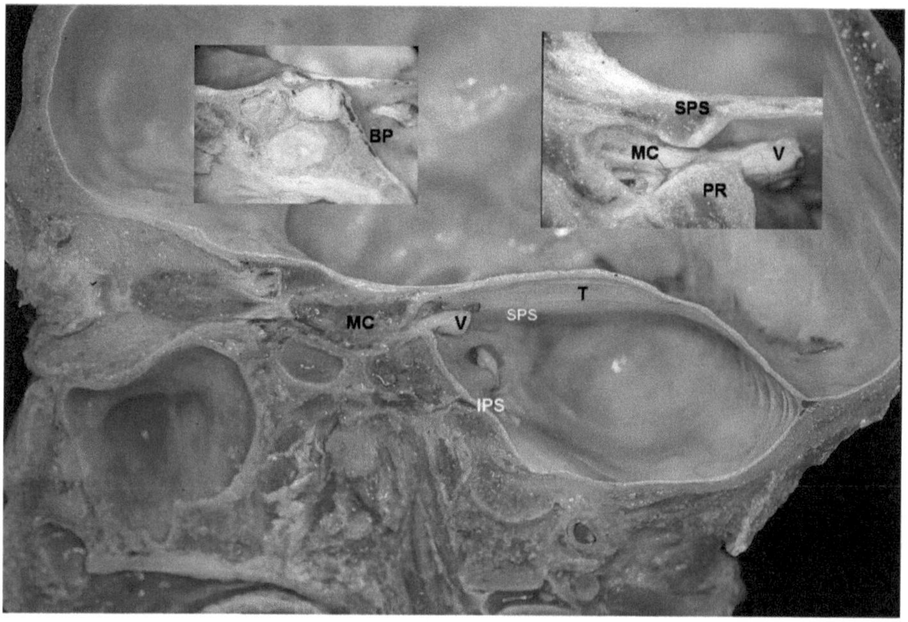

Fig. 8. Sagital section of a fresh specimen: to emphasize on Meckel's cave relationships. *MC* Meckel's cave; *V* 5th nerve; *SPS* superior petrosal sinus; *IPS* inferior petrosal sinus; *T* tentorium; *BP* basilar plexus; *PR* petrous ridge

without bone coverage in 16% of cases. It is nevertheless always in a depression in the bone surface.

Cochlea (Figs. 4 and 5). By drilling inside the first portion of the facial nerve, its knee and the geniculate ganglion, in the angle between the facial nerve and the greater petrosal nerve, the dense capsule of the cochlea is exposed to an average depth of 3–4.5 mm [30]. The bone then looks darker as one drills the highly dense cortical until penetration of the membrane covering of the fluid-filled cochlea. The average distance between the cochlea and the geniculate ganglion is 0.8 mm.

Intrapetrous carotid artery and carotid canal (Figs. 5, 6 and 9). The internal carotid enters the skull via a periosteous canal. The exocranial opening of the carotid canal is located just in front of the jugular foramen, and the endocranial opening is near the petrous apex. The artery can be easily dissociated at its adhesion points in the canal, except where it enters into the vertical segment, at which point it is attached by strong fibrous tissue. The intrapetrous carotid artery has two segments, one vertical and one horizontal joined at the carotid knee. The dimension of each segment is exactly the same according to Paullus, on average 5.2 mm [30]. The average length of the vertical segment is 10.5 mm, and that of the horizontal segment 20.1 mm [30]. The horizontal segment starts at the knee and continues in the antero-medial axis of the foramen lacerum, in front of the cochlea, eventually emerging at the apex. Its roof is exposed by drilling. The medial part of the horizontal portion of the carotid canal may be covered only by the dura mater or it may be covered in bone, elements which separate the carotid from the trigeminal ganglion. The carotid knee is separated from the cochlea which is located behind and above it in most cases, the average distance between the cochlea and the knee being 2.1 mm (range: 0.6–10 mm). Nevertheless, the cochlea covers part of the knee in 33% of cases [30]. These ideas make it possible to understand why it is difficult to expose the intrapetrous carotid – especially the knee and the vertical segment – without impairing hearing function [42, 43].

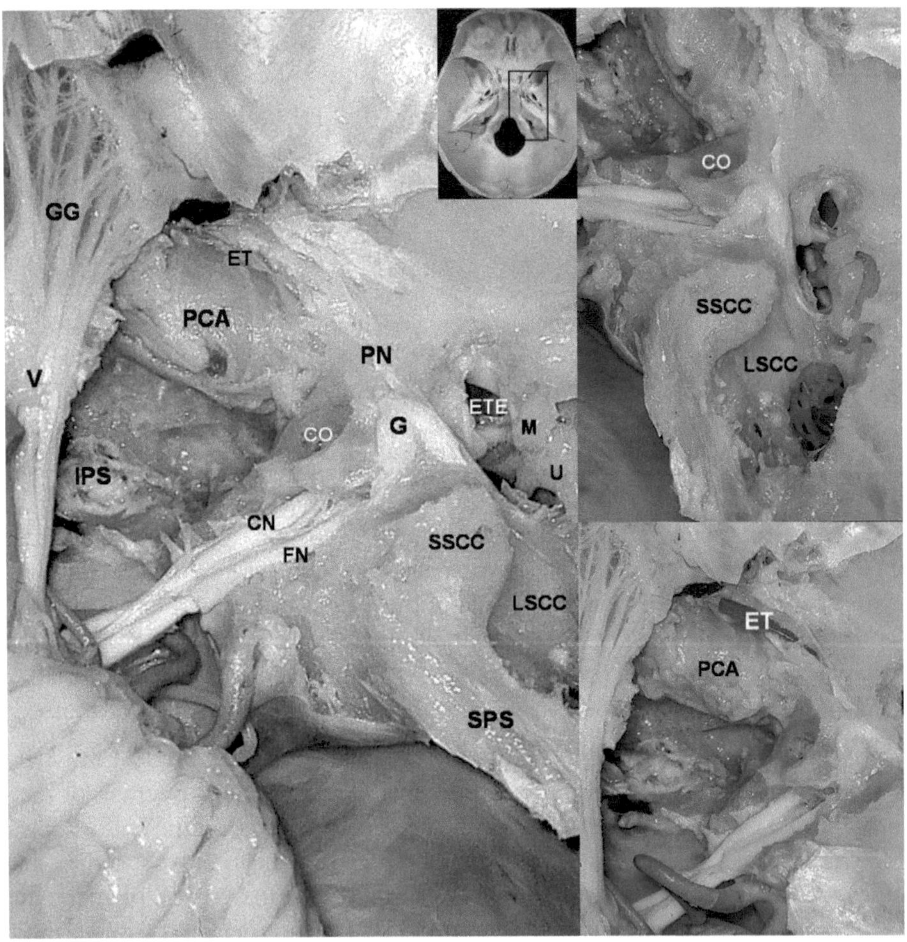

Fig. 9. Superior view of a right middle cranial fossa following drilling and dissection of the petrous bone: see the right tympanic cavity, and its relationships. *GG* Gasserian ganglion; *ET* Eustachian tube; *PCA* petrous carotid artery; *IPS* inferior petrosal sinus; *V* 5th cranial nerve; *PN* petrosal nerve; *CO* cochlea; *G* geniculate ganglion; *CN* cochlear nerve; *FN* facial nerve; *ETE* Eustachian tube entrance; *M* malleus; *U* uncus; *SSCC* superior semicircular canal; *LSCC* lateral semicircular canal; *SPS* superior petrosal sinus

Medial drilling of the horizontal segment in front of the cochlea reveals the vertical segment. Below, the drilling exposes a wide inferior petrosal sinus (Fig. 9) which goes as far as the jugular gulf between the glossopharyngeal nerve (nerve IX) and the vagus nerve (nerve X). The jugular tubercle separates this sinus from the canal of the hypoglossa and from the hypoglossal nerve. The pericarotid venous plexuses described by Paullus as sheathing the artery in its periosteous envelope are more numerous in its distal portion [30, 42, 43] although they were relatively under-developed in all our dissections.

In 50 carotid arteries, Paullus only observed collaterals of the intrapetrous carotid in 38% of cases, all of which arose in the horizontal segment [30]. He only observed one vidian artery and one periosteous artery. When present, these branches can be identified at the opening of the periosteum sheathing the carotid. They sometimes account for why the intrapetrous carotid is still supplied in a retrograde direction in some cases in which the cervical carotid is blocked.

There is major variation in the intrapetrous carotid artery which should be recognized and diagnosed before denudation of one or other of its segments. According to Lasjaunias [23], the intrapetrous segment is fenestrated in some carotid arteries, the summit of the fenestration being located at the knee. In addition, an abnormal path is known in the middle ear or abnormal flow through the ascending pharyngeal artery [14, 22, 23, 32]. This variation is rarely bilateral and is more commonly seen on the right, and may be suspected on clinical grounds (pulsating tinnitus or not, more or less constant, moderate and progressive hypoacusis). The diagnosis is made on the basis of CT scan and angiography results. TDM slices do not show the vertical segment adjacent to the cochlea and the floor of the middle ear is dehiscent. Angiography [22] uses the vertical vestibular line which should always be located outside of the carotid knee. In this type of arrangement, the flow uses the lower tympanic artery, a branch of the ascending pharyngeal artery, and the hyoid artery. In this case, the artery passes through Jacobson's canal or the tympanic canal rather than the vertical portion of the carotid canal which is atretic [23]. Other abnormalities may be associated, the most common being persistence of a stapedial artery substituting for the middle meningeal artery without any foramen spinosum present.

Middle ear, eustachian tube, tensor tympani muscle, posterior labyrinth and facial nerve (second portion) (Figs. 9 and 10). By drilling out the antero-medial side of the arcuate eminence, the upper semicircular canal can be exposed. Step-by-step drilling reveals the blue line corresponding to this canal in the surrounding compact bone at a depth of about 2 mm (between 1 and 3.5 mm according to Pellet [31]). Lateral drilling exposes the horizontal semicircular canal. By drilling the tegmen in front and outside of the horizontal semicircular canal, one penetrates the cavity of the middle ear. The opening is completed by drilling laterally through to the geniculate ganglion. The tympanic opening of the eustachian tube is easy to identify in front of the cochleariform process, and the insertion of the tensor tympani muscle. Also seen is the head of the malleus, the uncus and its short branch. Our dissections show the close relationship between the second portion of the facial nerve and the anterior branch of the horizontal semicircular canal. This is a key landmark for the second portion. It should be noted that this second portion is located on the medial or labyrinthine wall of the tympanic cavity where it projects out to the dorsal wall and penetrates into the mastoid. This projection of the canal of the facial forms the separation between the medial wall of the tympanic cavity and that of the aditus ad antrum.

The eustachian tube and the tensor tympani muscle are located in front of and parallel to the horizontal segment of the petrous carotid (Fig. 10), below the bony floor. The muscle may be above, in front of or behind the eustachian tube [28]. Both are covered in bone – in all cases according to Paullus [30]. The ostium of the eustachian tube and the tympanic cavity are located just behind the carotid knee in 63% of cases [30]. In 20% of cases according to the same

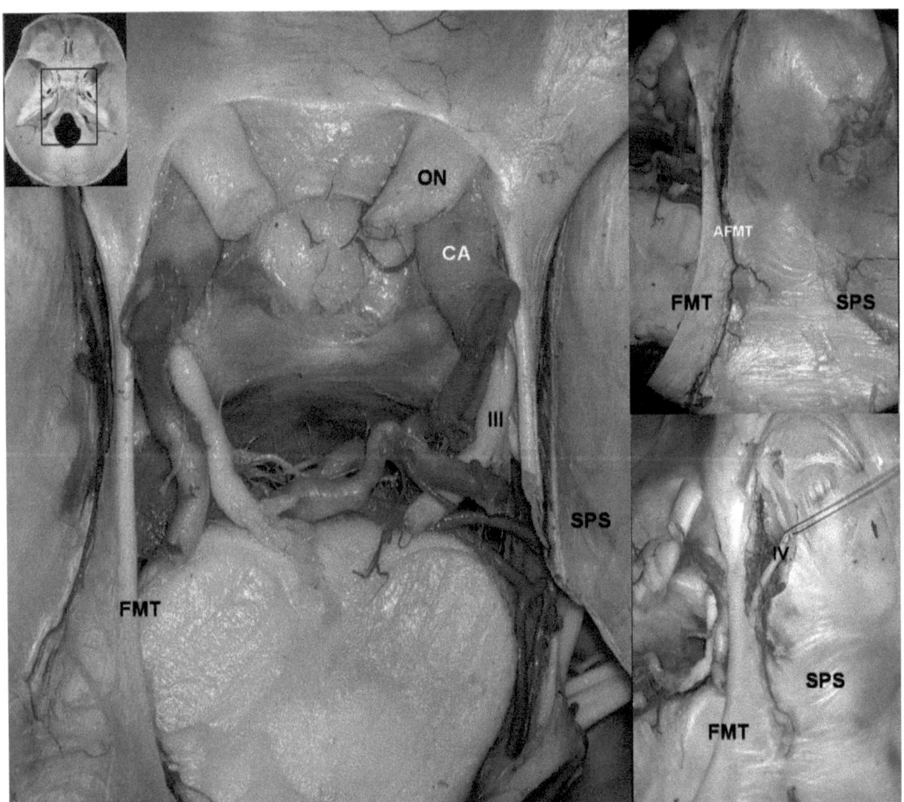

Fig. 10. Superior view of a cadaver skull base: see dural vascular supply from cavernous carotid artery. *ON* Optic nerve; *CA* carotid artery; *FMT* free margin of the tentorium; *SPS* superior petrosal sinus; *III* 3rd cranial nerve; *AFMT* artery of the free margin of the tentorium; *IV* 4th cranial nerve

expert, this ostium is located laterally to the vertical segment of the carotid and the knee. The average thickness of the bone separating the ostium from the carotid knee is 3.2 mm [30]. The eustachian tube and muscle are separated by the inter-musculo-tubar septum.

The dura mater of the middle, posterior levels (Figs. 6, 8 and 10). This lies simply on the floor of the middle cranial fossa, not posing any detachment problem apart from a few adhesion points. It covers the trigeminal nerve increasingly intimately as one moves laterally away from the apex, becoming less easy to dissociate close to where this nerve branches off, notably to form V3. It is nevertheless possible to devise a detachment plan which exposes the true lateral wall of the cavernous sinus, which will be described in the next chapter. It covers the horizontal segment of the petrous carotid, the petrosal nerves and – as we have seen in some cases – the geniculate ganglion if it is not protected by a bony covering. We have also noticed that it can form an invagination under the trigeminal ganglion to separate it from the medial portion of the horizontal carotid. It only consistently invaginates in the foramen spinosum, and sometimes in the sulcus of the petrosal nerves. At the posterior face of the pyramid, it invaginates and spreads around nerves in their respective openings.

The dura mater lines the endocranial face of the clivus, only leaving a single opening for passage of the abducent nerve under the petro-sphenoidal or petro-clinoid ligament marking the entry of the nerve's canal (Dorello's canal) (Fig. 6). We will see that there can be two distinct openings on each side for the nerve to pass through the dura. In the normal configuration, the two foramina (right and left) are separated by a distance of 20 mm (17–27 mm) [21]. The basilar venous plexuses located in the thickness of the clival dura mater can be extensively developed (Fig. 8). They are linked to the marginal sinuses of the greater foramen [25, 43].

This dura mater is prolonged by a roof which closes the petroclival region at the top in the tentorium, a thick, double sheet which is an extension of the anterior petroclinoid ligament.

This dura mater is composed of several layers which let veins and sinuses of variable dimensions through at various spots. We have mentioned the SPS, the SPI and the basilar plexus. This dura mater is vascular with meningeal branches coming from the intracavernous carotid and from the ascending pharyngeal artery (Fig. 10). These arteries take on special importance when the tumor has developed from the dura mater, notably in meningioma. The surgeon's ability to expose this dura mater as extensively as possible is one of the key features of transpetrosal approaches. About the dura of the petroclival region, V. Dolenc [6] made the following statement, "Where the layered dura at the petrous apex joins the tentorium, the lateral wall of the parasellar space, and especially, dural layers in the vicinity of Meckel's cave constitutes the richest, most complex junction of intracranial dural structures".

The superior petrosal sinus (Figs. 1, 8 and 10). This runs along the petrous crest at the junction of the upper and posterior faces of the pyramid, rejoining the cavernous sinus at the elbow of the sigmoid sinus near the sinuso-dural angle (Citelli's angle). At its origin, it is linked to the inferior petrosal sinus by the transverse sphenoidal sinus [34]. It overlies the trigeminal nerve when this crosses the petrous apex without adhering to the nerve. Its main afferent is represented by the group of upper petrosal veins [25] including the always-present upper petrosal vein which runs along the lateral edge of the nerve up till the sinus. The sinus is at least 3 mm from the porus and from the roof of the internal acoustic meatus [31]. This sinus may be prolapsed (10%), reducing the size of this space.

The inferior petrosal sinus (Figs. 8 and 10). Always very wide (and with a diameter which is often under-estimated), it runs along in a very broad sulcus cut by the petro-occipital suture, uniting the cavernous sinus at the gulf of the jugular vein. It is easy to understand that this bulky sinus could considerably hinder drilling of the petrous apex, and it has been proposed that it be embolized prior to surgery [11, 12].

Venous sinuses and the concept of petroclival venous confluence (PVC). This concept has been developed in a main paper by Destrieux *et al.* [7]. Briefly the PVC is located at the junction of the posterior part of the cavernous sinus, the SPS, the IPS and the basilar plexus. This part of the PCR includes not only the venous sinuses but also the abducens nerve and the clival arteries. Ozveren [28] have reported two types of trabecula inside the PVC. A delicate type, fragile, transparent and membranous, and a tough fibrous type forming structures that bridge the two layers of the dura.

Contents of the petroclival region (Figs. 5, 6 and 11)

The cisterns

The PCR is a cisternal space represented by the association of several arachnoid sheets which form the neighbouring cisterns. In practice, there is no petroclival cistern as such but inside and in front there is a prepontine cistern which adheres to and communicates with the cerebellopontine cistern outside and behind.

Oculomotor nerve (Fig. 11)

The third nerve is a very fragile nerve which is highly complex in functional terms, lying outside the petroclival region which forms its upper boundary. Manipulation of the nerve usually leads to severe palsy of the whole components of the nerve. Ptosis and pupillary function are usually recovered but some oculomotor function may be reduced. Exiting from the interpeduncular space, it passes intracisternally at a horizontal, slightly oblique laterally and enters the cavernous sinus at the top of the lateral wall. Its entry point in the lateral wall of the parasellar

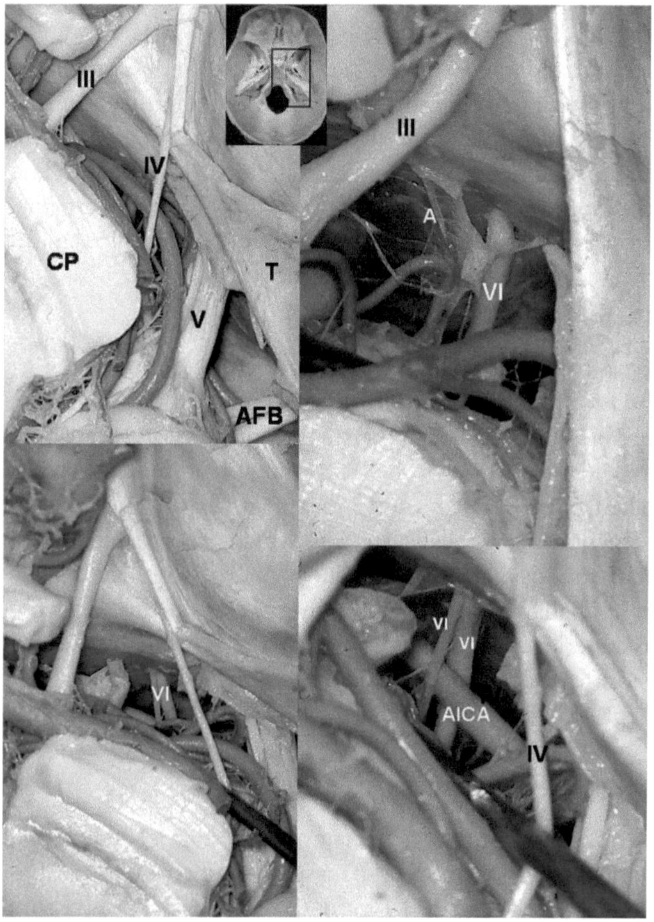

Fig. 11. Superior views of the right cisternal petroclival area and its contents: *CP* cerebral peduncle; *AFB* acousticofacial bundles; *T* tentorium; *A* arachnoid; *AICA* anterior inferior cerebellar artery; *III* 3rd cranial nerve; *IV* 4th cranial nerve; *V* 5th cranial nerve; *VI* 6th cranial nerve

space is a key surgical spot because it comes with a very limited sheath of arachnoid at the porus oculomotorius and an oblique groove at the upper surface of the nerve can always be distinguished. This oculomotorius porus gives access to a canal that can be opened far to the anterior pole of the lateral wall at the point where the trochlear nerve joins the third nerve at the entry of the superior orbital fissure. The nerve is usually safe with PC tumors but involvement of the cavernous sinus may modify the anatomy. Usually the tumor exits from the CS by the porus oculomotorius and pushes the nerve upwards.

The average cisternal course of nerve III is 20 mm in length and that of nerve IV is 32.6 mm [21].

Trochlear nerve (Fig. 11)

The forth nerve is a very small, fragile nerve, purely motor and supplying a single muscle. Localized at the upper part of the petroclival field in its cisternal course. Closely related to the inferior surface of the free edge of the tentorium. Fused to the free edge in a porus before it enters the lateral wall of the CS. The point of fusion is variable from one subject to another. In pathology, the nerve is shifted upwards and to the side making it more accessible for manipulation.

Trigeminal nerve (Figs. 5 and 6)

The PC region is centered by the root of the trigeminal nerve, the course of which is close to the horizontal and anteroposterior. This bulky root comes from Meckel's cave which lies in the gasserian cistern, a depression located on the upper surface of the petrous portion of the temporal bone. Meckel's cave is formed by a double-walled portion of the dura mater and is occupied by an arachnoid extension of the pontocerebellar cistern in which cerebrospinal fluid circulates – which is perfectly visible in MRI sequences. This root enters the PCR by passing into an oval-shaped fold of the dura mater constituted at the top by the canal of the superior petrosal sinus and at the bottom by a sheet which lines the depression formed by the porus trigeminus (Fig. 8).

On average it runs for 12.3 mm (range: 9–17 mm) within the cistern [21].

Abducens nerve (Fig. 11)

The sixth nerve arises from the ponto-medullary junction from a single trunk or two distinct trunks [1]. As emphasized by Brassier, three types of configuration of this nerve have been observed. Type I (86.5%) corresponds to a single trunk of the nerve from its origin as far as where it penetrates the dura in Dorello's canal. Type II (6%) corresponds to one origin in a single trunk which soon divides to form two branches which enter the clival dura mater separately. Type III (7.5%) corresponds to two trunks of origin with two different dural entry points. We have observed a nerve with dual origin, the two roots of which pass either side of the AICA and use the same dural entry point (Fig. 11). This type of configuration does not correspond to any of the three above-described types. Mercier reports one case of fenestration of nerve VI [26]. When the configuration is of the conventional Type I form, the nerve runs more or less vertically from the bottom up and slightly outside, flattened against the arachnoid which it crosses perpendicularly to enter Dorello's canal under the petroclinoid ligament (Fig. 6). Its average length in the cistern is 16.5 mm (12.5–21 mm) [21].

The nerve leaves the posterior fossa by piercing the meningeal dura over the clivus approximately 1 cm below and medial to the trigeminal root. The relationships between Dorello's canal and inferior petrosal sinus are very closed.

For the first few millimeters of its intradural course, this nerve is sheathed by the arachnoid and bathed in CSF [28]. It can be deduced that the petroclival portion of the abducens nerve does not belong to the extradural space. This is an important observation because, at the level of the petrous apex, it twists round horizontally under the petroclival ligament (Gruber's ligament) to pass over the dorsal and lateral surface of the internal carotid artery as it enters the posterior cavernous sinus.

Ozveren [28] described two anatomic variations (lateral or medial) in the course of the abducens nerve in the petroclival region, depending on the nerve's angles and attachment points. The proximity of the abducens nerve to the petrous ridge in the lateral type (57% in the study from Tokyo) might have surgical importance in the anterior transpetrosal approach. The abducens is a small nerve which supplies a single muscle. Usually shifted downward and distorted between two fixed points. Sometimes involved and encased by the tumor if the lesion is an external one like a chordoma.

Acousticofacial bundles (Figs. 5 and 6)

The cochleo-vestibulo-facial bundle has been studied in detail by Mercier [26] and Rhoton [33]. It runs in an almost frontal plane as it crosses the cistern of the pontocerebellar angle (*cisterna cerebellopontis*). The relationships it has with the loop of the AICA are variable and have been reviewed by Lang [21]. In our preparation, the AICA crosses the nervous bundle by its dorsal face, the loop being fixed by the dura mater above the porus (6% according to Lang) [21]. The average cistern length of nerve VII is 16 mm (10–26 mm), and that of nerve VIII 15 mm (8.5–22 mm) [21].

This neurovascular structure transversally crosses the cerebellopontine angle and is protected by the arachnoid sheath of its individual cistern. Even though it is outside the petroclival region, it is exposed in the surgical field laid open by a number of common approaches to the PCR. Tumors originating from the PCR usually push the cerebellopontine cistern and its contents backwards.

The brain stem

The petroclival region is defined medially by the lateral aspect of the brain stem in its middle protuberant part. In practice, the lower boundary is the bulbo-pontine sulcus and the upper boundary is the ponto-mesencephalic sulcus.

Surgical anatomy

The surgical anatomy of the petroclival region is detailed in each of the approaches we describe below. Here, we consider two complementary concepts dealing with the systematization of the lateral skull base.

Skull base anatomy and triangles (Fig. 12)

When detailing the anatomy of the base of the skull, it is possible to find reliable permanent landmarks that are helpful to delineate operative corridors. Since these corridors are broadly speaking triangular in shape, several authors have systematized the triangulation of skull base landmarks as follow [4, 8, 9, 13, 42].

The triangles from the parasellar subregion

- Anteromedial triangle (Dolenc): the limits are the lateral border of the optic canal, medial surface of the third nerve within the sheath of the dura entering the superior orbital fissure, and the distal dural ring.
- Medial triangle (Fukushima): the limits are the lateral wall of the intradural carotid artery, posterior clinoid process and porus oculomotorius. An intradural intracisternal space.
- Superior or paramedial triangle: the limits are located in the lateral wall of the cavernous sinus between the third and the fourth nerve. The anterior apex is formed by the point at which nerve IV crosses over nerve III.

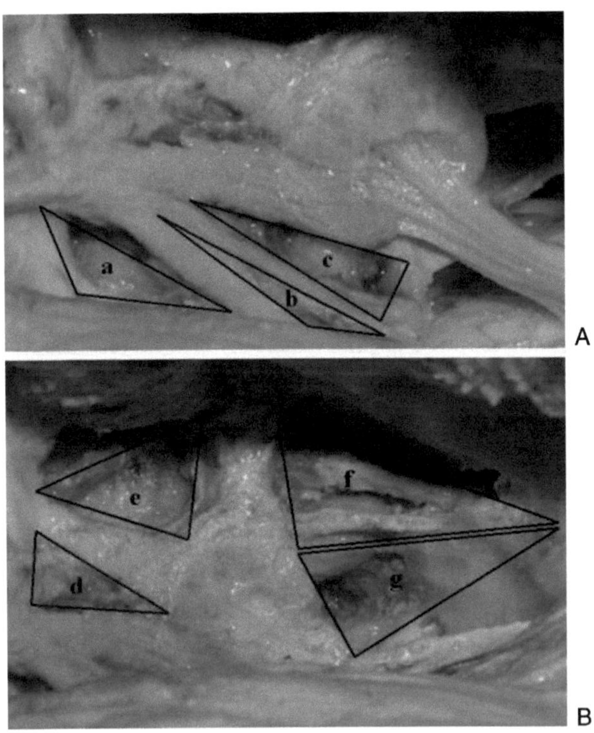

Fig. 12. Systematization of the main skull base triangles: (A) Triangles of the parasellar subregion: *a* anteromedial triangle, *b* paramedial triangle, *c* lateral triangle. (B) Triangles of the middle cranial fossa subregion: *d* anterolateral triangle, *e* far lateral triangle, *f* posterolateral triangle, *g* posteromedial triangle

- Oculomotor trigone (Dolenc): the three summits of the triangle are the ACP, the PCP, the petrous apex.
- Lateral triangle (Parkinson): the limits are the lateral wall of the cavernous sinus between the trochlear nerve and the ophthalmic division of the trigeminal nerve, and the dura between and behind these two nerves. Provides direct access to the intracavernous carotid artery.

The limits of the triangles from the middle cranial fossa subregion

- Anterolateral triangle (Mullan): between the ophthalmic and the maxillary branches of the trigeminal nerve.
- Far lateral triangle (Dolenc): between the foramen rotundum and the foramen ovale (or between the second and third division of the trigeminal nerve).
- Posterolateral triangle (Glasscock): posterior rim of foramen ovale and third branch of the trigeminal nerve (anterior border), the line from the arcuate eminence to the posteromedial corner of gasserian ganglion, and the line between the foramen spinosum and arcuate eminence. Through this triangle, the following important structures may be accessed: the great superficial petrosal nerve, the intrapetrous carotid artery (C6), the tensor tympani muscle and the eustachian tube.
- Posteromedial triangle (Kawase): the line connecting the arcuate eminence and the postero-medial corner of the geniculate ganglion – nerve V – the line connecting the arcuate eminence and posterior aspect of nerve V where it crosses the crest of the petrous apex.

The triangles from the petroclival subregion

- Inferomedial triangle (Dolenc): this triangle is formed by the apex of the Posterior clinoid process, the dural entry point of nerve IV into the tentorium, and the dural entry point of nerve VI [8].
- Inferolateral (trigeminal) triangle: this triangle is defined by the dural entry point of nerve IV into the tentorium (upper point), the entry point of nerve VI into the dura of the clivus (medial point), and the entry point of the petrosal vein into the SPS (lateral point).

The petrous bone segmentation

Pellet *et al.* [31] formulated the concept of petrous bone segmentation. The surface of the petrous pyramid carries several landmarks and is covered in critical neurovascular structures that can be easily identified during surgery. The internal carotid artery, the internal auditory canal, the fallopian canal and the semicircular canals are used as the boundaries in this concept. This segmentation is

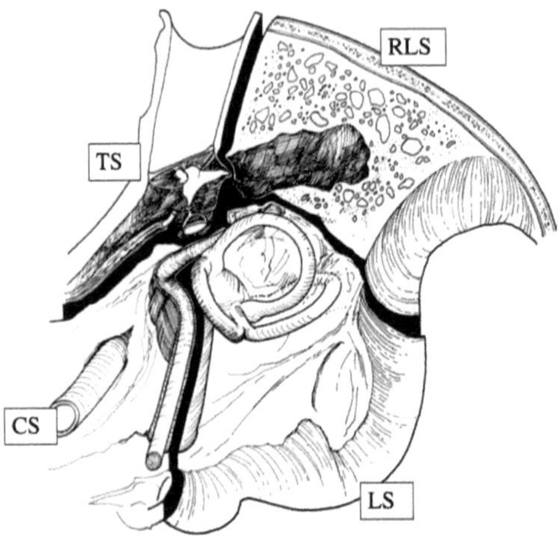

Fig. 13. Petrous bone segmentation (from Pellet *et al.*): *CS* carotid segment, *LS* labyrynthine segment, *RLS* retrolabyrynthine segment, *TS* tympanic segment

particularly applicable when it comes to the posterolateral approach to the petrous bone. This concept is illustrated in Fig. 13.

- The posterolateral segment is also named the retrolabyrinthine or mastoid segment. Superficially, it is limited by the posterior margin of the external auditory canal in front and by the sigmoid sinus behind. This segment contains mastoid air cells particularly the antrum. Horizontal removal of this area gives access to the third portion of the intrapetrous facial nerve and the semicircular canal.
- The postero-medial segment is also named the labyrinthine segment. The anterior limit is the posterior margin of the internal auditory canal and the medial limit is the dura of the posterior fossa. This segment is a logical progression from the mastoid segment, accessed by drilling the semicircular canals and the vestibule.
- The anterolateral segment also called the tympanic segment corresponds to the middle ear and is rarely exposed in current approaches to the petroclival region.
- The anteromedial segment or carotid segment corresponds to the petrous apex. It is limited medially by the petrous ridge, laterally by the intrapetrous carotid, in front by the porus trigeminus and behind by the anterior border of the internal auditory canal.

Classification of the approaches

Many different approaches have been described for the removal of petroclival tumors. There is no single ideal approach and which is the most suitable will depend on several parameters. Ongoing progress in neuroimaging techniques are making it easier to identify the origin and spread of the lesion which are important parameters when it comes to choosing the approach route. Extradural tumor masses are mainly represented by chordomas, chondrosarcomas, epidermoid cysts and cholesterol granulomas. Tumors originating from the dura are mainly meningiomas while intracisternal lesions are schwannomas of the trigeminal nerve or epidermoid cysts. For all these lesions it is also necessary to consider relationships with the cranial nerves and the brain stem. Ideally, surgeons who operate at the base of the skull should be familiar with all the relevant approaches but in practice, most have more experience with a limited number of routes: this will also influence their surgical decision.

Briefly we can describe three kinds of approaches to the PCR: anterior transmaxillary or transfacial approaches; intradural cisternal approaches; and approaches via the base of the skull. In this paper we will focus on lateral skull base approaches because we consider that these facilitate resection with very moderate invasiveness and are associated with relatively low level postoperative morbidity. However, here are a few comments about the other two types of approach:

Anterior transmaxillary or transfacial approaches need two-team expertise and are recommended for midline clival tumors (preferably extradural). The operative field that is created is deep and narrow, laterally limited by both carotids and the cavernous sinus [18]. The angle of approach is thus reduced, vascular control is hazardous, and closure is compromised (particularly when the dura is opened).

Intradural cisternal approaches were historically the way to gain access to the PCR. These routes use the natural spaces afforded by the cistern to advance towards the target. Their main advantages are short exposure time and rapid identification of neurovascular structures. However, in many respects they are not specific to the PCR because they do not give direct, close access to this region and require intradural retraction of the parenchyma.

The pterional-trans-sylvian approach was first popularized by Yasargil. The sylvian fissure opening gives access to the pericarotid and optochiasmatic cisterns. Working corridors are between the optic pathway and carotid artery, and between carotid artery and the third nerve. The posterior clinoid process has to be drilled and then opening of the Liliequist membrane gives access to the upper pole of the petroclival tumor, particularly when the tumor is inserted close to the posterior clinoid process. Although the usefulness of this approach is limited, it can offer many advantages when included in a more complex strategy involving an epidural transcavernous approach to the parasellar and suprasellar extensions of some petroclival tumors.

The subtemporal transtentorial approach was developed by Drake for basilar trunk aneurysms, particularly for basilar tip vascular lesions. In this approach, the third and fourth temporal gyri are directly retracted upwards to gain access to the free edge of the tentorium. This approach can be convenient for resection of tentorial and falcotentorial meningiomas but affords poor PCR exposure. Direct temporal lobe retraction and venous problems constitute serious limitations.

The retrosigmoid – lateral suboccipital approach is still routinely used by many experienced surgeons to reach the PCR. The disadvantages are that the acousticofacial bundle is always in the way and that the working corridor is narrow and deep. Moreover, it is difficult to control lesions that are located close to the basilar trunk and in front of it [35]. Control is compromised if the tumor has a supratentorial portion, in which case the trochlear nerve is at risk when the tentorium is encroached upon. Possibilities for resection of the dura and underlying bone tissue are very limited.

Lateral skull base approaches (Fig. 15)

These approaches offer the shortest distance to the PCR. Coming from an extradural route means less brain retraction and better preservation of veins. It also means earlier interruption of the tumor vascular supply, earlier tumor detachment and more radical resection. However it should be kept in mind that extra time is needed to perform this approach and a collaborative team is often required. Moreover, a good knowledge of the anatomy of the lateral skull base

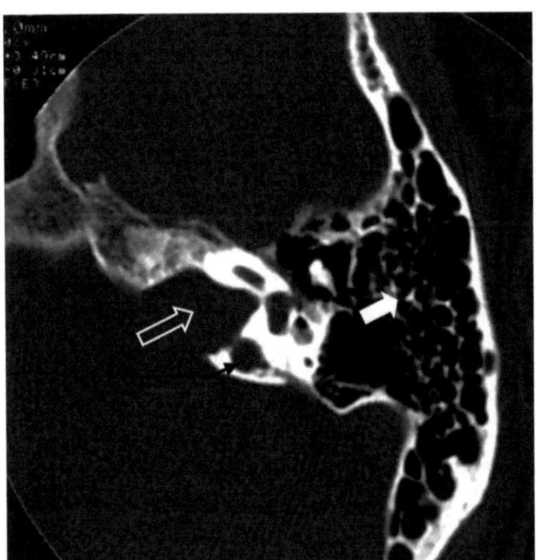

Fig. 14. Axial CT scan of a left petrous bone (bone window) showing several individual variations: the bold white arrow shows the high degree of the pneumatization. The black small arrow shows a high jugular bulb positioned close to the posterior lim of the internal auditory meatus. The empty white arrow shows the widening of the internal auditory canal

is required as well as sustained training and practice if these approaches are to be successfully exploited. As mentioned above, careful analysis of neuroradiologic images will provide a satisfactory estimate of the origin, insertion and development of the lesion and will show individual anatomical variations that may influence the operation (Fig. 14). From a technical point and regardless of the approach that is selected, the following general principles should always be applied: use constant anatomical landmarks for the drilling step, optimize dura exposure and opening, take care with the retractors to preserve veins, induce clotting meticulously one step at a time, protect and preserve critical neurovascular structures, perform reconstruction with care, and hermetically close the dura.

Epidural subtemporal approaches (from above). Anterior & lateral skull base approaches (1 & 2 from Fig. 15)

Middle fossa anterior transpetrosal approach (anterior petrosectomy)

Background

This approach was developed by Kawase in 1985 to treat two aneurysms at the vertebro-basilar junction [20]. It was adapted by House in 1986 to treat advanced or extensive lesions in the ventro-superior part of the cerebellopontine angle [16], and then by Velut in 1988 to excise a petroclival meningioma [44]. In 1991, Kawase reported using this approach to excise a series of ten spheno-

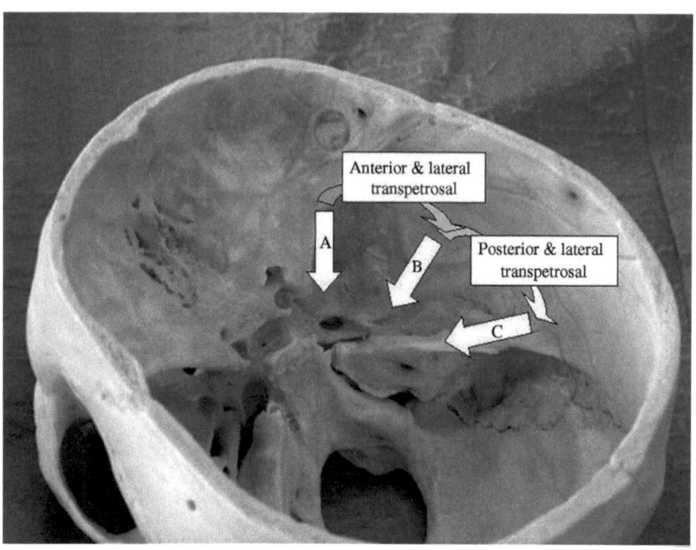

Fig. 15. Lateral skull base approaches: *A* Operative trajectory when the petroclival area is approached from the epidural temporopolar transcavernous route. *B* The arrow indicates the operative trajectory using an anterior petrosectomy. *C* The arrow simulates the surgical trajectory when using a retrolabyrinthine route

petroclival meningiomas [19]. Fournier proposed using this approach to gain access to prepontile lesions (after preliminary embolization of the IPS) [11, 12].

The principle of this approach is to perform, via a sub-temporal extradural route, petrectomy of the petrous apex, in front and medial to the horizontal segment of the intrapetrous carotid, preserving the cochlea and therefore hearing. This approach affords access to the brain stem in front of the cranial nerve plane.

Technique

The patient is placed in a supine position with the head turned to an angle of 50° on the opposite side to where the approach is to be made, with the cervical spine in slight extension. The sagittal plane is then horizontalized by rotating the operating table (Figs. 16–20). The authors recommend a crossbow incision with a fronto-temporal line in the hairline together with a dorsal incision over the auricle to reach the retro-mastoid line behind. The fronto-pterional scalp is lifted leaving the superficial temporal fascia and the galea in the same plane. The temporal scalp releases the roof of the external acoustic meatus. A stalked temporal flap is created in its lower ventral part on the temporal muscle and trimmed flush to the base. With microscopic guidance, extradural basi-temporal detachment is begun, extending from the sinuso-dural angle behind to the foramen spinosum in front

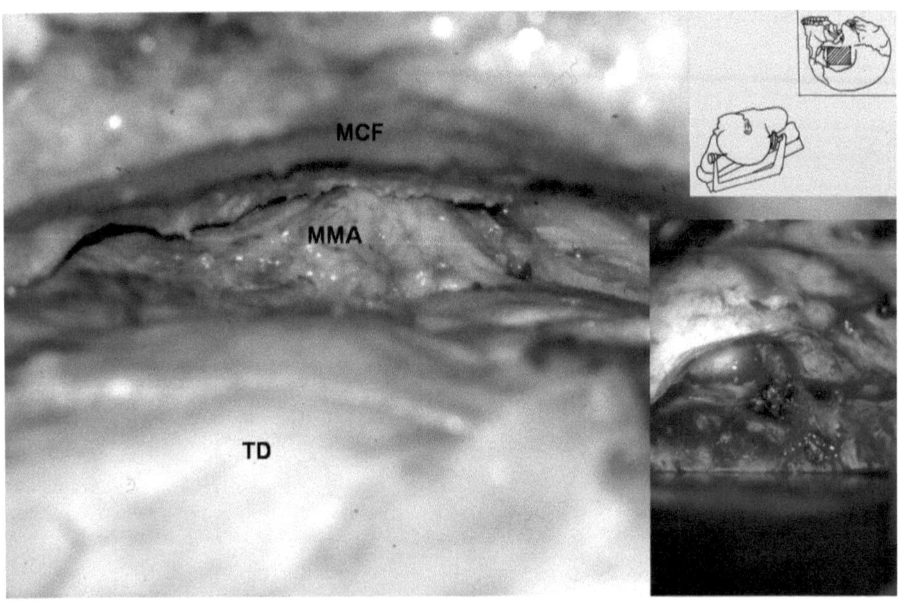

Fig. 16. Right sided anterior petrosectomy on a cadaver dissection: identification of the main anatomical landmarks. *MCF* Middle cranial fossa; *MMA* middle meningeal artery; *TD* temporal dura. See on the right lower corner of the figure the correlation with a clinical case

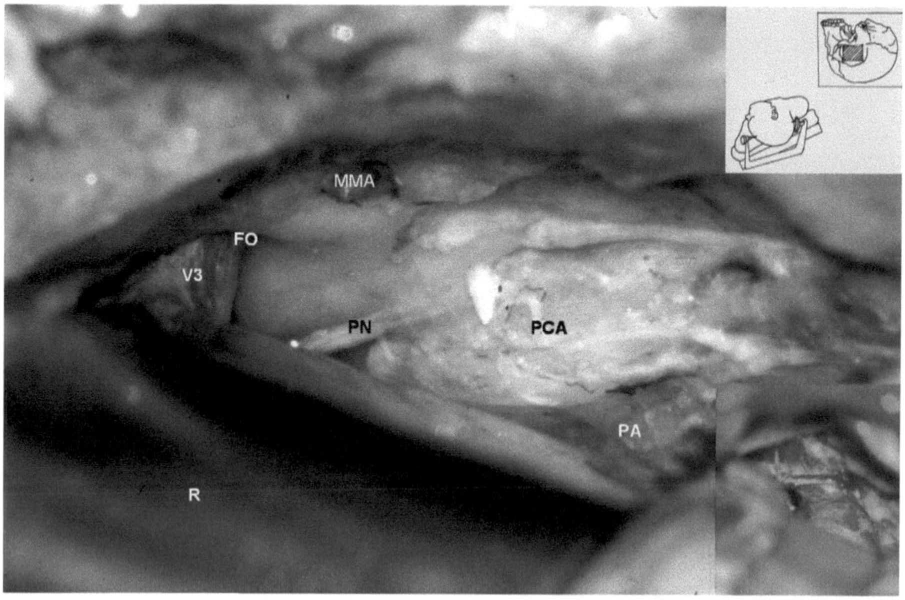

Fig. 17. Right sided anterior petrosectomy on a cadaver dissection: exposure of the horizontal segment of the petrous carotid artery (*PCA*). *MMA* Middle meningeal artery; *FO* foramen ovale; *V3* 3rd branch of the Vth nerve; *PN* petrosal nerve; *R* retractor; *PA* petrous apex

(Fig. 16). Coagulation is performed and the middle meningeal artery is sectioned, as well as the petrosal nerves in order to prevent traction on the geniculate ganglion [43, 44] (Fig. 17), although Kawase recommends preserving these nerves in order to prevent inhibiting homolateral tears secretion [19]. Identify the foramen ovale. If the foramen lacerum is covering it, the horizontal carotid can be localized by means of two landmarks as we have previously seen (Fig. 17): the axis of the petrosal nerves and the axis joining the middle points of the foramen ovale and the foramen spinosum which are parallel to the horizontal segment. When the roof of the horizontal carotid is denuded by a long or relatively non-covering foramen lacerum, the dura mater which separates it from the temporal lobe can be detached fairly easily. As we have pointed out, there may be inconvenient venous bleeding which will be all the more abundant as one comes closer to the distal part of the horizontal segment. Drilling of the portion covering the foramen lacerum may also be hindered by this venous bleeding. Lifting of the dura is restricted in front by the mandibular nerve. An attempt must be made to detach the superior petrosal sinus from its sulcus before drilling is begun. This is performed medially over the entire exposable length of the horizontal carotid without going further back than the plane passing through the hiatus of the petrosal nerves in order to avoid the cochlea and the first portion of the facial nerve (Fig. 18). Despite the obstacle

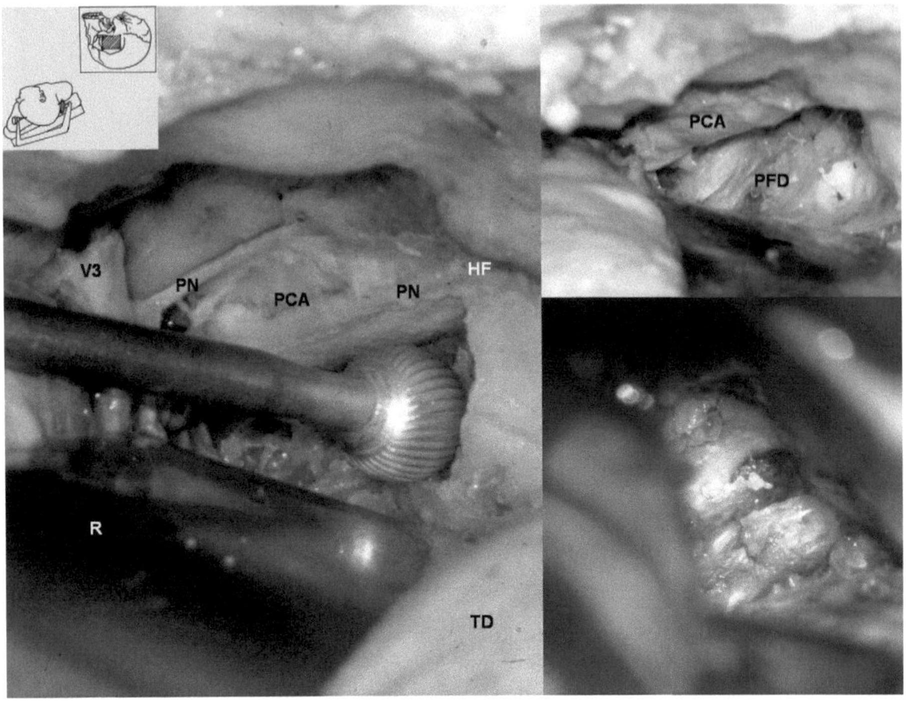

Fig. 18. Right sided anterior petrosectomy on a cadaver dissection: drilling of the petrous apex following carotid artery identification. *V3* 3rd branch of the Vth nerve; *PN* petrosal nerve; *R* retractor; *PCA* petrous carotid artery; *HF* hiatus Falopi; *TD* temporal dura; *PFD* posterior fossa dura

of the dural lifting and as long as embolization is performed beforehand, we propose extending the drilling beyond the inferior petrosal sinus [10–12].

This releases a triangle of the dura mater located between the upper and inferior petrosal sinuses, respectively at the top and at the bottom, going behind as far as to denude the ventral dural wall of the internal acoustic meatus (Fig. 18). The dura mater of the posterior fossa is open behind from the top down.

Exposure (Fig. 19) [10]

The photograph shows the operative field.

- The ventral side of the pons is exposed from nerve V as far as the origin of nerve VI.
- Also exposed: the homolateral V, the entire path of the homolateral VI, and the origin of the homolateral acoustico-facial bundle in its cisternal passage. Only the contralateral VI will be seen in the distal portion of its cisternal passage.
- The basilar artery is exposed over a little more than one centimeter as well as the AICA from its origin as far as the ventral part of its loop.

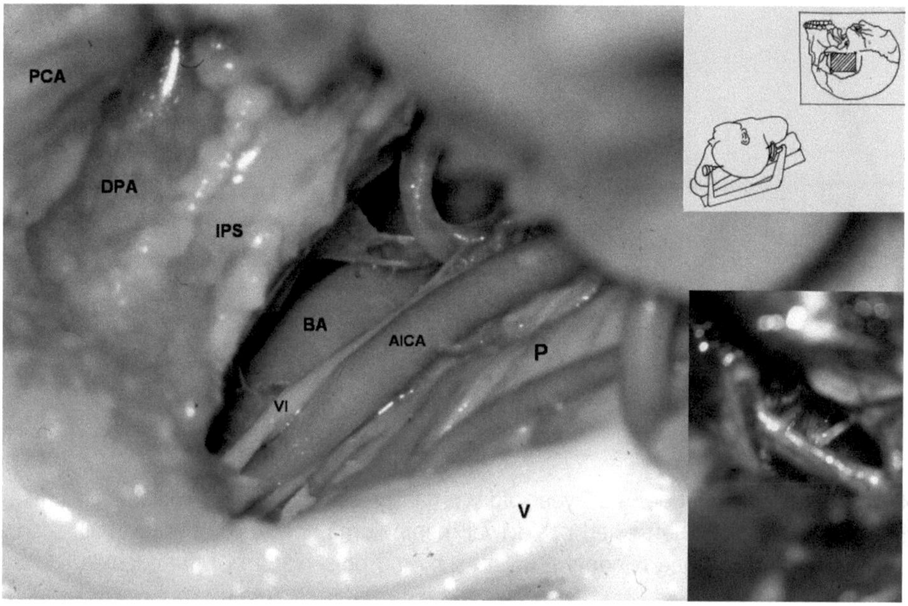

Fig. 19. Right sided anterior petrosectomy on a cadaver dissection: intradural exposure and operative field. *PCA* Petrous carotid artery; *DPA* drilled petrous apex; *IPS* inferior petrosal sinus; *BA* basilar artery; *VI* 6th cranial nerve; *AICA* anterior inferior cerebellar artery; *P* pons; *V* 5th cranial nerve

A clinical example is proposed (Fig. 20), namely a right petroclival meningioma operated upon via this approach.

Reconstruction

Limited. If petrosal cells have been opened, they should be filled with powdered bone or muscle. The surgical cavity can be filled with fat, being aware of the risks of septic necrosis. Kawase proposes lining the floor of the temporal fossa by rotation of the temporal muscle, the edges of the dural defect being sutured on the muscular fascia [19].

Pros and cons

Pros:

- Principally access to the ventral side of the pons, in front of the plane of VII and the lower cranial nerves.
- With preserved hearing function.
- Extradural access, protecting the temporal lobe, is considered as an advantage by all experts.

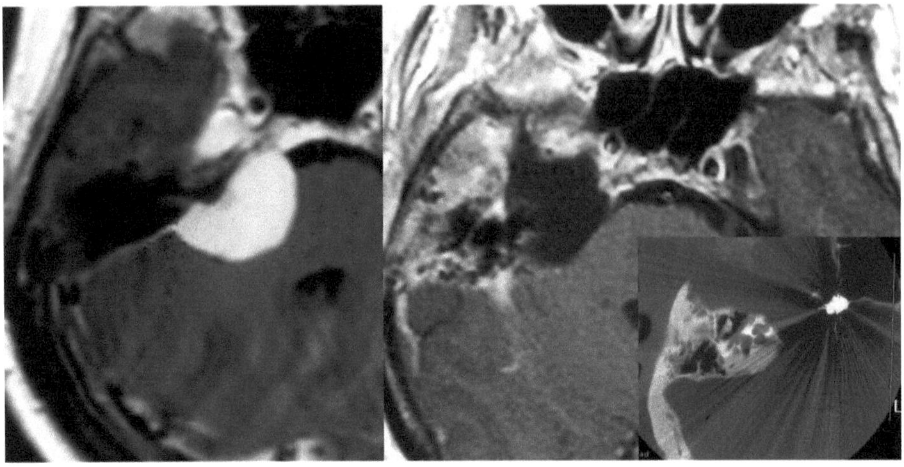

Fig. 20. Case illustration: a 30-year-old woman presenting with headaches and mild hearing loss. See the left sided petroclival meningioma, with postoperative MR scan, and postoperative bone window CT scan showing preservation of the cochlea

- Access can be gained to the contralateral apex if the lesion is pushing all the axial structures back.
- Finally, as will be described further on, transtentorial extension as needed can afford access beyond V and the upper pontile sulcus.

Cons:

- Some temporal retraction is unavoidable.
- The mandibular nerve restricts retraction of the dura, drilling down and drilling under the lower dorsal angle of the trigeminal ganglion and thus hinders access to the cavernous sinus.
- The "useful" access to the foramen magnum is practically impossible via this approach. Drilling of the carotid knee via this approach almost always means sacrificing the cochlea with very little gain.
- This approach permits no real control of the petrous carotid and does not afford either the repair or the bypassing that might be necessary.
- Access to the pontocerebellar angle is limited.
- No access is afforded to either the cerebello-medullary angle or the lower cranial nerves.

Transtentorial extension

The dural opening can be extended, if desired. The dura mater is cut into on either side of the superior petrosal sinus which is interrupted (e.g. using clips) in front of the point where it joins the upper petrosal vein and behind where nerve IV enters the dura (at least one centimeter behind the posterior clinoid process). These landmarks are difficult to discern without the intradural control image of the free edge of the tentorium. The dura mater of the middle cranial fossa is open in parallel to the superior petrosal sinus. The tentorium is cut. This extension makes it possible to control the pons above nerve V at the top at the expense of more extensive temporal retraction.

Anterior petrosectomy as an extension of the epidural temporopolar transcavernous approach (Fig. 21)

This anterior petrectomy can represent the second stage of a broader approach described in the next chapter. It may be further extended by drilling outside the cavernous carotid. This stage will make it possible to go lower, mobilizing the cavernous carotid but virtually always entails opening the cochlea. This type of drilling is very useful in the context of surgery to treat chordoma.

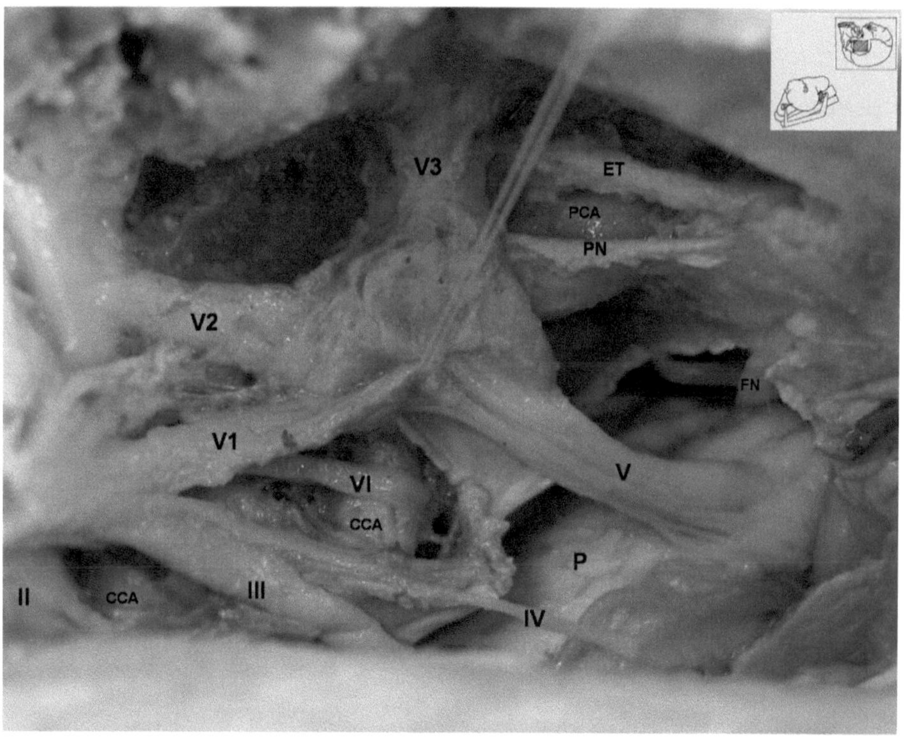

Fig. 21. Extension of an anterior petrosectomy with achievement of an epidural temporopolar transcavernous approach in a cadaver dissection: *V* 5th cranial nerve with first (*V1*) second (*V2*) and third (*V3*) divisions; *II* Optic nerve; *III* 3rd cranial nerve; *IV* 4th cranial nerve; *VI* 6th cranial nerve; *CCA* cavernous carotid artery; *P* pons; *ET* Eustachian tube; *PCA* petrous carotid artery; *PN* petrosal nerve; *FN* facial nerve

Epidural temporopolar transcavernous middle fossa approach

We detail here a widened lateral skull base approach that combines an epidural temporopolar transcavernous (Dolenc, Fukushima, Hakuba, Day) approach with a middle fossa anterior transpetrosal approach (Kawase) [2, 5, 9, 13, 15, 16, 19, 20]. Of course, this extended option is not always necessary to remove tumors from the PCA but is very useful for tumors which occupy the posterior fossa at the level of the petrous apex and clivus and reach the middle fossa (Meckel cave, posterior cavernous sinus, superior orbital fissure, optic canal, suprasellar region).

Installation (patient lying in the supine position)

The head is rotated to a 45° lateral position and maintained in a 3 pin Mayfield frame. Care should be taken to avoid compression of the contralateral jugular vein. Neuromonitoring of the cranial nerves and a CSF closed drainage system are prepared.

Skin incision (Fig. 22)

Is performed in the shape of a question mark starting anterior to the tragus at the level of the zygomatic arch, passing over the external ear and coming into the frontal region. This incision can be modified according to the extent of the planned drilling. The frontotemporal pericranial flap is dissected and the temporal muscle is turned back in a posteroinferior direction. Identification of the root of the zygoma is an important step for the future drilling of the middle fossa but usually, orbitozygomatic deposit does not give additional exposure to petroclival tumors.

Bone flap (Fig. 22)

A frontotemporal craniotomy is performed as far as the floor of the middle fossa below. The pterional region is drilled to flatten both the orbital roof and the lateral wall of the orbit. Opening of the frontal sinus and of the periorbital fascia should be avoided during this step. The pterion (lateral portion of the great sphenoid wing and lesser sphenoid wing) is drilled with a cutting drill until the meningo-orbital band is seen. There is no need for an orbitozygomatic osteotomy as seen in literature [17].

Exposure of the epidural temporopolar space (Fig. 23)

The external border of the superior orbital fissure (SOF) is exposed by shaving the lateral wall of the orbit anteriorly and by gently retracting the temporopolar dura back after the meningo-orbital band has been cut. At this point, it is necessary to shave the anterolateral (Mullan) triangle between V1 and V2 and then

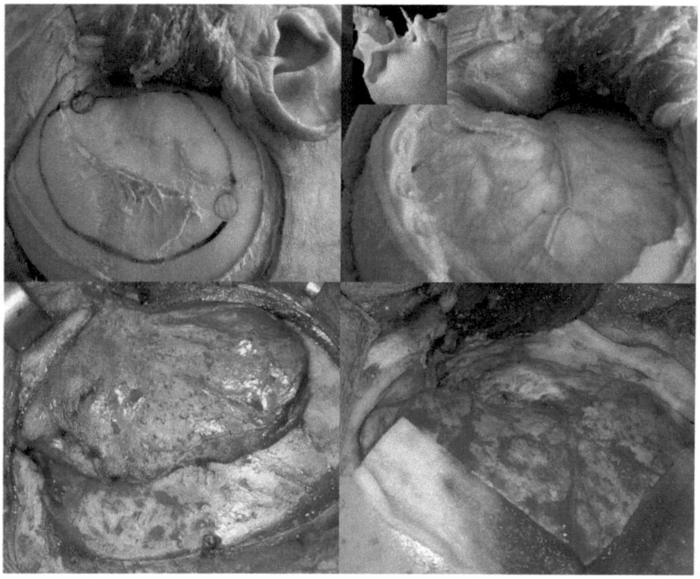

a b c d

Fig. 22. Superficial steps of the anterolateral skull base approaches: head cadaver, right side. (a) Design of the skin incision & delineation of the bone flap. (b) The bone flap is achieved and the frontotemporal dura mater is exposed. Operative case, right side. (c) Incision of the temporal muscle. Note that a muscle cuff is kept on the bone in order to improve the stitching at the end of the procedure. Just under the retractor, the zygomatic arch is shown (d) Exposure of the dura that is elevated from the middle fossa. Note the red point as the key hole

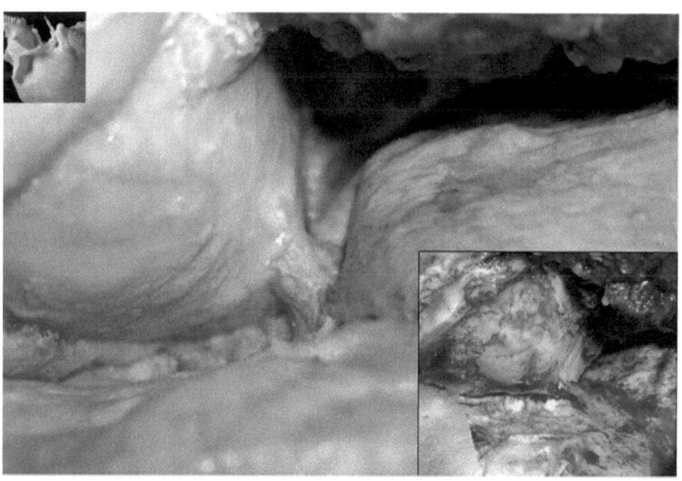

Fig. 23. Exposure of the epidural temporopolar space (Head cadaver dissection, right side): the meningoorbital band is the thick fibrous band that connect the periorbital fascia to the temporopolar dura. At the right bottom corner, the same view is shown in an operative case

the far lateral triangle between V2 and V3. This step is facilitated by drilling the foramen rotundum and foramen ovale. In order to generate more room for the drilling of the far lateral triangle, the dura from the floor of the great sphenoid wing. This entails identification, cutting and coagulation of the middle meningeal artery at the foramen spinosum. Some venous bleeding from the posterior margin of the ovale foramen is normal because the dura at that point is filled by bridging veins that connect the lateral cavernous sinus with the pterygoid venous plexus. Such bleeding is easily stopped by gentle packing with small pieces of oxidized cellulose. These steps are necessary for exposure of the true lateral wall of the cavernous sinus but also make it possible to work backwards to the anterior petrosectomy.

Extradural Anterior clinoid process (ACP) removal and optic canal exposure (Fig. 24)

Whether or not this step is undertaken will depend on the extent of the tumor. If the tumor has spread to the suprasellar space and optic canal, this step is indicated.

In order to generate space in the direction of the anterior clinoid process, it is helpful to cut the meningo-orbital band in first, to release CSF from the lumbar drain, and then to install a rigid, extradural self-retaining retractor. The unroofing of the optic canal provides a good landmark to avoid injuring the nerve intradurally while drilling the ACP. This roof is exposed after lifting the dura away from the orbital roof and pushing it in a medial direction towards the planum sphenoidale. Once it has been clearly identified, the ACP is removed

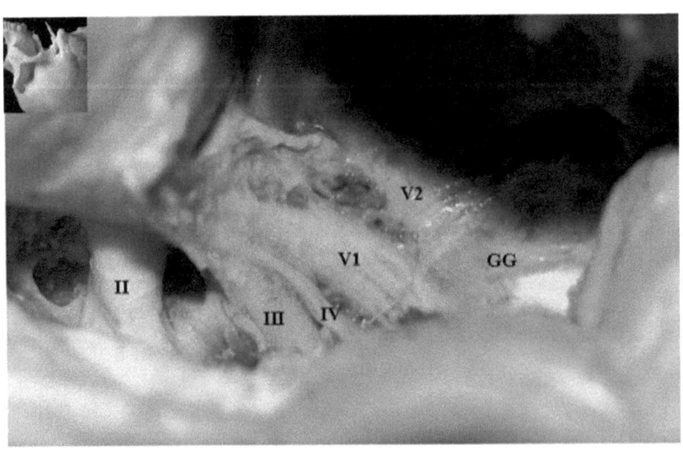

Fig. 24. Extradural removal of the anterior clinoid process and exposure of the optic canal. *II* Optic canal, *III* third nerve in the lateral wall of the cavernous sinus, *IV* fourth nerve, *V1* ophtalmic division of the trigeminal nerve, *V2* maxillary division of the trigeminal nerve, *GG* Gasserian ganglion

using the eggshell technique (hollowing out the inside by drilling) and peripheral dissection outside using a thin, sharp, rigid dissector (Fukushima's instrumentation). The final step is one-piece removal of the "tooth-like" skeleton of the ACP. It is now possible to expose the optic canal through 270° of its circumference by drilling the floor of the optic canal also named the optic strut.

Anterior petrosectomy

The dura is now retracted from the subtemporal middle fossa below V3. It is necessary to identify the thin bone of the tegmen tympani, the eminencia arcuata, and the fibers from the GSPN. It is always possible to preserve these fibers. The GSPN actually adheres to the middle fossa dura but sharp dissection using a 15 blade knife or a thin dura elevator will separate it, from the Fallopian Hiatus and geniculate ganglion on the lower side of the Meckel's cave. It is important to mobilize V3 and to lift the dura of the Meckel's cave in order to proceed medially toward the petrous apex. The GSPN overlies the horizontal portion of the intrapetrous carotid artery (C6). These two structures are important landmarks when it comes to defining the boundaries of Glasscock's triangle. One should keep in mind that the medial segment of the bony roof of C6 is usually dehiscent which is why we recommend first flattening the middle fossa using a diamond drill until the carotid has been clearly identified. Glasscock's triangle should be drilled if the surgeon wishes to mobilize the C6 carotid segment laterally. Such a step requires identification of the tensor tympani muscle and the Eustachian tube underneath. Both structures lie at the lateral surface of C6 and may be sacrificed during this procedure. When lifting the dura, the surgeon will reach the petrous ridge and the groove of the superior petrosal sinus. The limits of Kawase triangle are delineated as follow: C6 laterally, petrous ridge medially, Meckel cave and V3 anteriorly. At this point, some authors recommend unroofing the internal auditory canal that defines the posterior limit of the petrous apex. Whatever the technique used to locate the IAC, it is necessary to expose the dura of the anterior border of the porus. Attempting to unroof the whole canal, particularly the fundus, may damage the geniculate ganglion and the deeper cochlea.

Once the landmarks of the posteromedial triangle have been identified, the petrous apex is drilled. Drilling is facilitated by a high pneumatization in some cases but if this is not possible, the fatty aspect of the bone is usually helpful. In cases of petrous apex meningiomas, the osteoma needs to be resected using a cutting drill. Approaching the cortical bone of the inner surface, close to the dura, needs more cautious drilling to avoid opening the dura at too early a stage. The operator should drill downwards until the blue color of the inferior petrosal sinus is seen. If the IPS is torn, bleeding is always abundant and the sinus lumen should be gently packed with small pieces of oxidized cellulose. This type of problem can be prevented by pre-operative embolization of the

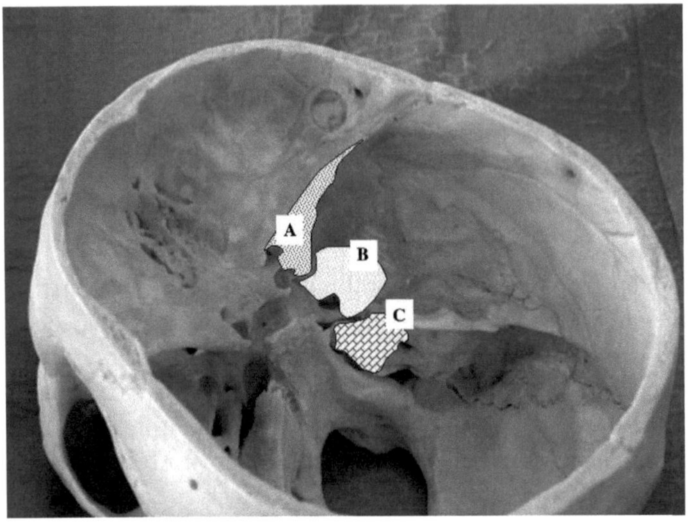

Fig. 25. Extent of the skull base resection during the anterolateral skull base approach: *A* Resection of the lesser sphenoid wing and anterior clinoid process, *B* drilling of the anterolateral and far lateral triangles, *C* resection of the posteromedial triangle

sinus, as recommended by Fournier *et al.* [11, 12] but the proximity of the abducens means that this technique entails a risk of nerve palsy. It is sometimes quite difficult to reach the extreme tip of the petrous apex and upward retraction of the Meckel cave is then needed. Usually the apex can be removed in the same way followed by the anterior clinoid process. Once drilling is finished, careful hemostasis of the dura and epidural space is important before the dura is opened. At the end of the procedure and before opening the dura, the extent of the skull base resections is shown on Fig. 25.

Opening the dura (Fig. 26)

As we have previously seen, the anatomy of the petroclival dura is particularly complex. Optimal opening of the dura should be systematically matched to pre-existing bone exposure. Insufficient dura opening may narrow the operative corridor and entail unnecessary retraction. Care should be taken to proceed in a methodical, meticulous way to avoid damaging the underlying cranial nerves, prevent excessive bleeding from the venous sinuses, and preclude closure problems.

Step 1. Lifting of the dura propria from the lateral wall of the cavernous sinus (Fig. 24): A cleavage plane exists at the junction of the temporal dura and the periorbital fascia, at the apex of the superior orbital fissure. Gradual lifting of the dura propira will allow identification of the true cavernous membrane of the lateral wall – a loose tissue sheathing the oculomotor nerves and V1.

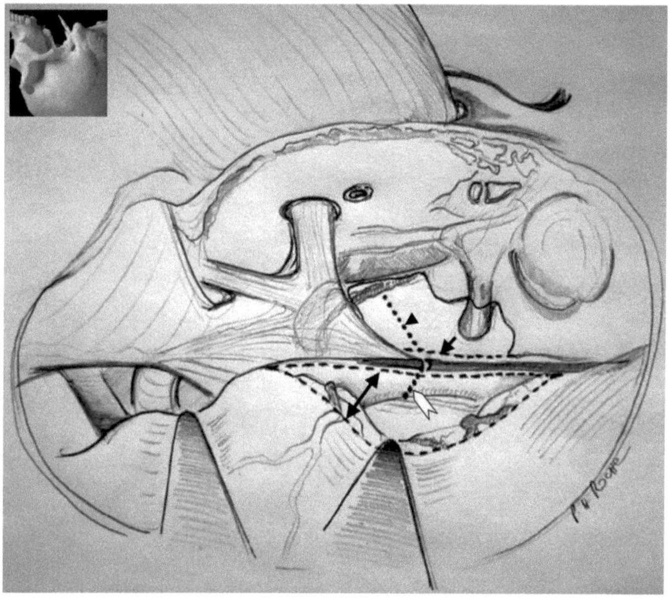

Fig. 26. Artistic drawing showing the process of dura opening (right side): the double arrow shows the horizontal incision of the temporal dura above the superior petrosal sinus. The black arrow indicates the horizontal section of the posterior fossa dura under the superior petrosal sinus. The arrow head shows the vertical incision of the posterior fossa dura between the superior and inferior petrosal sinuses. The chevron arrow shows the transversal section of the tentorium until the free edge is reached

Extradural lifting of the temporal lobe preserves the veins. Lifting behind exposes the trigeminal ganglion and is blocked in the medial direction by the edge of the tentorium.

Step 2. Opening the dura over the sylvian fissure and as far as the optic canal – using a T-shaped configuration. Following these two steps (1 and 2), the dura can be removed from the lateral wall of the cavernous sinus when necessary, e.g. if there is a meningioma encroaching upon the lateral wall. Here the temporal veins draining into the sphenoparietal sinus may be sacrificed.

Step 3. Opening the dura of the posterior fossa (Fig. 26). Clear identification of the SPS. Horizontal section of the basitemporal dura parallel and just above the SPS from the Meckel cave to the suprameatal area behind. Horizontal section of the posterior fossa dura just under the SPS, from the porus trigeminus to the suprameatal area behind. Coagulation and transverse section of the SPS. It is usually necessary to push oxidized cellulose into the SPS to induce hemostasis. Suture of both edges of the cutting section and traction lifting of the threads to broaden the surgical field. Progression medially to the free edge of the tentorium but not too close to the posterior wall of the cavernous sinus (to avoid damaging nerve IV). If the tentorium is involved by

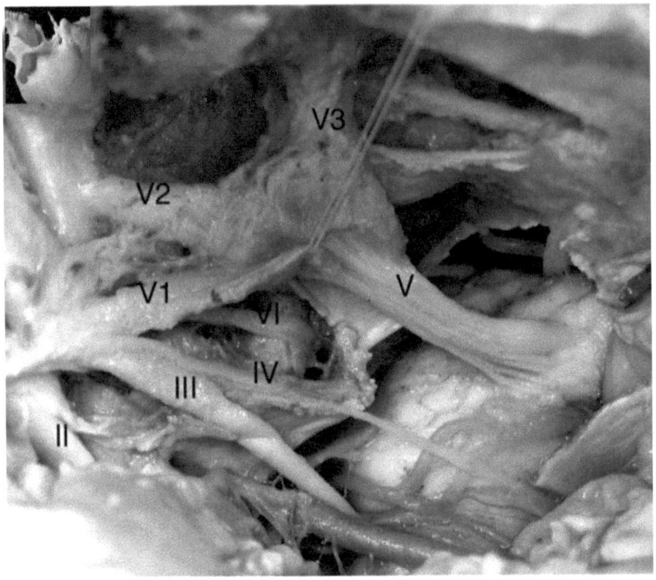

Fig. 27. Exposure of the cranial nerves from the optic nerve to the acousticofacial bundle after achievement of the epidural temporopolar transcavernous approach: *II* The optic nerve is shown in its intracranial compartment and coursing in the optic canal. *III* The third nerve is shown in its intracisternal portion and in the lateral wall of the cavernous sinus. The same aspect is shown for the fourth nerve (*IV*). *VI* The sixth nerve is shown while its cross the carotid artery inside the cavernous sinus. *V3* Mandibular division of the trigeminal nerve. *V* Sensitive root of the trigeminal nerve

the tumor, it is easily removed providing a direct communication between the supra and infratentorial spaces and exposing the cranial nerves from the optic nerve to the acousticofacial bundles (Fig. 27).

Tumor removal

This approach offers various operative corridors from the middle to the posterior fossa. Usually, the tumor is removed not in its entirety but in fragments. The microsurgical technique used will of course depend on the origin and nature of the tumor. During the removal of chordomas or chondrosarcomas, the extradural step is essential because most of the tumor is resected before opening of the dura; usually the tumor consists of soft tissue which can be removed using ring curettes and forceps under controlled suction. For meningiomas, the surgeon alternates extracapsular devascularization and detachment maneuvers with intracapsular debulking.

The surgical problems will of course depend on the lesion being resected.

– Vessels. The middle and upper cerebellar arteries and, inside, the basilar trunk are often in contact with bulky tumors. Particular difficulties are linked to meningiomas in which vessels are sometimes totally surrounded by the tumor (which can be predicted from the pre-operative images). The veins at risk are at the interface between the tumor and the trunk. Usually the petrous veins can be preserved but it is much more difficult to save the integrality of the pontine subpial veins in cases of large tumors because of adhesion.

- Nerves. The fourth nerve is at the external pole of the tumor, flattened up against the free edge of the tentorium. The sixth nerve is below and is visible at the end of thc procedure at the bottom and in front. Sometimes, it is not identified in the course of resection and remains at a distance. The trigeminal is in the middle of the field and is usually easily dissected being strong and large-caliber.
- Brain stem. The lateral side of the pons is exposed over its entire height during the approach, centered by the entry point of the trigeminal nerve.

Closure

The closure procedure should be meticulous, hermetic, helped by abundant use of grafting material (particularly fat or temporal muscle). In some cases, when

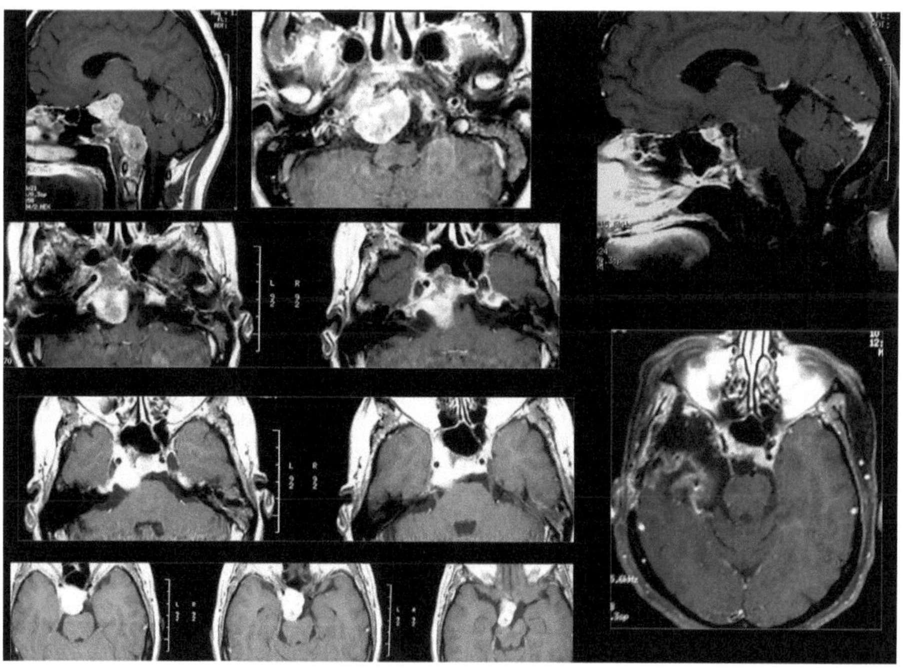

Fig. 28. Case illustration: a 40-year-old woman presenting with a recurrent clival chordoma, chordoma which was operated on 2 years ago elsewhere and treated subsequently by proton beam therapy. She complained of headaches, gait disturbances, and diplopia. Pre and post operative (using an epidural temporopolar transcavernous middle fossa approach) MR scan are presented

the sinuses have been extensively opened up or if there is parapharyngeal exposure, reconstruction with a vascularized muscle flap will be necessary: in this case, it is useful to ask a plastic surgeon to help with reconstruction. If special tissues are used, the patient should be warned and derails should be given in the operative chart because post-operative MR control results may be misinterpreted if this information had not been communicated beforehand. Extradural drainage should be avoided so that no CSF channel is created. If drainage is unavoidable, install superficial layers with low-pressure aspiration. There is a need for an extensive peripheral holding of the dura. Meticulous reapplication and stitching of the temporal muscle is required and the skin is stitched in two layers.

A clinical case is presented on Fig. 28. A 40-year-old woman was referred to us with a recurrent clival chordoma. The patient was operated on 2 years ago and underwent proton beam therapy before recurrence.

Subtemporal preauricular infratemporal fossa approach (inferolateral)

Principle

Technically more difficult than anterior petrectomy, this fully mobilizes the petrous carotid.

This approach was first described by Sekhar to expose and control the upper cervical carotid and the entire intrapetrous carotid, in the course of surgery to address bulky lesions at the base of the skull [40]. It is used for the excision of extradural, originally exocranial lesions of the skull base (possibly extending into the cranium on the median line) [27, 36–39]. It was then adapted to approach intradural structures in the petroclival region located in front of the brain stem [41]. The principle underlying this approach is to expose the ventral side of the pons and the prolonged medulla from nerve V to the petrous apex at the top as far as nerve XII at the greater foramen below, by completely drilling out the anterior part of the petrous pyramid, preserving the cochlea and remaining outside the pharynx in front. The infra-temporal approach makes it possible to work underneath the temporal lobe without any retraction, as a result of total ablation of the floor of the middle cranial fossa; it also means that the bone can be drilled as far as the hypoglossal canal. Most importantly, it affords access to the brain stem in front of the plane of nerve VII and the mixed nerves.

Technique

The patient in installed in a supine position, with the head in a bone-gripping frame turned to an angle of 45° away from the side of the incision, in slight extension. An arc-shaped, fronto-temporal incision is made at the hairline, extending in front of the tragus, running around the lobule of auricle and terminating at the anterior edge of the sternocleidomastoid muscle. To preserve the frontal, temporal and zygomatic branches, the incision should be made flush with the tragus and should allow sub-periosteal detachment of the posterior root.

The trunk of the facial nerve is identified directly above the ventral edge of the cartilage of the external acoustic meatus, and is followed up until its entry into the parotid. Then superficial parotidectomy is performed allowing identification of the nerve's branches.

The zygomatic arch is sectioned using an oscillating saw in front at the root of the temporal process of the zygomatic bone and behind just in front of the mandibular fossa in front of the transverse root. It is displaced downwards.

The temporal muscle is taken out of the temporal fossa and also displaced downwards.

One exposes at the neck the internal jugular vein with nerve XI running along its lateral face. It is then followed at the top as it passes medially to the diagastric to cross the facial nerve. The muscle is sectioned and the occipital

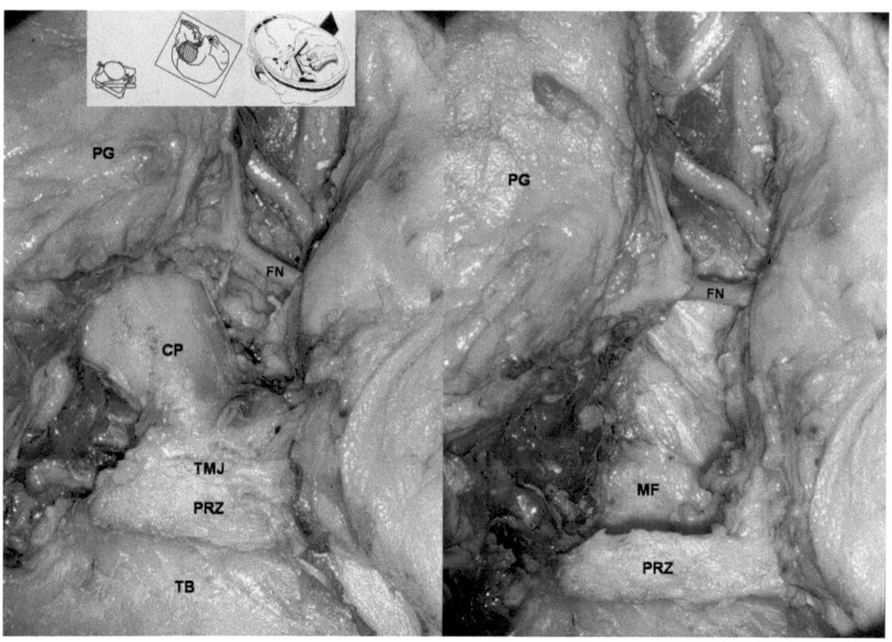

Fig. 29. Right sided inferolateral approach on a cadaver dissection: see exposure of the condylar process (*CP*) and temporomandibular joint (*TMJ*) on the right part of the figure, and resection of the condylar process with exposure of the mandibular fossa (*MF*) on the left. *PG* Parotid gland; *FN* facial nerve; *PRZ* proximal root of zygoma, *TB* temporal bone

artery is interrupted where it crosses the internal carotid which allows dissection of nerve XII from where it emerges from the base to pass between the internal carotid and the jugular vein (Fig. 29).

Then the styloid process is exposed which is ablated together with the vaginal process after removal of the elements of the stylian diaphragm. The internal carotid is then exposed up till about one centimeter from where it enters the carotid canal.

The capsule of the temporomandibular joint is opened. The condyle process is luxated. Better exposure is obtained by resection of the condyle process and from the upper third of the mandibular ramus, the only option for formaldehyde-fixed preparations. This resection can be extended down to the mandibular incisure without any risk of damaging the lower alveolar nerve which penetrates the mandible at the mandibular foramen located about one centimeter under the incisure. This exposes the mandibular fossa (Fig. 29).

Temporal craniotomy extended in front flush with the pterion and behind to the top of the roof of the external acoustic meatus. The posterior root of the zygoma is ablated from the mandibular fossa and the floor of the temporal fossa as far as the foramen spinosum and the foramen ovale to expose nerve V3 (Fig. 30).

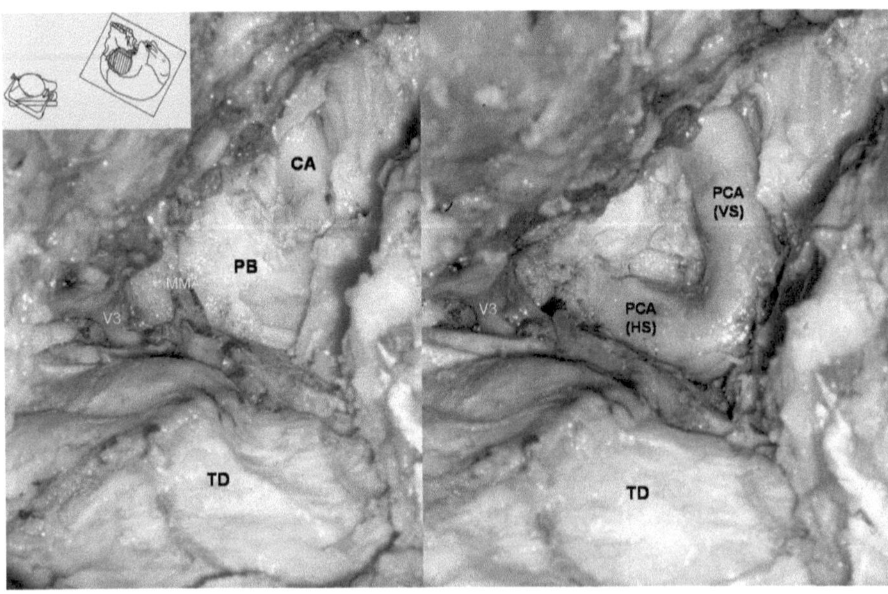

Fig. 30. Right sided inferolateral approach on a cadaver dissection: progressive exposure of the entire petrous carotid artery: *CA* cervical carotid artery; *PB* petrous bone; *TD* temporal dura; *MMA* middle meningeal artery; *V3* 3rd branch of Vth nerve; *PCA (VS)* petrous carotid (vertical segment); *PCA (HS)* petrous carotid (horizontal segment)

The dura is detached from behind forwards and from the outside inwards. The middle meningeal artery and the petrosal nerves are interrupted.

The eustachian tube and the tensor tympani muscle are exposed and resected. The eustachian tube will be filled in subsequently.

Then the lateral covering of the intrapetrous carotid is drilled without going beyond the knee located inside the section of the eustachian tube. The pericarotid venous plexuses are found developed mainly at the distal portion of the horizontal segment. The periosteum of the carotid canal adheres to a fibroacartilaginous annulus which encircles the carotid at the point at which it enters the canal. This annulus must be opened in order to be able to mobilize the artery. This is dissected in its high cervical portion above nerve VII in the downward direction. The petrous carotid is then released with its periosteal envelope and displaced forwards and laterally (Fig. 31).

Then the petrous bone is drilled medially to the carotid and the cochlea as far as the anterior edge of the internal acoustic meatus (Fig. 31). In front and without interrupting nerve V3 by virtue of its approach from below up, the drilling can expose the medial carotid at the lower dorsal angle of the trigeminal ganglion. The drilling field retracts down because of the canal of the hypoglossa and the jugular foramen. This exposes a triangle of the dura mater at the subtemporal base. The drilling will go below the inferior petrosal sinus which should be first embolized.

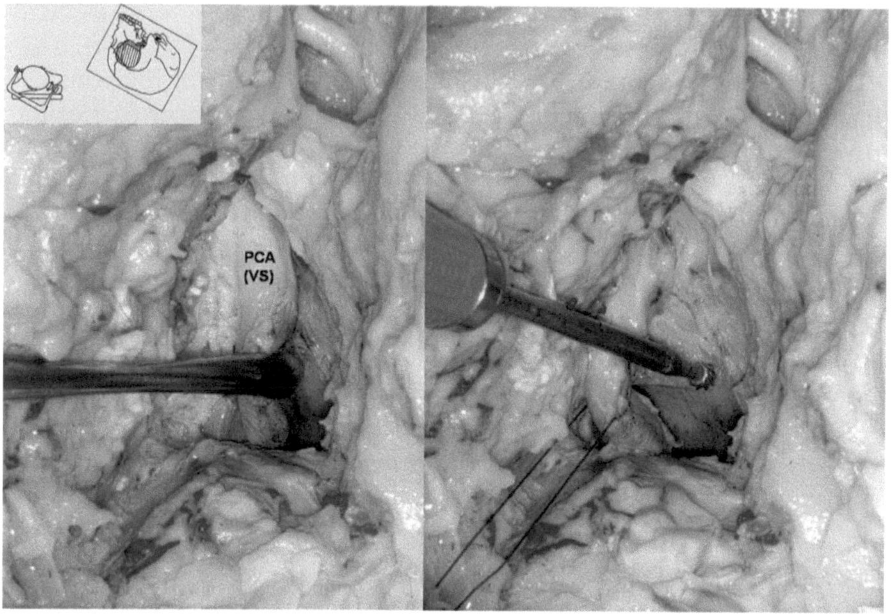

Fig. 31. Right sided inferolateral approach on a cadaver dissection: Mobilization of the petrous carotid artery and drilling of the petrous apex: *PCA (VS)* petrous carotid (vertical segment)

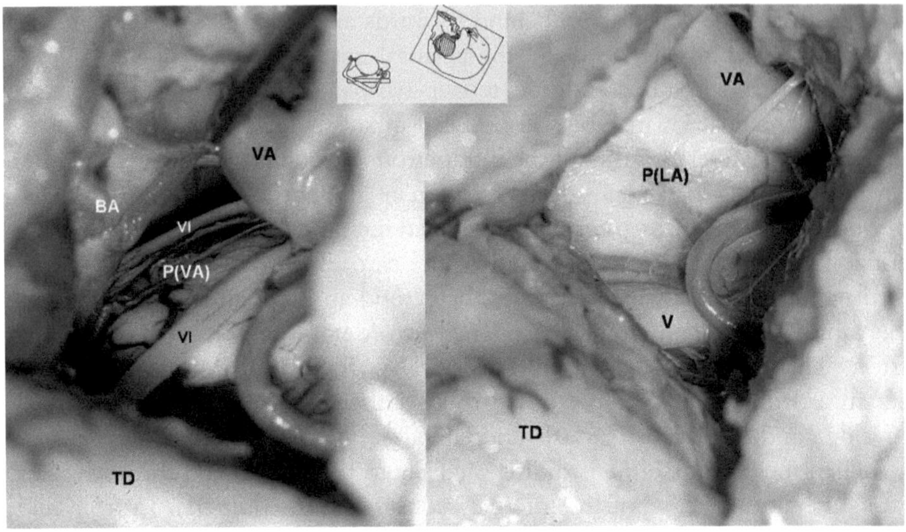

Fig. 32. Right sided inferolateral approach on a cadaver dissection: intradural exposure and operative field. See both VIth nerves (VI) and ventral aspect of the pons (PVA). *BA* Basilar artery; *VA* vertebral artery; *TD* temporal dura; *V* 5th nerve

Exposure

The following structures are exposed: (Fig. 32) [10]

- The brain stem – more specifically the ventro-lateral side of the pons below nerve V, the lower pontile sulcus, the oliva and the upper part of the pyramid.
- The cranial nerves from nerve V at the top to nerve XII at the bottom without visualizing the lower cranial nerves (the homolateral nerve V from the pons to the petrous apex, the homolateral nerve VI from its origin to its dural entry point, the contralateral nerve VI over one-third of its cisternal passage, the homolateral cochleo-vestibulo-facial bundle from its origin as far as the open porus in front, and the rootlets of the homolateral nerve XII.
- The basilar artery, the vertebro-basilar junction if it is ipsilateral or median, the homolateral AICA from its origin to the anterior part of the pontocerebellar angle.

Reconstruction

All the dural incisions must be scrupulously closed by direct suturing or by interposition of a pericranial flap. The cavity is then filled using fat (e.g. taken from the abdomen). If the approach has created communication channels between the intradural space and air-filled cavities (the nasopharynx, the paranasal sinuses, etc.), a vascular flap must be used to protect the dura mater and the major vessels. If dehiscence is limited and the vascularization of the temporal muscle has been preserved, the latter can be used in rotation (knowing the angle is limited). Some experts recommend using a fragment of rectus abdominis muscle stalked on deep epigastric vessels. Other flaps may be used.

Pros and cons

Pros:

- The whole carotid (intra-petrous and high cervical) is controlled meaning grafting and reconstruction, if necessary.
- The contralateral petroclival region can be accessed if the lesion is involving axial structures behind.
- The approach can be extended in front or up at the same time. Notably, it will be seen that access up to nerve V is obtained by combination with an intradural, sub-temporal approach. In this way, exposure of the posterior clinoid processes from nerve II to nerve IV can be added.

Cons:

- Interruption of the eustachian tube will entail permanent tympanostomy.
- Apart from reconstruction, the loss of a condyle process in the event of resection is responsible for trismus, malocclusion and contralateral pain, at least temporarily.

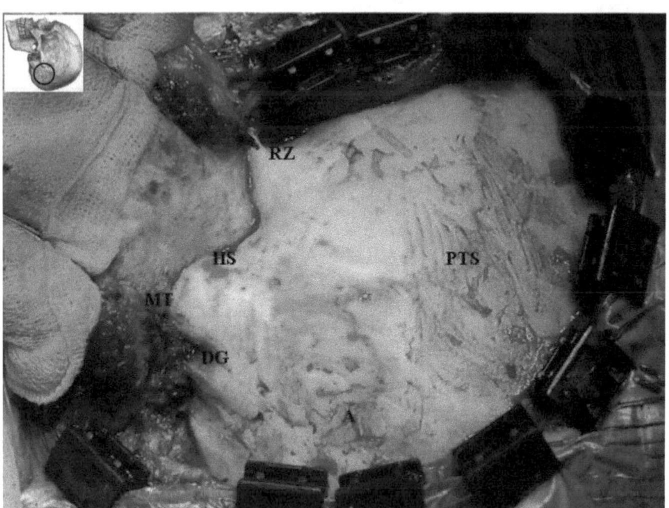

Fig. 33. Combined petrosal approach (left side). The skin and muscle have been elevated and the main bony landmarks are identified. *A* Asterion, *MT* Mastoid tip, *PTS* parietotemporal suture, *RZ* root of zygoma, *SH* spine of Henle

Combined petrosal approaches

For large tumors growing from the petroclival region and extending behind into the cerebellopontine angle, pure lateral or anterolateral approaches are insufficient to provide total resection. A few skull base teams have developed combined approaches that reach the petroclival by temporal craniotomy combined with a varied degree of removal of the petrous bone. These approaches provide the surgeon a multifocal extensive operative corridor extending from the posterior to the middle fossa. We have chosen to detail the least invasive of these approaches, one that allows the preservation of neuro-otologic structures.

The combined retrolabyrinthine (Anterior Sigmoid)-middle fossa approach [2, 3, 11, 13]

Head positioning and the skin incision

The head is secured with three-point pin fixation and placed in the lateral position facing away from the surgeon. A periauricular skin incision in the

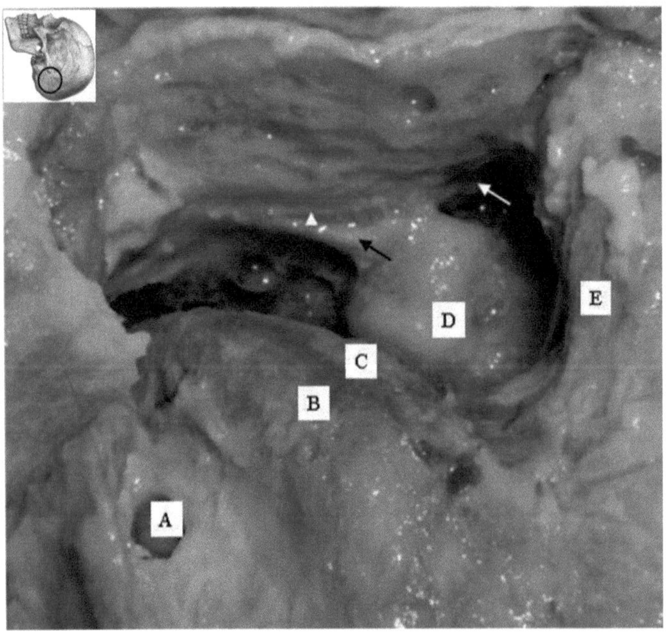

Fig. 34. Head cadaver dissection (left side) showing the final exposure of the retrolabyrinthine step of the approach: *A* Retrosigmoid dura, *B* sigmoid sinus, *C* presigmoid dura at the level of the endolymphatic sac, *D* semicircular canals at the level of the common crus, *E* temporobasal dura. The black arrow indicates the facial nerve in the Fallopian canal at the junction between the second and the third portion. The arrow head shows the corda tympani. The white arrow indicates the ossicles in the tympanic cavity

shape of a question mark or an L is made. Continue as far as possible in the anterior direction in order to retract the temporal muscle down and forwards. The following bony landmarks are now exposed (Fig. 33): Mastoid tip, spine of Henle, asterion, parietotemporal suture, root of zygoma.

Bone drilling and bone flap

A retrolabyrinthine mastoidectomy is then performed. This will superficially expose the sigmoid sinus and the jugular bulb, the presigmoid dura and the dura under the temporal lobe. In the depth, after removal of the mastoid air cells, the shape of the semicircular canals can be identified. The yellowish compact bone of the lateral semicircular canal is first identified at the medial surface of the mastoid antrum, once this air cell has been broadly drilled out using a diamond drill. The loop of the lateral semicircular canal is a constant landmark for the fallopian canal because the second portion of the facial nerve passes just underneath. It is necessary to expose the relief of the posterior labyrinth properly in order to improve the angle of vision (Fig. 34). A large temporo-occipital bone flap is then created, exposing the retrosigmoid and temporobasal dura (Fig. 35). This step allows lifting of the dura from the middle fossa, proceeding

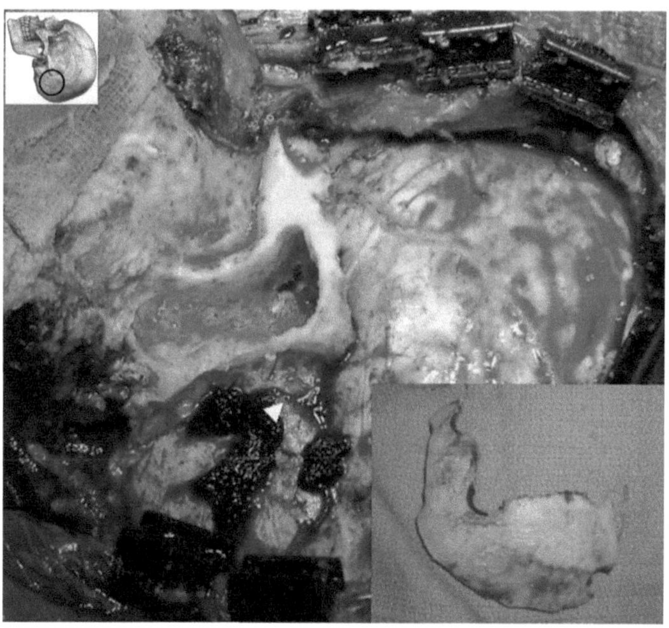

Fig. 35. Combined petrosal approach (left side): the temporo-occipital bone flap has been elevated (small window), exposing the dura and the transverse sinus. The junction between transverse and sigmoid sinus is shown by the small white arrowhead. The early step of the mastoidectomy has been undertaken. Note that in this case, the bone flap has been performed before the mastoidectomy

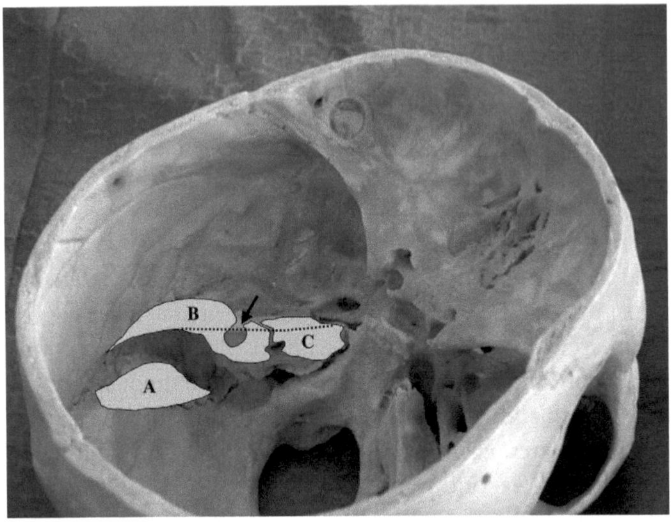

Fig. 36. Combined petrosal approach (left side): on the dry skull, the skull base is viewed from inside and the A letter indicates the retrosigmoid part of the resection, the B shows the retrolabyrinthine part and the C the anterior part of the bony resection. The black arrow indicates the position of semicircular canal that has not been drilled. The dotted line represents the junction between the superior and posterior surfaces of the petrous bone (petrous crest)

gradually from the arcuate eminence to the Meckel cave forward and medially. The retromeatal triangle (between the superior semicircular canal and internal auditory canal) and the posteromedial (Kawase) triangle are then drilled and the internal auditory canal is unroofed. Care should be taken to follow and resect the petrous ridge, proceeding forwards in the direction of the porus trigeminus after lifting of the dura out of the superior petrosal sinus. The extent of bony resection from the skull base is illustrated by the Fig. 36.

Opening of the dura (Fig. 37)

As mentioned above, opening and management of the dura is a key step of skull base approaches particularly in the present approach. Opening of the presigmoid dura from the sinodural angle to the jugular bulb. Cutting of the basitemporal dura just above the sinodural angle toward the geniculate ganglion, parallel to the superior petrosal sinus. It is important not to cut the dura too far back in order to preserve the posterior temporal vein of Labbe. Then the superior petrosal sinus is cut and coagulated, the dura of the tentorium is incised proceeding toward the free edge medially and anteriorly, avoiding damage to the trochlear nerve. It becomes possible to resect a large portion of the tentorium if this dural structure is involved by the tumor. This approach offers multiple angles of vision of the petroclival region and related structures (depending

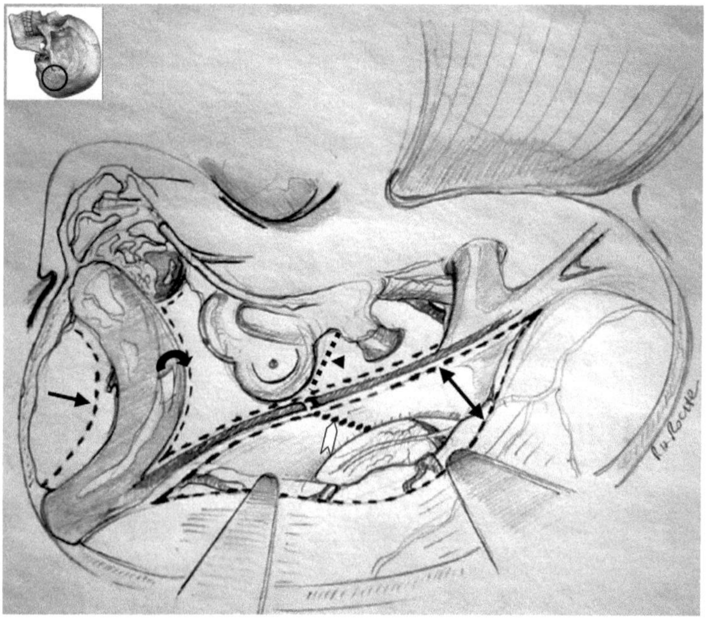

Fig. 37. Artistic drawing showing the process of dura opening during the combined petrosal approach (left side): the double arrow shows the horizontal section of the temporal dura. The arrow head indicates the vertical section of the posterior fossa dura. Note that the location of this section can be modified anteroposteriorly. The chevron arrow shows the transversal section of the tentorium. The black arrow shows the opening of the retrosigmoid dura while the circular arrow shows the incision of the presigmoid dura

on the positioning of the extradural triangular retractors) (Fig. 38). It is particularly easy to control the cerebellopontine angle and also the lower cranial nerves behind and below. Now, the ipsilateral cranial nerves can be identified from nerves III to XII. Tumor removal proceeds in the same way as described above, and the principles of closure are also the same. The dura is to be stitched and immobilized in a meticulous way. The bone flap is positioned and fixed. A clinical case is presented on Fig. 39.

This approach offers quite similar exposure to the wider transcochlear approaches but it remains conservative because intrapetrosal neuro-otologic structures (i.e. labyrinth and facial nerve) are unopened or unmobilized. The main disadvantage is indisputably the extra time entailed by this approach.

Other combined approaches

Instead of a retrolabyrinthine approach, a translabyrinthine approach can be combined with anterior petrosectomy. In this procedure, quasi-total petrosectomy is achieved and the operative corridor is widened. This technique is of particular interest when there is already deafness in the ipsilateral

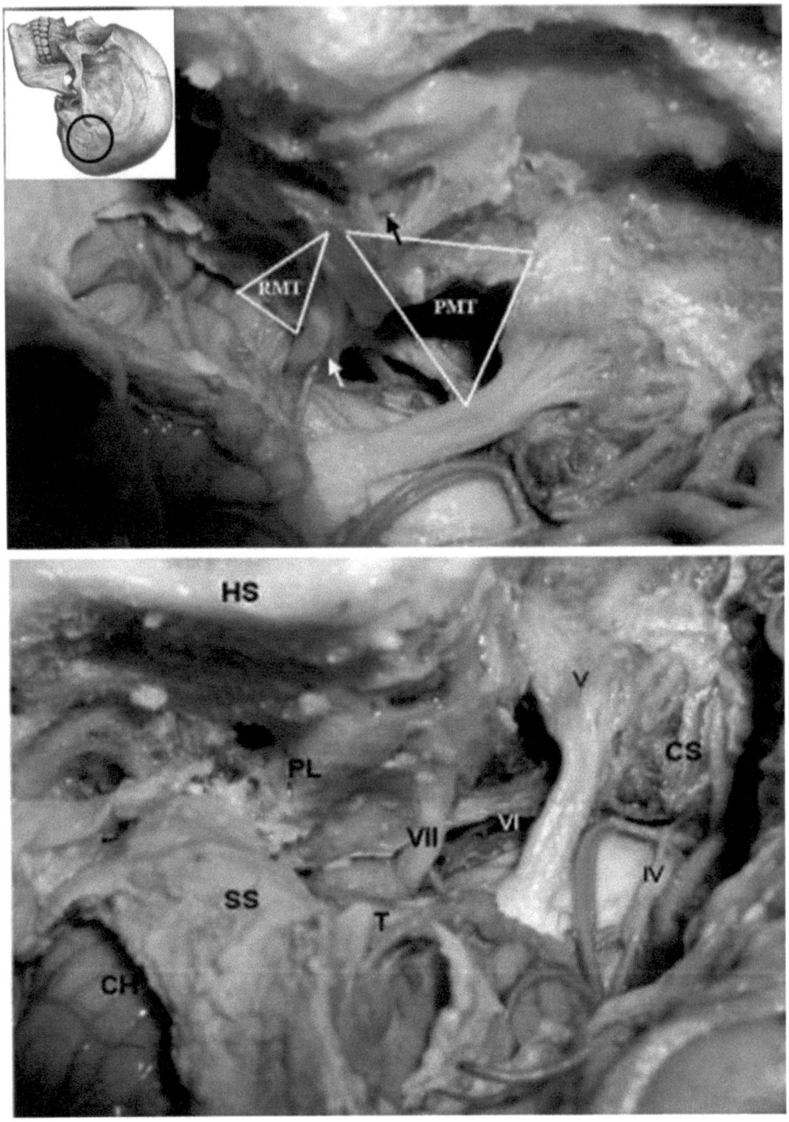

Fig. 38. Injected head cadaver dissection (left side). The combined petrosal approach has been achieved and the dura has been removed in order to show the main intradural structures. (a) The petroclival region is approached from above. The white arrow shows the acousticofacial bundle and the black arrow indicates the middle ear ossicles after opening the tegmen tympani. The RMT triangle is the retromeatal triangle and the PMT triangle is the premeatal triangle. (b) The petroclival region is approached from the back. *CH* Cerebellum hemisphere, *CS* cavernous sinus, *HS* henle spike, *PL* posterior labyrinthe, *SS* sigmoid sinus, *T* tentorium

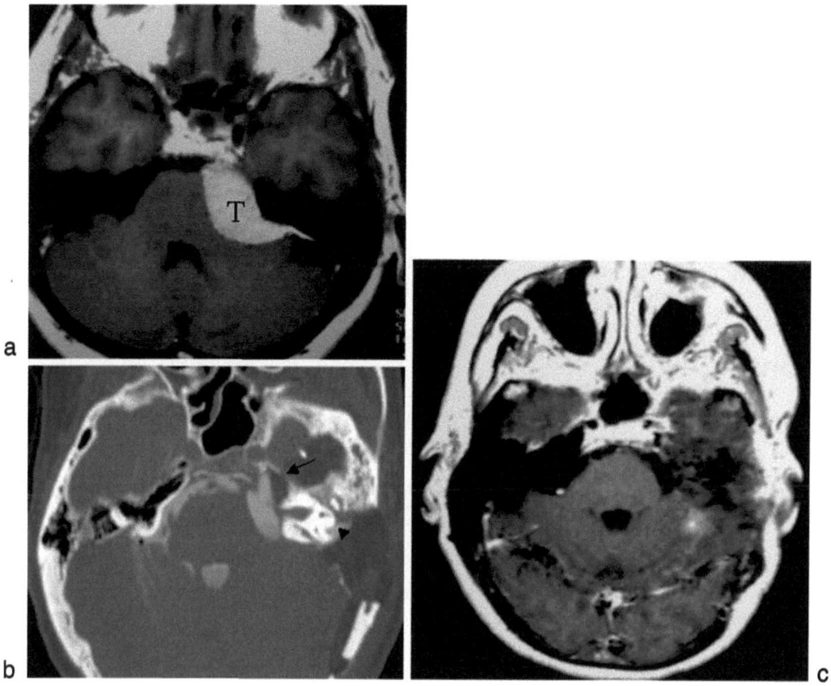

Fig. 39. Case illustration: a 49-year-old woman presenting with headaches, moderate gait ataxia and hypoacousia on the left side. (a) Preoperative MR imaging shows a left petroclival tumor (*T*) that is homogeneously enhanced after gadolinium administration. This feature is in favour of a petroclival meningioma. (b) The combined petrosal approach is visualized by this CT scan cisternography using bony window. Black arrow indicates the anterior petrosectomy while the black arrowhead shows the lateral semicircular canal that has been skeletonized during the retrolabyrinthine step of the approach. (c) Axial postcontrast MRimaging at 3 years following the surgery. The petroclival area is devoid of any residual or recurrent meningioma

ear. Dura opening, tumor removal and closure are conducted following the same principles. Another solution is to associate a partial labyrynthectomy to the apicectomy. In this approach, a large segment of the SCC and of the PCC is resected at the level of the common crus. This canalicular defect is immediately obtured by bone wax, thereby theoretically preventing the deafness.

Indications

The purpose of this paper is not to give a flow chart of surgical strategies for the removal of petroclival tumors. Moreover, given the complexity of the parameters to betaken into account, each situation is different. Many variables are related to the patient: age, general condition, neurological status (peripheral nerve, axial structures, hydrocephalus), prior treatments, factors that may influence treatment. Tumor-dependent variables include histology and anatomical origin of the lesion (from the bone, the dura, the cranial nerves, etc.), growth potential, insertion, volume, extension, relationship to critical structures. Of course, the experience of the surgical team and the availability of effective adjunctive techniques (e.g. radiosurgery or conformational radiation therapy) may influence the therapeutic strategy and the approach.

Conclusions

Despite considerable progress in non-invasive therapeutic modalities, many lesions that involve the petroclival region still require surgical treatment. This treatment remains challenging due to many characteristics: the depth of the PCR, the propensity for many tumors to engulf nerves and blood vessels, the invasion of neighbouring areas and extension to multiple cranial fossae and foramina.

The goals of this chapter are to provide the basics of the comprehensive surgical anatomy that is required to treat the lesions occupying the PCR, and to illustrate our purpose by detailing the most important approaches via the lateral skull base. These approaches are conservative insofar as they preserve intrapetrosal neuro-otologic structures. However, in many cases, attempts at total resection may risk impaired function. That is the reason why the trend these days is towards selective, tailored surgery rather than radical resection. Surgery is one component in a global multimodal management strategy in which less invasive techniques have their place. In this field, outcomes of combined microsurgical and radiosurgical techniques should be promising for petroclival tumors.

References

1. Brassier G (1984) Anatomie microchirurgicale du sinus caverneux. Thèse Méd, Rennes, 154 p
2. Cho CW, Al-Mefty O (2002) Combined petrosal approach to petroclival meningiomas. Neurosurgery 51: 708–718
3. Day JD, Fukushima T, Giannotta SL (1997) Cranial base approaches to the aneurysms of the posterior circulation. J Neurosurg 87: 544–554
4. Day JD, Fukushima T, Giannotta SL (1994) Microanatomical study of the extradural middle fossa approach to the petroclival and posterior cavernous sinus region: description of the rhomboid construct. Neurosurgery 34: 1009–1016
5. Day JD, Gianotta SL, Fukushima T (1994) Extradural temporopolar approach to lesions of the upper basilar artery and infrachiasmatic region. J Neurosurg 81: 230–235
6. De Oliveira E, Rhoton AL Jr, Peace D (1985) Microsurgical anatomy of the region of the foramen magnum. Surg Neurol 24: 293–352
7. Destrieux C, Velut S, Kakou MK, Lefrancq T, Arbeille B, Santini JJ (1997) A new concept of Dorello's canal microanatomy: the petroclival venous confluence. J Neurosurg 87: 67–72

8. Dolenc VV (2003) Microsurgical anatomy and surgery of the central skull base. Springer, Wien New York, 185 p
9. Dolenc V, Skrap M, Sustersic J (1987) A transcavernous-transsellar approach to the basilar tip aneurysms. Br J Neurosurg 1: 251–259
10. Fournier HD, Mercier PH, Menei P, AlHayek G, Guy G (1995) Transpetrosal approaches to the clivus: surgical anatomy, pretentions and limits. Neurochirurgie 41(1): 6–28
11. Fournier HD, Pasco-Papon A, Mercier P, Menei P, Hayek G, Guy G (1997) The anterolateral transpetrosal approach to the clivus and the pons. Preoperative embolisation of the inferior petrosal sinus. Interventional Neuroradiol 3: 255–260
12. Fournier HD, Mercier P (2000) A limited anterior petrosectomy with preoperative embolisation of the inferior petrosal sinus for ventral brainstem tumor removal. Surg Neurol 54: 10–18
13. Fukushima T, Day JD, Hiraha K (1996) Extradural total petrous apex resection with trigeminal translocation for improved exposure of the posterior cavernous sinus and petroclival region. Skull Base Surg 6: 95–103
14. Goldman C, Singeton GT, Holly EH (1971) Aberrant internal carotid artery presenting as a mass in the middle ear. Arch Otolaryng 94: 269–273
15. Hakuba A, Nishimura S, Inoue Y (1985) Transpetrosal-transtentorial approach and its application in the therapy of retrochiasmatic craniopharyngiomas. Surg Neurol 24: 405–415
16. House WF, Hitselberger WE, Horn KL (1986) The middle fossa transpetrous approach to the anterior-superior cerebellopontine angle. Am J Otolo 7(1): 1–4
17. Ikeda K, Yamashita J, Hashimoto M, Futami K (1991) Orbitozygomatic temporopolar approach for a high basilar tip aneurysm associated with a short intracranial internal carotid artery: a new surgical approach. Neurosurgery 28: 105–110
18. Jackson IT, Laws ER Jr, Martin RD (1983) A craniofacial approach to advanced recurrent cancer of the central face. Head Neck Surg 5: 474–488
19. Kawase T, Shiobara R, Toya S (1991) Anterior transpetrosal transtentorial approach for sphenopetroclival meningiomas: surgical method and results in 10 patients. Neurosurgery 28: 869–876
20. Kawase T, Toya S, Shiobara R, Mine T (1985) Transpetrosal approach for aneurysms of the lower basilar artery. J Neurosurg 63: 857–861
21. Lang J (1991) Anatomy of the posterior skull base. Rivista di Neuroradiologia 4 [Suppl] 1: 125–134
22. Lapayowker MS, Liebman EP, Ronis ML, Safer JN (1971) Presentation of the internal carotid artery as a tumor of the middle ear. Radiology 98: 293–297
23. Lasjaunias P, Berenstein A (1987) Surgical Neuroangiography, vol 1, functional anatomy of craniofacial arteries. Springer, Berlin Heidelberg New York, 426 p
24. Lasjaunias P, Merland JJ, Theron J, Moret J (1977) Dural vascularization of the middle cranial fossa. J Neuroradiology 4: 361–384
25. Matsushima T, Rhoton AL Jr, De Oliveira E, Peace D (1983) Microsurgical anatomy of the veins of the posterior fossa. J Neurosurg 59: 63–105
26. Mercier Ph, Cronier P, Mayer B, Pillet J, Fischer G (1982) Microanatomical study of the arterial blood supply of the facial nerve in the ponto cerebellar angle. Anat Clin 3: 263–270
27. Mickey B, Close L, Schaeffer S, Samson D (1988) A combined frontotemporal and lateral infratemporal fossa approach to the skull base. J Neurosurg 68: 678–683
28. Ozveren MF, Uchida K, Aiso S, Kawase T (2002) Meningovenous structures of the petroclival region: clinical importance for surgery and intravascular surgery. Neurosurgery 50: 829–837

29. Pait TG, Zeal A, Harris FS, Paullus WS, Rhoton AL Jr (1977) Microsurgical anatomy and dissection of the temporal bone. Surg Neurol 8: 363–391
30. Paullus WS, Pait TG, Rhoton AL Jr (1977) Microsurgical exposure of the petrous portion of the carotid artery. J Neurosurg 47: 713–726
31. Pellet W, Cannoni M, Pech A (1989) Otoneurochirurgie. Springer, Berlin Heidelberg, 237 p
32. Poncet P, Miller P (1979) Le trajet aberrant de la carotide interne intrapétreuse dans la caisse du tympan. Ann Otolaryng (Paris) 96: 793–804
33. Rhoton AL (1974) Microsurgery of the internal acoustic meatus. Surg Neurol 2: 311–318
34. Rhoton AL, Hardy DG, Chambers SM (1979) Microsurgical anatomy and dissections of the sphenoid bone, cavernous sinus and sellar region. Surg Neurol 12(1): 63–104
35. Roche PH, Régis J (2005) Cerebellopontine angle meningiomas. Neurosurgical forum, letter to the editor. J Neurosurg 103: 935–937
36. Sekhar LN, Estonillo R (1986) Transtemporal approach to the skull base: an anatomical study. Neurosurgery 19: 799–808
37. Sekhar LN, Janecka IP, Jones NF (1988) Subtemporal-infratemporal and basal subfrontal approach to extensive cranial base tumors. Acta Neurochir (Wien) 92: 83–92
38. Sekhar LN, Schramm VL Jr, Jones NF (1987) Subtemporal preauricular infratemporal fossa approach to large lateral and posterior cranial base neoplasms. J Neurosurg 67: 488–499
39. Sekhar LN, Schramm VL Jr, Jones NF (1987) Operative management of large neoplasms of the lateral and posterior cranial base. In: Sekhar LN, Schramm VL Jr (eds) Tumors of the cranial base: diagnosis and treatment. Futura, Mt Kisco, NY, pp 655–682
40. Sekhar LN, Schramm VL, Jones NF, Yonas H, Horton J, Latchaw RE, Curtin H (1986) Operative exposure and management of the petrous and upper cervical internal carotid artery. Neurosurgery 19: 967–982
41. Sen CN, Sekhar LN (1990) The subtemporal and preauricular infratemporal approach to intradural structures ventral to the brain stem. J Neurosurg 73: 345–354
42. Sen C, Chen CS, Post KD (1997) Microsurgical anatomy of the skull base and approaches to the cavernous sinus. Thieme, New York, 42 p
43. Uttley D, Moore A, Archer DJ (1989) Surgical management of midline skull-base tumors: a new approach. J Neurosurg 71: 705–710
44. Velut S, Jan M (1991) Anterior petrosectomy during approach to the petroclival area. In: Schmidek HH (ed) Meningiomas and their surgical management. W.B. Saunders, Philadelphia, pp 435–450

Offprint from
Advances and Technical Standards in Neurosurgery, Vol. 32
Edited by J.D. Pickard

Percutaneous destructive pain procedures on the upper spinal cord and brain stem in cancer pain: CT-guided techniques, indications and results

Y. KANPOLAT

Department of Neurosurgery, School of Medicine, Ankara University, Ankara, Turkey

With 16 Figures

Contents

Abstract

In the century of science and technology, the average life span has increased, bringing with it an increase in the incidence of degenerative and cancer disease. Intractable pain is usually the main symptom of cancer. With the advancement in technology, there is a large group of patients with intractable pain problems who can benefit from special help medically or surgically. Destructive pain procedures are necessary to control the cancer pain and are based on the lesioning of the pain conducting pathways. Percutaneous cordotomy, trigeminal tractotomy and extralemniscal myelotomy are special methods based on lesioning of the pain conducting pathways. The procedure consists of obtaining direct morphological appearance of the upper spinal cord and surrounding structures by computed tomography (CT). The next step is functional evaluation of the target and its environment by impedance measurement and stimulation. The final step is terminated with controlled lesioning obtained by a radiofrequency system (generator, needles, electrode system).

In the last two decades, CT-guided destructive procedures were used as minimally invasive procedures as follows: percutaneous cordotomy (207 patients), trigeminal tractotomy-nucleotomy (65 patients), and extralemniscal myelotomy (16 patients). Most of these patients had cancer pain.

Minimally invasive CT-guided destructive pain procedures are still safe and effective operations for relieving intractable cancer pain in selected cases.

Keywords: Intractable cancer pain; percutaneous cordotomy; trigeminal tractotomy-nucleotomy; extralemniscal myelotomy.

Introduction

In the last two decades, the impact of technology in medical practice has highly dominated our lives. In this period, the terms quality of life, minimally invasive, robotic, high technology, high-tech, neuromodulation, and neurostimulation have become widely accepted. As a result, those surgical treatment methods utilizing high technology and appearing to be minimally invasive have gained widespread acceptance. Unfortunately, as a consequence of this process over time, some less technological but highly effective methods are neglected or discounted and become generally perceived as dangerous.

In pain surgery, some of the very important and effective procedures have basically been abandoned in developed western literature because of their risky application. Some pain-relieving procedures are currently described as destructive, minimally invasive, safe and effective, but they are rarely preferred in intractable pain treatment in cancer patients [38]. These procedures are usually described as "classically ablative" procedures. Definition of the term "ablation" according to Webster's Third New International Dictionary as "removal of an organ or part by surgery" does not reflect the true purpose of this technique [48]. Procedures destroying the pain pathways can be performed with the help of minimally invasive stereotactic methods in our daily practice.

The century of science and technology has witnessed an increase in our average life span. In other words, in the age of science and technology, we are living in a society of advanced age. Thus it is not surprising that the incidence of cancer in this society is higher than was observed in younger societies. It is commonly held that pain is the most classical symptom of cancer disease and is dominant in the terminal stages [10]. As scientists and neurosurgeons we must propose some effective and rational solutions for these patients. Recent technological improvement has facilitated the development of some effective and simple procedures in the treatment of cancer pain, yet they are still not widely used. In this paper, contrary to established opinion, we will present some safe and effective destructive procedures targeting a unique part of the human body for achieving control of intractable cancer pain. The described methods are based on destruction of pain-conducting pathways, but the most important difference is demonstrating the target and destructive elements of the pain destructive equipment (Kanpolat cannula and electrode kits and lesion generator, Cosman Company, Burlington, MA, USA) [18]. For this reason, we have termed this group of procedures as computed tomography (CT)-guided pain procedures [15, 17–19]. In this group, CT-guided percutaneous cordotomy, CT-guided trigeminal tractotomy-nucleotomy and CT-guided extralemniscal myelotomy are presented.

CT-Guided percutaneous cordotomy

The pain-conducting tractus was discovered in clinical observations. Müller was the first to report an isolated analgesia observed after lesion of the spinal cord [35]. In this case, the whole of one half of the spinal cord and both dorsal columns had been damaged by a stab wound. The results of the lesion were anesthesia to touch on both sides and analgesia of the side opposite to the lesion. A few years later, Gowers reported a case of localized injury to the anterolateral column at the level of the 3rd cervical segment, which resulted in complete analgesia with preservation of tactile sensation on the opposite half of the body. From this case, Gowers concluded that the afferent pathway for pain was located at the anterolateral column of the spinal cord [45]. The existence of the spinothalamic tract was evidenced in 1889 by Edinger based on degeneration experiments in amphibians and newborn cats. Schüller performed sectioning of the anterolateral tract in monkeys, and named the procedure chordotomie [41]. It was used for the first time for relief of intractable pain in humans in 1911 by open technique as proposed by Spiller and performed by Martin [46]. The procedure was independently performed by Foerster and Tietze in 1913 [6]. In 1920, Frazier published a series of six cordotomy patients [7]. After this publication, cordotomy was accepted as an important method of pain surgery. Traditionally, cordotomy was an effective method using a posterior approach. The anterior approach in the lower cervical region was described by Cloward and Collis, but has not been widely utilized [2, 3].

Cordotomy is predominantly performed in cancer patients who cannot tolerate open surgery because of their poor clinical condition. Thus, surgeons have searched for noninvasive modalities in the treatment of these patients. In 1963, Mullan *et al.* described and performed percutaneous cordotomy using radioactive-tipped strontium needle [32]. Because of the uncontrolled effect of the radioactive source, Mullan *et al.* later tried unipolar anodal electrolytic lesions in 1965 [34]. In the same year, Rosomoff *et al.* described the technique of percutaneous cordotomy using radiofrequency (RF) electrode system [40]. In the following years, this system was used with impedance measurements and some contrast agents for visualization [9, 47]. Percutaneous cordotomy was routinely performed with the help of X-ray. In 1986, together with my colleagues, I attempted to use CT visualization for pain surgery in the CT unit for extralemniscal myelotomy [15]. We published the first paper regarding CT-guided extralemniscal myelotomy two years later, in 1988 [15]. In the following years, we used CT guidance as a classical visualization method in percutaneous stereotactic pain procedures [15, 17, 19, 23–27].

Anatomic target

The main anatomic target is the lateral spinothalamic tractus located in the anterolateral part of the spinal cord. Anatomical details of the pain-conducting tractus and especially of the lateral spinothalamic tractus have been presented by us in many papers [24–27]. This target is approached at the C1–2 level (Figs. 1 and 2). Localization of the target is defined by CT visualization (Fig. 4). In our experimental and clinical studies, it has been demonstrated that diametral measurements of the spinal cord are not standard. For this reason, diame-

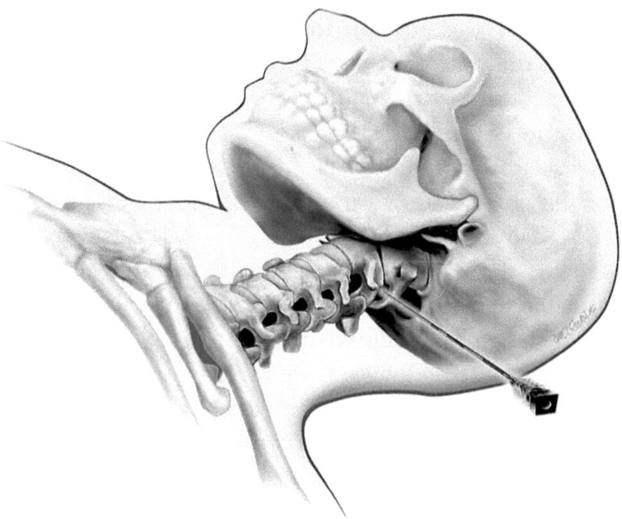

Fig. 1. Schematic drawing of percutaneous approach at the C1–2 level

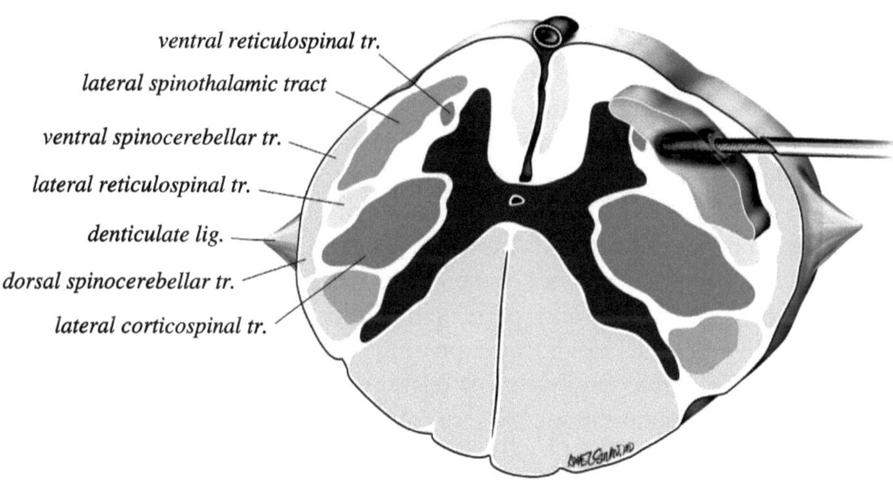

Fig. 2. Schematic drawing of the target-electrode relation and main anatomical structures in percutaneous cordotomy

tral measurements of the spinal cord are determined for each patient before the procedure and calibration of the inserted part of the active electrode is obtained with the help of these measurements [14].

Indications and contraindications

Cordotomy operation is principally based on the lesioning of the lateral spinothalamic tractus, which carries pain and temperature sensation. This fiber decussates in the spinal cord. For this reason, the procedure is performed contralateral to the pain site. In the past, the procedure was widely performed for benign and malignant intractable pain patients. In our daily practice, CT-guided percutaneous cordotomy is performed especially for cancer patients. The best candidates are those with unilateral localized intractable cancer pain, as seen in mesothelioma of the chest wall or carcinoma of the lower extremities, and those with unilateral localized pain problems [16, 17, 23]. Bilateral CT-guided cordotomy is chosen for the patient with intractable pain localized in the lower extremities [22]. Bilateral upper body pain is not accepted because of complication risk. There is a generally accepted opinion that cordotomy is chosen just after morphine therapy [10]. However, we recommend cordotomy just prior to initiation of narcotic agents, even if the patient's survival is less than six months. In the practice of intractable cancer pain treatment, there is a consensus dictating selection of these procedures usually in the terminal stage [50]. Our experience has shown, however, that if we are confident regarding the effectiveness of the procedure for intractable cancer pain, CT-guided percutaneous cordotomy before morphine therapy is a reasonable choice. The rationale of this strategy is based on the effectiveness and safety of the procedure observed over the course of our 20 years of clinical experience. Patients with severe pulmonary dysfunctions and in whom partial oxygen saturation is lower than 80% are not suitable candidates for cordotomy. We also do not employ percutaneous cordotomy if a patient's survival is less than three months. The most important consideration in percutaneous bilateral cordotomy is pain location. I personally do not perform bilateral cordotomy for bilateral upper body cancer pain. Another important contraindication for the procedure is the behavior of the patient and his/her family. The procedure should be considered carefully, particularly in patients receiving long-term treatment with opiate alkaloids, who possibly developed a dependency, and in cases of psychopathic family-patient relations [27].

Indications-contraindications of cordotomy have been summarized in Table 1.

Table 1

	Indications	Contraindications
Cordotomy	– Unilateral malignancies	– Behavior of the patient and her/his family
	– Lower extremities' pathologies (unilateral/bilateral)	– Bilateral upper extremities' pathologies
	– Failed back syndrome	– Severe pulmonary dysfunction
	– Chronic nociceptive painful conditions	

Technique

Preparation of the patient

The patient should be fasted for five hours before the procedure. The required dose of analgesics is given parenterally. The patient is informed before the procedure by the surgeon. Iohexol (7–8 mL of 240 mg/mL) is given 20–30 minutes before the operation by lumbar puncture. After injection of the contrast medium, the table is repositioned to trendelenburg position and it is kept 15 minutes to see the contrast in cervical region. If the general condition of the patient does not permit lumbar puncture, contrast material is injected during the procedure at the C1–2 level [17, 22, 27].

Positioning

As stated before, CT-guided cordotomy is performed in the CT unit. After the administration of contrast material, the patient is taken to the CT unit and placed on the CT table in the supine position [24–27]; the head is positioned on the headrest, flexed and fixed with band. The shoulders must be held low. The maximum comfort of the patient must be obtained; if necessary, some neuroleptic analgesics can be given [24–27]. Midazolam 0.5 mg/kg and fentanyl 1 μg/kg are used for neurolept anesthesia.

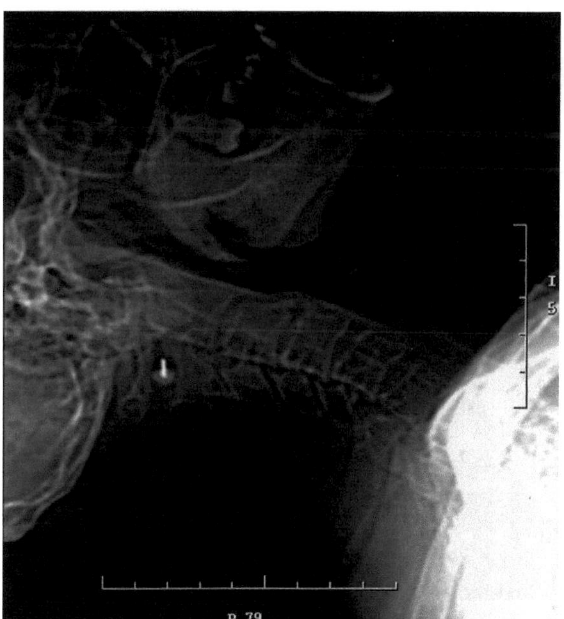

Fig. 3. Lateral radiograph of percutaneous cordotomy

Anatomic localization with CT

Before each procedure, routine cranial CT scan is obtained to exclude any intracranial mass lesions (metastasis, etc.). If such lesions are visualized, the procedure was not done. Routine lateral radiograph and axial CT slices of the C1–2 level are obtained. Diametral measurements of the spinal cord are taken, and distance between skin and dura is measured at the C1–2 level. The importance of these measurements described before [14]. The inserted portion of the active electrode is calibrated using diametral measurements of the spinal cord. Local anesthetic is given by separate inserted needle and cordotomy needle is inserted to approach the anterolateral part of the spinal cord at the C1–2 level. Ideal placement of the needle is initially just localized in the anterolateral part of the dura of the upper spinal canal. After every step of cannula movement, new CT slices are taken with lateral scanogram (Fig. 3). The new CT slices are not only for demonstrating the final position of the cannula but also for orienting where the tip of the cannula locates. In some cases, especially in cancer patients, who had radiotherapy before, the dura is very thick and difficult to puncture. If the puncture is painful, additional local anesthetic is given. Repeat CT slices can aid the surgeon in preventing improper puncturing. After the dural puncture, ideal localization of the tip of the cannula (Figs. 4 and 5) is 1 mm anterior to the dentate ligament for lumbosacral fibers and 2–3 mm anterior to the dentate ligament for thoracic and cervical fibers. After achieving the ideal positioning of the needle tip, the straight or curved electrode is inserted [17, 22–27].

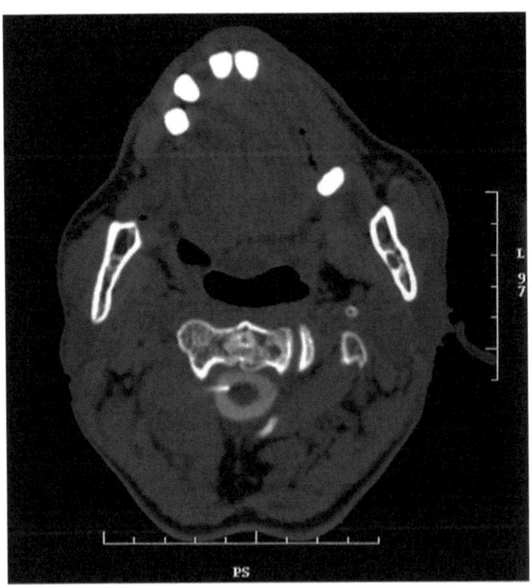

Fig. 4. Final position of the cannula on axial CT scan at the C1–2 level in percutaneous cordotomy

Physiologic localization

With the help of neurophysiological confirmation via impedance measurement and stimulation, functional response of the target is confirmed. Impedance measurements are taken to identify whether the active electrode tip is in the cerebrospinal fluid (CSF) (around 100 Ω), in contact with the spinal cord (around 300 or 400 Ω) or inside the spinal cord (more than 700 Ω). The target-electrode relationships are easily detected by direct visualization of the needle-electrode system under CT guidance [24, 27]. Figure 6a and b present the generator (Cosman RFG-1A) and needle-electrode system used.

Lesions

With our needle electrode system, permanent lesions can usually be achieved at a tip temperature of greater than 60 °C within 30 seconds. Energy and tip temperature of the active electrode are continuously monitored on the generator and both are gradually increased. During and after the lesioning, motor functions and pain perception and discrimination of hot and cold sensation are tested. Usually, the final lesion is made at 70–80 °C for 60 seconds. If the required level of analgesia is not obtained, the lesion is repeated using the same parameters. We prefer a maximum of three 60-second lesions for unilateral cordotomy. In bilateral cordotomy, we prefer to minimize the number of the lesions, but sometimes use two or three lesions for the dominant pain side [17, 22].

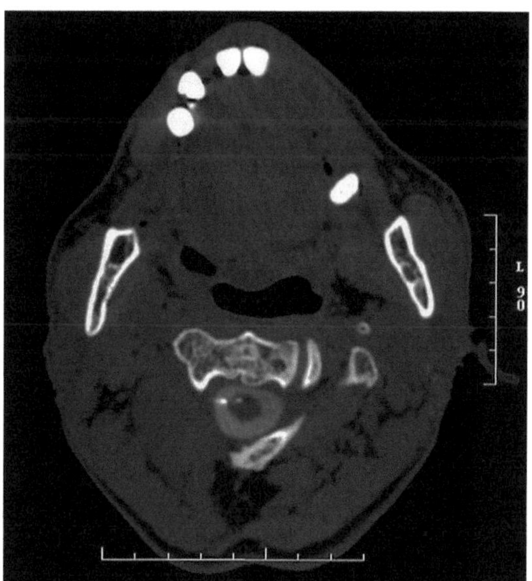

Fig. 5. Final position of the electrode on axial CT scan at the C1–2 level in percutaneous cordotomy

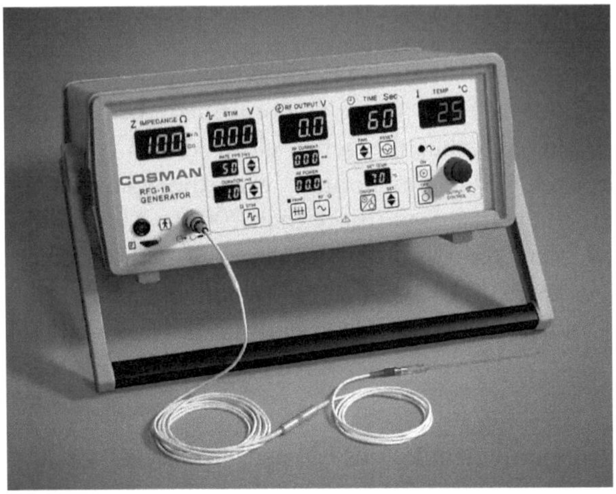

a

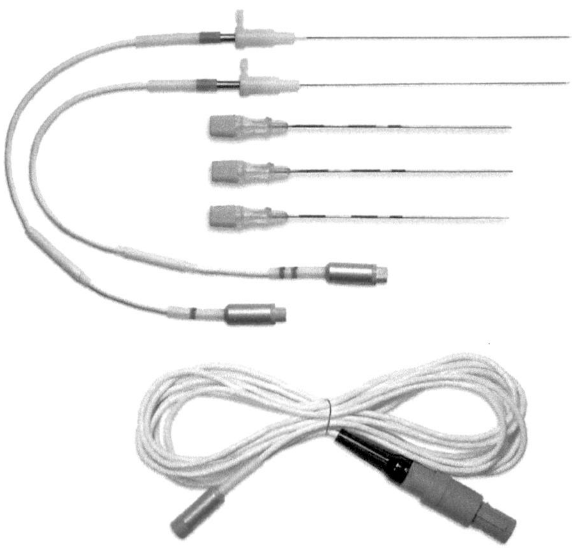

b

Fig. 6a and b. The generator (Cosman RFG-1A) (a) and the needle-electrode system used (b)

Postoperative

After the procedure, patients are usually monitored in the intensive care unit (ICU). If the patient's vital parameters are sufficient, the patient can be sent home 5 or 6 hours after the procedure. We usually inform the patient regarding his/her post-cordotomy life. If the patient has special dependency on some narcotic drugs, the doses will be gradually decreased; there is no standard.

Mooij *et al.* have described some causes of failure in high cervical percutaneous cordotomy [33]. In bilateral cordotomy, the patient is usually monitored at least one night in the ICU [23, 27].

Results and complications

Between 1987 and 2006, we performed 232 CT-guided percutaneous cordotomies in 207 patients. Most (193 cases) suffered from intractable pain related to malignancy. In 12 cases, CT-guided cordotomy was performed bilaterally with a one-week interval. In 181 cases, CT-guided cordotomy was performed unilaterally. In the malignancy group, pulmonary malignancies [58], mesothelioma [23] and Pancoast tumors [15] represented the majority of cases (49.7%). In addition, there were 23 patients with gastrointestinal carcinoma, 21 with metastatic carcinoma, and 53 patients with other types of malignancy. The procedure was also applied to 14 cases with benign pain. The initial success rate of CT-guided percutaneous cordotomy was 95%. The success rate was slightly higher in the malignancy group. In the cancer group, only the painful region of the body was relieved from pain in 83%, thus achieving selective cordotomy. In 12 cases, bilateral selective percutaneous cordotomy was successfully applied [22–27]. Due to respiratory complication risks, 12 bilateral cordotomies were performed in cases of pain only below the chest region. Nevertheless, in bilateral cordotomy Ondine's curse may be a problem. However, the appearance of arrest of nightly breathing (Ondine's curse) is dramatically minimized if between the first and the second side a time lag of one week to ten days is left.

Nowadays, percutaneous cordotomy is often referred to as an old and ablative technique and is usually criticized regarding its success rate, complications and failures. Even in the age of science and technology, based on my own experience I can confirm that cordotomy with CT guidance is a safe and effective method for selected intractable pain patients. After performing more than 300 CT-guided procedures, we can report no mortality and major complications. In 207 percutaneous cordotomy series, there was no mortality or major morbidity. We observed only five cases (2.4%) of temporary motor

Table 2

Patients in Cordotomy (Total: 207)
Pulmonary malignancies (58)
Mesotheliama (23)
Pancoast tumor (15)
Gastrointestinal carcinoma (23)
Metastatic carcinoma (21)
The other malignancies (53)
Benign pain (14)

Table 3

Complications
Mortality (0%)
Major morbidity (0%)
Temporary motor complication (2.4%)
Temporary ataxia (2.4%)
Hypotension (1.4%)
Temporary urinary retention (0.9%)
Dysesthesia (1.9%)

complication and five cases of temporary ataxia. These complications usually resolved within three weeks. In the bilateral cordotomy series, there were three cases (1.4%) of temporary hypotension and two cases (0.9%) of temporary urinary retention; these also returned to normal. The only true complication post-cordotomy in our series was dysesthesia, seen in four cases (1.9%).

The numbers of the patients and complications have been presented in Tables 2 and 3.

CT-Guided trigeminal tractotomy-nucleotomy (TR-NC)

Destruction of the descending trigeminal tract in the medulla is known as trigeminal tractotomy. The procedure was first performed in 1938 by Sjöqvist [45]. In 1969, Sweet observed hypoalgesia in the regions innervated by the 7th, 9th, and 10th cranial nerves after trigeminal tractotomy [49]. In 1965, Kunc developed a high cervical approach for cutting the tractus and used the procedure selectively to relieve glossopharyngeal neuralgia, with a high rate of success [28]. Crue *et al.* and Hitchcock independently developed a stereotactic percutaneous technique using RF thermocoagulation that enabled them to perform the first stereotactic trigeminal tractotomies [4, 13]. Schvarcz used this technique and named the procedure trigeminal nucleotomy to emphasize the significance of creating lesions primarily in the second-order neurons at the oral pole of the nucleus caudalis [43]. In 1990, Nashold *et al.* described an open surgical technique to destroy the whole substantia gelatinosa of the nucleus caudalis and named the procedure nucleus caudalis DREZ operation [36, 37]. We adapted the CT-guided system to the trigeminal tractotomy in 1989, terming it CT-guided trigeminal tractotomy-nucleotomy (TR-NC) [19, 21], and have routinely performed the procedure since that time.

Anatomic target

The main anatomic target is the lateral descending trigeminal tractus located in the posterolateral part of the spinal cord. Anatomical details of the pain con-

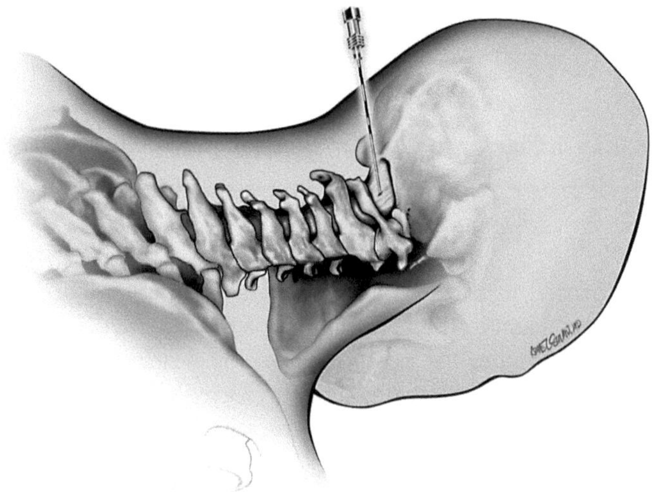

Fig. 7. Schematic drawing of percutaneous TR-NC approach at occiput-C1 level

ducting tractus and especially of the descending trigeminal tractus and nucleus caudalis have been presented by us in several papers [23–26]. This target is approached at the occiput-C1 level (Fig. 6). Localization of the target is defined by CT visualization (Fig. 7). As stated previously, diametral measurements of the spinal cord are taken for each patient before the procedure and calibration of the inserted part of the active electrode is obtained with the help of these measurements.

Indications and contraindications

Trigeminal TR-NC operation is principally based on the lesioning of the descending trigeminal tractus and nucleus caudalis, which carry pain and temperature sensation fibers of the face, ear and throat. Pertinent anatomy and physiology of the system have been described in previously published papers. These targets are optimum sites for lesioning of the tractus and nucleus. The best candidates for the procedure are patients with unilateral localized intractable central and peripheral 5th, 7th, 9th, and 10th painful areas of the face, ear and throat. In this group, those appropriate for treatment with trigeminal TR-NC operation include patients with anesthesia dolorosa, post-herpetic dysesthesia, atypical facial pain, dysesthetic squeal after previous trigeminal surgery, post-traumatic neuropathy, and head, neck or facial pain duc to malignancy, and those with vagal, glossopharyngeal or geniculate neuralgia [19, 21, 24–26]. Occipitocervical bone abnormalities would preclude application of the procedure, but this has not been encountered in our limited practice. Patients with short neck and highly obese patients are also not suitable for TR-NC.

Technique

Preparation of the patient

Preparation of the patient is similar to the preparation for percutaneous cordotomy.

Positioning

CT-guided TR-NC is performed in the CT unit. After the administration of contrast material, the patient is taken to the CT unit and placed on the CT table in the prone position [24–26]; the head is positioned on the headrest, slightly flexed and fixed with band. The chest is elevated and supported with soft pads. A nasal catheter is placed to provide oxygen during the procedure [24–26].

Anatomic localization with CT

Before each procedure, routine cranial CT scan is obtained. Routine lateral scanogram and axial CT slices of the occiput-C1 level are obtained. Diametral measurements of the spinal cord are taken, and distance between skin and dura is measured at the occiput-C1 level. A 20 or 22 gauge cannula is preferred following injection of the local anesthetic agents; the cannula is inserted at the occiput-C1 level via posterior parasagittal route, 7–8 mm lateral from the midline. Placement of the cannula at the occiput-C1 level can be visualized in the lateral scanogram and the direction of the needle can be manipulated toward the occipitocervical space with the help of axial CT sections (Fig. 8). The needle

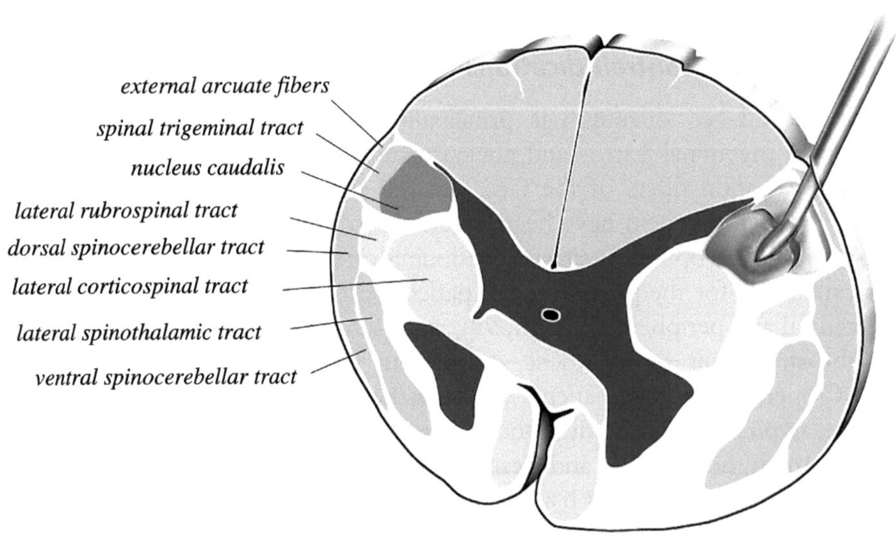

Fig. 8. Schematic drawing of the target-electrode relation and main anatomical structures in percutaneous TR-NC

is positioned posterolaterally to the spinal cord (Fig. 9). The best place for the electrode tip is toward the lateral third of the transverse diameter (equator) of the semi-cord (Fig. 10). After achieving the ideal position of the needle tip, the straight or curved electrode is inserted [24–26]. Curved electrode provides a 1 mm more anterior, posterior and lateral, medial extensions in the area.

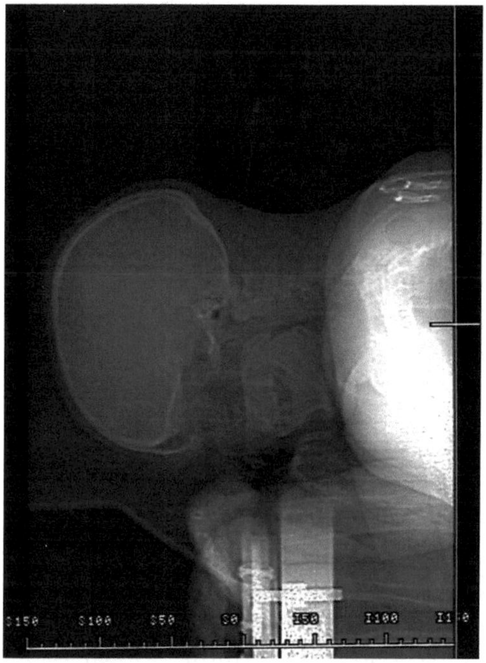

Fig. 9. Lateral radiograph of TR-NC

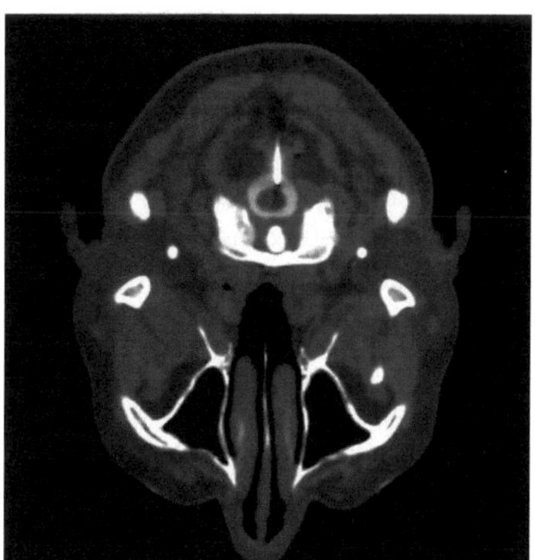

Fig. 10. Final position of the cannula on axial CT scan at occiput-C1 level in TR-NC

Physiologic localization

With the help of neurophysiological confirmation via impedance measurement and stimulation, functional response of the target is confirmed. Impedance measurements are taken to identify whether the active electrode tip is in the CSF (around 100 Ω), in contact with the spinal cord (around 300 or 400 Ω) or inside the spinal cord (more than 700 Ω). The target-electrode relationships are easily detected by direct visualization of the needle-electrode system by CT-guidance [24–26]. Puncture of the tractus nucleus complex is painful. The patient must be informed in this regard and a neuroleptic anesthetic is mandatory before the insertion. Electrical stimulation with low (2–5 Hz, 0.3–0.5 V) and high (50–100 Hz, 0.2–0.3 V) frequencies is used. Paresthesia of the ipsilateral half of the face can be observed with stimulation in most patients. Geniculate, glossopharyngeal and vagal fibers are usually located posterolaterally to the targets and the patient describes some dysesthetic sensation in the throat or inside the ear, indicating that the tip is in the nociceptive fibers of the 7th and 10th cranial nerves [24–26].

Lesions

With our needle electrode system, permanent lesions can usually be achieved at a tip temperature of greater than 40–45 °C within 10–20 seconds. Lesioning of the tractus nucleus complex is painful. Energy and tip temperature of the active electrode are continuously monitored on the generator and both are gradually increased. Some patients cannot tolerate high temperatures around 70 °C. If the patient tolerates 65–70 °C, two or three lesions are performed. Each lesion is of 60 seconds duration [19, 21, 24–26].

Postoperative

After the procedure, patients are usually monitored in the ICU. If the patient's vital parameters are sufficient, the patient can be sent home 5 or 6 hours after the procedure. We usually inform the patient regarding his/her post-TR-NC life. If the patient has special dependency on some narcotic drugs, the dose will gradually be decreased; there is no standard [24–26].

Results and complications

Between 1987 and 2006, we performed 65 CT-guided trigeminal TR-NC in 61 patients. Complete or partial satisfactory pain control was obtained in 52 patients (88.1%). The first and largest group consisted of 19 patients with atypical facial pain. Total or partial pain control was obtained in 17 patients; in the remaining two, nucleus caudalis DREZ operation was partially effective.

Good results were obtained from the group with glossopharyngeal (n: 16) or geniculate (n: 4) neuralgia. In the glossopharyngeal group, pain control was obtained partially or completely in 14 of the 16 cases. In this group, a small lesion was effective. In two cases, the procedure was ineffective. Recurrence was seen in six cases – in two repeated tractotomy, in two additional rhizotomies and in the last two nucleus caudalis DREZ operation controlled the pain attacks. In the geniculate group, we treated four patients with TR-NC. In three of them, the procedure was effective, and in one TR-NC did not control the pain attack. We performed nucleus caudalis DREZ operation. The pain was controlled but the patient died because of severe pulmonary edema on the postoperative 2nd day.

The third largest group consisted of 12 patients with craniofacial and oral cancer pain. In this group, 11 of 12 patients were successfully treated by TR-NC. In one case, pain relief was not complete and in one invasive hypophisial tumor, the pain was not controlled. For these two patients, nucleus caudalis DREZ operation was used but pain control was obtained in only one.

In unilateral post-herpetic neuralgia of the craniofacial region, four cases were treated with TR-NC; in two cases, pain control was obtained, and in one case, nucleus caudalis DREZ was performed but neuropathic pain was not completely controlled. No further treatment was attempted in the fourth case.

Two cases of multi-operated trigeminal neuralgia and one of bilateral trigeminal neuralgia were treated with nucleus caudalis DREZ operation. The procedure was partially effective in all of them.

There was no mortality in CT-guided TR-NC; only six cases (approximately 10%) of transient ataxia were observed. Transient motor complication was observed in two cases at a rate of approximately 3%. All of these complications disappeared in two weeks.

CT-Guided extralemniscal myelotomy

Extralemniscal myelotomy is a stereotactic lesioning of the central cord at the cervical medullary junction. The procedure was first performed by Hitchcock in 1968 to destroy the upper cervical commissural fibers and attain analgesia in a patient suffering from pain in his neck and both arms caused by esophageal adenocarcinoma [12]. Later procedures on the central cord show that the lesions caused relief of pain not only in the upper body and extremities but also in the lower body and extremities, as well as relief of visceral cancer pain. In 1976, Schvarcz stated that "The procedure, however, was not aimed at severing segmental decussating fibers, but at interrupting selectively the extralemniscal system. That is an ascending nonspecific polysynaptic pathway" [42]. He named the procedure "extralemniscal myelotomy". Gildenberg and Hirshberg performed limited myelotomy with an open technique at the T-10 level for similar purposes [8, 11]. Nauta *et al.* used central cord lesioning by an open method at the T-7 and T-4 levels using a punctate incision with a 16-gauge needle [11]. In the past, percutaneous extralemniscal myelotomy has conventionally been performed with the aid of radiographic visualization at the occiput-C1 level, although we have recommended later using CT-guided technique since 1988. In 1997, Nauta *et al.* reported punctate midline myelotomy for destruction of midline dorsal column visceral pathway as demonstrated by Hirshberg *et al.* [8, 11]. The same procedure was repeated by Becker *et al.* for visceral cancer pain [1]. All of these procedures were performed in the central cord region percutaneously or via open procedure.

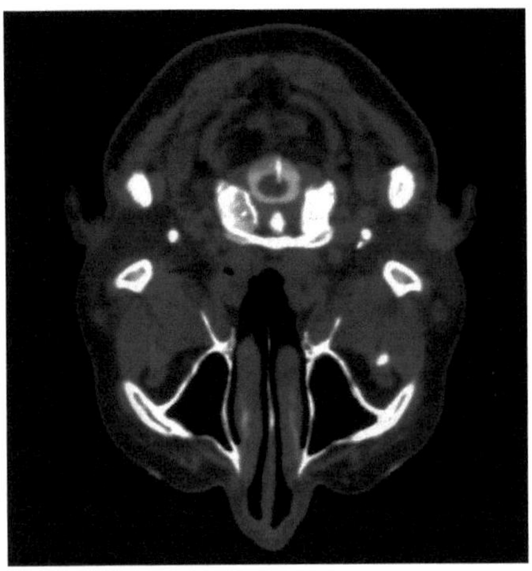

Fig. 11. Final position of the electrode on axial CT scan at occiput-C1 level in TR-NC

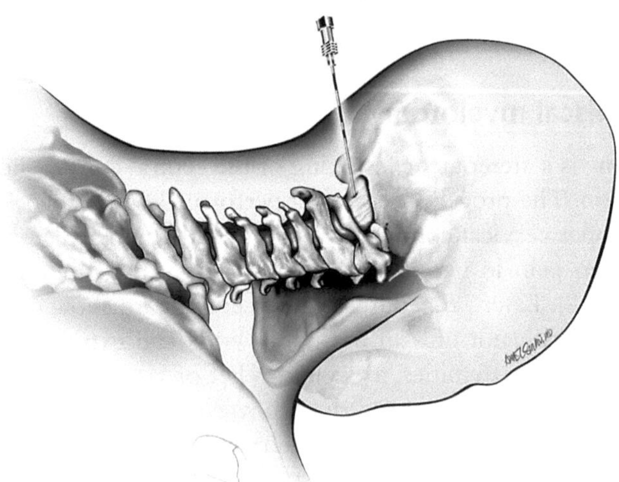

Fig. 12. Schematic drawing of percutaneous extralemniscal myelotomy approach at occiput-C1 level

Since 1986, we have used CT guidance for stereotactic upper cervical central cord lesioning and have named the procedure stereotactic extralemniscal myelotomy [15, 20].

Anatomic target

The main anatomic target is in the central part of the spinal cord. Anatomical details of the central spinal cord and ascending multi-synaptic pathway have been presented by us in many papers [24–26]. This target is approached at the occiput-C1 level (Fig. 11). Localization of the target is defined by CT visualization (Fig. 12). Diametral measurements of the spinal cord are taken for each patient before the procedure and calibration of the inserted part of the active electrode is obtained with the help of these measurements.

Indications and contraindications

CT-guided extralemniscal myelotomy operation is principally based on the lesioning of the central cord area at the occiput-C1 level [24–26]. The mechanism of the procedure is not properly known. In my limited experience, the best candidates for the procedure are those with visceral chronic cancer pain of lower abdominal and perianal regions [24–26].

Technique

Preparation of the patient

Preparation of the patient is similar to the preparation for percutaneous cordotomy.

Positioning

CT-guided extralemniscal myelotomy is performed in the CT unit. After the administration of contrast material, the patient is taken to the CT unit and placed on the CT table in the prone position; the head is positioned on the headrest, slightly flexed and fixed with band. The chest is elevated and supported with soft pads. A nasal catheter is placed to provide oxygen during the procedure [24–26].

Anatomic localization with CT

Before each procedure, routine cranial CT scan is obtained. Routine lateral scanogram and axial CT slices of occiput-C1 level are obtained. Diametral measurements of the spinal cord are taken, and distance between skin and dura is measured at occiput-C1 level. A 20 or 22 gauge cannula is preferred following

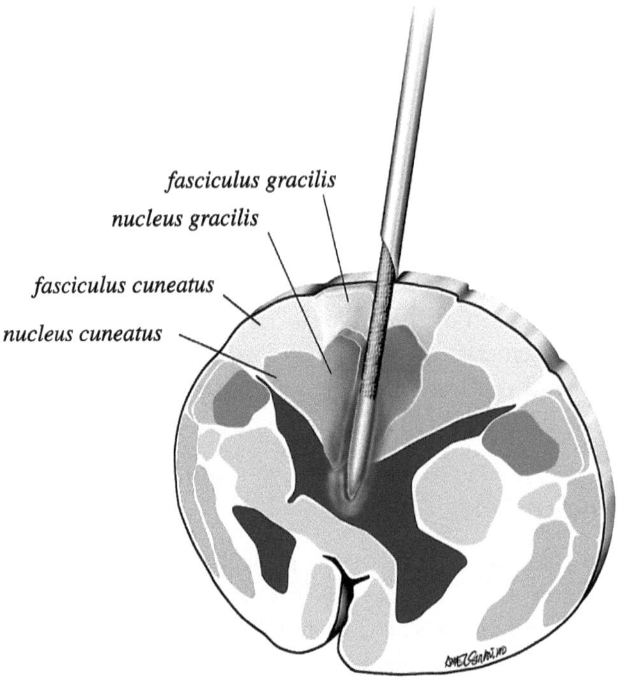

Fig. 13. Schematic drawing of the target-electrode relation and main anatomical structures in percutaneous extralemniscal myelotomy

injection of the local anesthetic agents; the cannula is inserted at the occiput-C1 level, posterior parasagittal route at the midline. Placement of the cannula at the occiput-C1 level can be seen in the lateral scanogram and the direction of the needle can be manipulated towards the occipitocervical space with the help of axial CT sections (Figs. 13–15). The needle is positioned at the posterior midline of the spinal cord at the occipitocervical level. The best position for the electrode tip is the medial part of the occipitocervical junction of the spinal cord. After localization of the cannula at the posterior part of spinal cord at the occipitocervical junction, the active straight electrode is inserted to the midline [24–26].

Physiologic localization

With the help of neurophysiological confirmation via impedance measurement and stimulation, functional response of the target is confirmed. Impedance measurements are taken to identify whether the active electrode tip is in the CSF (around 100 Ω), in contact with the spinal cord (around 300 or 400 Ω) or inside the spinal cord (more than 700 Ω). The target-electrode relationships are easily detected by direct visualization of the needle-electrode system by CT-guidance [24–26]. Puncture of the posterior part of the spinal

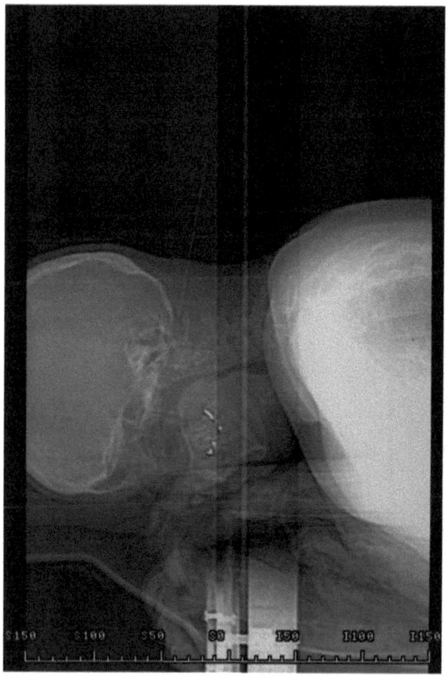

Fig. 14. Lateral radiograph of extralemniscal myelotomy at occiput-C1 level

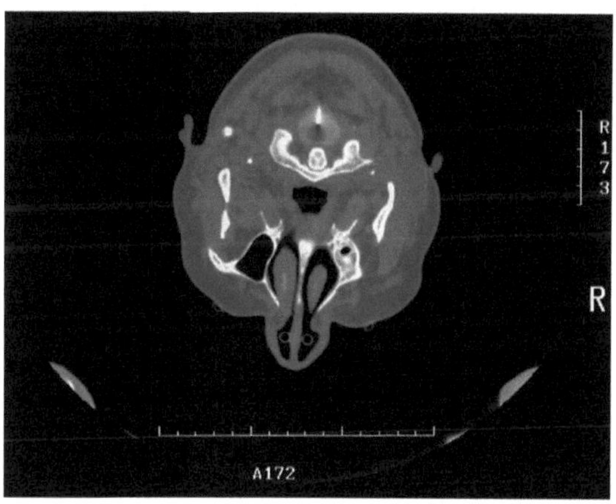

Fig. 15. Final position of the cannula on axial CT scan at occiput-C1 level in extralemniscal myelotomy

cord in the midline is not painful. Electrical stimulation with low (2–5 Hz, 0.3–0.5 V) and high (50–100 Hz, 0.2–0.3 V) frequencies is used. Paresthesia of bilateral lower extremities indicates that the electrode is in the proper target [24–26].

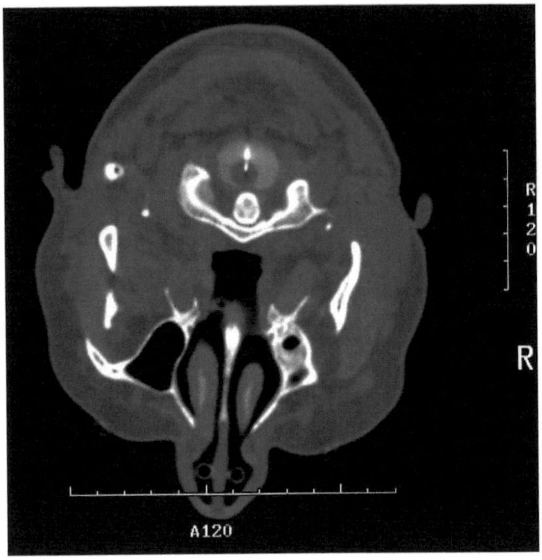

Fig. 16. Final position of the electrode on axial CT scan at occiput-C1 level in extralemniscal myelotomy

Lesions

With our needle electrode system, permanent lesions can usually be achieved at a tip temperature of greater than 60 °C within 30 seconds. Lesioning of the central cord is not painful. Energy and tip temperature of the active electrode are continuously monitored on the generator and both are gradually increased. Two or three lesions can be performed around 70–80 °C to the same location [24–26].

Postoperative

After the procedure, the patient is usually monitored in the ICU. If the patient's vital parameters are sufficient, the patient is sent home 5 or 6 hours after the procedure [24–26].

Results and complications

Between the years 1987 and 2006, we treated 16 cases with CT-guided extralemniscal myelotomy. Complete or partial satisfactory pain control was obtained in 11 cases. In five cases, no contribution to pain status was obtained. We are not aware of the mechanism of the lesioning of the central cord and for this reason can offer no special comment about this procedure and its results. No particular complication or mortality was seen.

Conclusions

Destructive pain surgery is usually applied using stereotactic localization principals. Stereotactic principals and proper localization are needed for morphological target. Morphological localization was not properly obtained in the past, but given the scientific advances in the last two decades, application of direct visualization systems (like CT or magnetic resonance imaging, MRI) have become routine for safe application [5, 15, 17, 19, 31]. The second step of the procedure is physiological localization, which indicates which anatomical structure locates in the target area. This localization is properly obtained using impedance measurements and stimulation. Impedance measurement only provides information about the tissues, but stimulation reveals the function of the target where the tip of the active electrode is located. Another difference in stereotactic destructive pain procedures is the possibility it provides to observe neurological functions of the patient during the procedures. This interactive observation serves as a guide to the surgeon throughout the procedure. In other words, if the surgeon's experience and knowledge about the morphology of the system are adequate and if the physiological evaluation of the target is observed by him/her, the procedures are applied safely and effectively. Despite these great advantages, such procedures have nearly disappeared in current neurosurgical practice. As mentioned previously, despite the availability of new drugs and pump and stimulation techniques, the use of destructive pain procedures is still an option in neurosurgical practice. Aside from their safety and efficacy, their most important advantage is that routine visits to the hospital or doctors for refilling or calibration of systems are no longer necessary. These independent patients are sometimes able to return to their normal life if the primary disease is under control. The other advantage of this destructive procedure is that it is much cheaper than paying for pump or a stimulator. For these reasons, these procedures should be learned by specialist neurosurgeon and must be criticized and evaluated by experienced scientists.

The most important procedure of this group is the cordotomy. Before the CT and MRI era, some criticism of the cordotomy as a destructive method was justified, but given the technological advances, the mortality risk today is nearly zero. We must refer to the procedures mentioned herein as minimally invasive as well. Cordotomy is the best method for controlling unilaterally localized chronic cancer pain states. There is no comparable alternative to it. From among the works of the last two decades, there have been very few large series about percutaneous cordotomy. Two important collected series were published by Lorenz and Sindou [30, 44]. They stated that cordotomy is an effective procedure, but carries high risk of mortality and morbidity, at 0–9%. In bilateral cordotomy, mortality rates increase dramatically, up to 50%. However, these mortality rates are given for the X-ray guided percutaneous cordotomy group [5, 26, 31, 39, 51]. These complications significantly drop, to nearly 0%, with CT guidance. In the very important work of Lahuerta *et al.* [29], it was reported that approximately 20% of the cord must be destroyed to achieve adequate pain relief. This is a very important point related with the efficiency and complications of percutaneous cordotomy. The most important part of this procedure is anatomically localizing how we approach this 20% of the spinal cord with a real-time, direct, morphologically-based visualization system in place of X-ray visualization. As stated before, the first step of the procedure is anatomical localization, the second must be neurostimulation, and the procedure is finalized with controlled lesioning [24]. Sindou criticized the procedure, citing diminished hypo-analgesia level and percentage of pain relief over time [44]. However, if pain recurs, it is easy to re-operate when necessary with the help of CT-guidance. In our series, in the case of five patients, even though their pain scores were satisfactory, they insisted on repeat cordotomy for the comfort it provided. This is perhaps one of the strongest testimonies to the value of the procedure.

The second procedure in this group (TR-NC) is unique, because with localization of only the 5th, 7th, 9th, and 10th pain fibers in the descending trigeminal tractus and nucleus caudalis; it is possible to denervate these pain nerve areas. In the practice of craniofacial cancer pain treatments, it is not easy to denervate the painful areas of the 5th, 7th, 9th, and 10th nerves. The descending trigeminal tractus and nucleus caudalis are the only targets that enable us to denervate painful areas of these nerves percutaneously [24–27]. This procedure is the exact alternative to nucleus caudalis DREZ operation as a first step in treatment of craniofacial or cranio-oral carcinogenic chronic pain states. In this group, because of the invasion of many cranial nerves, it is not feasible to approach each nerve separately and perform pain procedures. However, TR-NC makes possible the effective and easy control of these symptoms. If we compare the risk of the procedures, ataxia risk was limited and the mortality rate was 0% in our 65 procedures. One of the patients in this group also insisted on reapplication of the procedure despite satisfactory pain scores.

We do not have sufficient knowledge and experience about central cord lesioning, but I believe that the central cord area is an important target area for visceral cancer pain. In the near future, after gaining an understanding of real functions of visceral ascending systems, these procedures will be standardized and widely used in neurosurgical practice. Finally, I believe destructive pain procedures are highly effective in controlling some special intractable chronic cancer pain. These procedures must be performed by the neurosurgeon and must be popularized in view of their safety and effectiveness.

Acknowledgement

This work was partly supported by the Turkish Academy of Sciences. I express my gratitude to Mrs. Mukaddes Kurum Yucel for her assistance in writing the manuscript, Mrs. Corinne Logue Can for her language editing, and Dr. Ahmet Sinav for his creative illustrations. This paper is dedicated to the memories of Dr. Murat Rezaki and Dr. Gunfer Gurer Aydin.

References

1. Becker R, Sure U, Bertalanffy H (1999) Punctate midline myelotomy – a new approach in the management of visceral pain. Acta Neurochir (Wien) 141: 881–883
2. Cloward RB (1964) Cervical cordotomy by an anterior approach; report of a case. J Neurosurg 20: 445
3. Collis JS Jr (1963) Anterolateral cordotomy by an anterior approach; report of a case. J Neurosurg 20: 445
4. Crue BL, Carregal JA, Felsoory A (1972) Percutaneous stereotactic radiofrequency. Trigeminal tractotomy with neurophysiological recordings. Confin Neurol 34: 389–397
5. Fenstermaker RA, Sternau LL, Takaoka Y (1995) CT-assisted percutaneous anterior cordotomy: technical note. Surg Neurol 43(2): 147–149; discussion 149–150
6. Foerster O (1927) Die Leitungsbahnen des Schmerzgefühls und die chirurgische Behandlung der Schmerzzustände. Urban & Schwarzenberg, Berlin, p 360
7. Frazier CH (1920) Section of the anterolateral columns of the spinal cord for the relief of pain. A report of six cases. Arch Neurol Psychiat 4: 137–147
8. Gildenberg PL, Hirshberg RM (1981) Treatment of cancer pain with limited myelotomy. Med J St Jos Hosp (Houston) 16: 199–224
9. Gildenberg PL, Zanes C, Flitter M *et al* (1969) Impedance measuring device for detection of penetration of the spinal cord in anterior percutaneous cervical cordotomy. Technical note. J Neurosurg 30: 87–92
10. Gybels JM (1995) Indications for the use of neurosurgical techniques in pain control. In: Bond MR, Charlton JE, Wolf J (eds) Proceedings of the Sixth World Congress on Pain. Elsevier, Amsterdam, p 475
11. Hirshberg RM, Al-Chaer ED, Lawand NB *et al* (1996) Is there a pathway in the posterior funiculus that signals visceral pain? Pain 67: 291–305
12. Hitchcock E (1970) Stereotactic cervical myelotomy. J Neurol Neurosurg Psychiatry 33: 224
13. Hitchcock ER (1970) Stereotactic trigeminal tractotomy. Ann Clin Res 19: 131–135
14. Kanpolat Y, Akyar S, Caglar S (1995) Diametral measurements of the upper spinal cord for stereotactic pain procedures: experimental and clinical study. Surg Neurol 43: 478
15. Kanpolat Y, Atalag M, Deda H *et al* (1988) CT-guided extralemniscal myelotomy. Acta Neurochir (Wien) 91: 151
16. Kanpolat Y, Caglar S, Akyar S *et al* (1995) CT-guided pain procedures for intractable pain in malignancy. Acta Neurochir Suppl 64: 88–91
17. Kanpolat Y, Deda H, Akyar S *et al* (1989) CT-guided percutaneous cordotomy. Acta Neurochir Suppl 46: 67
18. Kanpolat Y, Cosman E (1996) Special RF electrode system for CT-guided pain procedures. Neurosurgery 38: 600–603
19. Kanpolat Y, Deda H, Akyar S *et al* (1989) CT-guided trigeminal tractotomy. Acta Neurochir (Wien) 100: 112

20. Kanpolat Y, Savas A, Caglar S, Akyar S (1997) Computerized tomography-guided percutaneous extralemniscal myelotomy. Neurosurg Focus 2, Article 5
21. Kanpolat Y, Savas A, Caglar S, Aydin V, Tascioglu B, Akyar S (1999) Computed tomography-guided percutaneous trigeminal tractotomy-nucleotomy. Tech Neurosurg 5: 244–251
22. Kanpolat Y, Savas A, Caglar S, Temiz C, Akyar S (1997) Computerized tomography-guided percutaneous bilateral selective cordotomy. Neurosurg Focus 2(1), Article 4
23. Kanpolat Y (2003) Cordotomy for pain. In: Schulder M (ed) Handbook of stereotactic and functional neurosurgery. Marcel & Dekker, New York, pp 459–472
24. Kanpolat Y (2004) Percutaneous cordotomy, tractotomy, and midline myelotomy, minimally invasive stereotactic pain procedures, seminars in neurosurgery, vol. 2/3. Thieme, Stuttgart, pp 203–220
25. Kanpolat Y (2002) Percutaneous stereotactic pain procedures: percutaneous cordotomy, extralemniscal myelotomy, trigeminal tractotomy-nucleotomy. In: Burchiel K (ed) Surgical management of pain. Thieme, Stuttgart, pp 745–762
26. Kanpolat Y (2004) The surgical treatment of chronic pain: destructive therapies in the spinal cord. Neurosurgery Clin N Am 15: 307–317
27. Kanpolat Y (1998) Percutaneous cervical cordotomy for persistent pain. In: Gildenberg PL, Tasker RR (eds) Textbook of stereotactic and functional neurosurgery. McGraw-Hill Inc, New York, pp 1485–1490
28. Kunc Z (1965) Treatment of essential neuralgia of the 9th nerve by selective tractotomy. J Neurosurg 23: 494–500
29. Lahuerta J, Lipton S, Wells JC (1985) Percutaneous cervical cordotomy: results and complications in a recent series of 100 patients. Ann R Coll Surg Engl 67: 41–44
30. Lorenz R (1976) Methods of percutaneous spinothalamic tract section. In: Krayenbühl H, Brihaye J *et al* (eds) Advances and technical standards in neurosurgery. Springer, Wien New York 3: 123–154
31. Mc Girt MJ, Villavicencio AT, Bulsara KR, Gorecki J (2002) MRI-guided frameless stereotactic percutaneous cordotomy. Sterotact Funct Neurosurg 78(2): 53–63
32. Mullan S, Harper PV, Hekmatpanahh J *et al* (1963) Percutaneous interruption of spinal-pain tracts by means of a strontium-90 needle. J Neurosurg 20: 931–939
33. Mooij JJ, Bosch DA, Beks JW (1984) The cause of failure in high cervical pecutaneous cordotomy. Acta Neurochir (Wien) 72: 1–14
34. Mullan S, Hekmatpanah J, Dobben G *et al* (1965) Percutaneous, intramedullary cordotomy utilizing the unipolar anodal electrolytic lesion. J Neurosurg 22: 548–553
35. Müller W (1938) Beiträge zur pathologischen Anatomie und Physiologie des menschlichen Rückenmarks. Leipzig 1871 in Olof Sjöqvist's Studies on pain conduction in the trigeminal nerve, Helsingors 1938. Mercators Tryckeri, p 85
36. Nashold BS, El-Naggar A, Abdulhak MM, Ovelman-Levitt J, Cosman E (1992) Trigeminal nucleus caudalis dorsal root entry zone: a new surgical approach. Stereotac Func Neurosurg 59: 45–51
37. Nashold BS, Rossitch E (1990) Anesthesia dolorosa and the trigeminal caudalis nucleus DREZ operation. In: Rovit RL, Murali R, Janetta PJ (eds) Trigeminal neuralgia. William & Wilkins, Baltimore, pp 223–237
38. Poletti CE (2006) Open cordotomy and medullary tractotomy. In: Schmidek, Sweet (eds) Operative neurosurgical techniques, 5th edn. Saunders & Elsevier, Philadelphia & Amsterdam, pp 1559–1572

39. Raslan A (2005) Percutaneous computed tomography-guided transdiscal low cervical cordotomy for cancer pain as a method to avoid sleep apnea. Stereotact Funct Neurosurg 83(4): 159–164
40. Rosomoff HL, Carroll F, Brown J *et al* (1965) Percutaneous radiofrequency cervical cordotomy: technique. J Neurosurg 23: 639–644
41. Schüller A (1910) Über operative Durchtrennung der Rückenmarksstränge (Chordotomie). Wien Med Wschr 60: 2291
42. Schvarcz JR (1976) Stereotactic extralemniscal myelotomy. J Neurol Neurosurg Psychiatry 39: 53–57
43. Schvarcz JR (1975) Stereotactic trigeminal tractotomy. Confinia Neurol 37: 73–77
44. Sindou M, Jeanmonod D, Merten P (1990) Ablative neurosurgical procedures for the treatment of chronic pain. Neurophysiol Clin 20: 399–423
45. Sjöqvist O (1938) Studies on pain conduction in the trigeminal nerve. A contribution to the surgical treatment of facial pain. Acta Psychiatr Neurol Scand Suppl XVII: 93
46. Spiller WG, Martin E (1912) The treatment of persistent pain of organic origin in the lower part of the body by division of the antero-lateral column of the spinal cord. JAMA 58: 1489
47. Taren JA, Davis R, Crosby EC (1969) Target physiologic corroboration in stereotaxic cervical cordotomy. J Neurosurg 30: 569–584
48. Webster's Third New International Dictionary. Springfield, Massachusetts: Merriam-Webster; 1993: 4
49. White JC, Sweet WH (1969) Pain and the neurosurgeon. Charles C. Thomas Publisher, Springfield, IL, pp 232–243
50. World Health Organization (1996) Cancer pain relief and palliative care, 2nd edn. WHO, Geneva
51. Yegul I, Erhan E (2003) Bilateral CT-guided percutaneous cordotomy for cancer pain relief. Clin Radiol 58(11): 886–889

Offprint from
Advances and Technical Standards in Neurosurgery, Vol. 32
Edited by J.D. Pickard

Carpal tunnel syndrome – a comprehensive review

J. HAASE

Department of Health Science and Technology, Aalborg University, Aalborg, Denmark

With 16 Figures

Contents

"Hands are an instrument, as the lyre is the instrument of the musician . . . every soul has through its very essence certain faculties, but without aid of instruments is helpless to accomplish what is by nature disposed to accomplish"

(*Galen*)

Abstract

Purpose. To provide a comprehensive review of the management of carpal tunnel syndrome.

Methods and results. A systematic literature review is provided of the history, anatomy, pathophysiology, epidemiology, diagnostic criteria, investigative surgical techniques, results and complications for carpal tunnel syndrome.

Conclusion. Surgery for carpal tunnel syndrome requires meticulous attention to history-taking, investigation, counseling, training and surgical technique if unsatisfactory results and complications are to be avoided.

Keywords: Carpal tunnel syndrome; median nerve; neurophysiology; magnetic resonance imaging; microsurgery; endoscopy; systematic review.

Median nerve entrapments

Introduction

Entrapment means, "To be caught in a trap". Therefore entrapped nerves involved in nerve compression syndromes are treated by increasing the free space surrounding the nerve with the intention of lowering the presumed pressure on and in the nerve.

One of the most common symptoms when a peripheral nerve is compressed/ pinched is paraesthesia. Paraesthesia is unfortunately a purely subjective phenomenon that is only experienced by the patient. Consequently – Medical Doctors (MD) – when patients complain of paraesthesia (tingling) – consult anatomy books seeking for a plausible diagnostic solution to their diagnostic problem. If a nerve pierces a membrane or turns around a muscle in the anatomy book, many surgeons assume that this is "in accordance with the symptomatology". Based on this purely hypothetical and non-valid scientific conclusion, they may suggest to the patient to "decompress" the nerve. This may result in a relief of symptoms but is also often followed either by no change in symptoms (because the nerve was not compressed), or by deterioration due to surgical trauma.

Surgical intervention is a kind of agreement between patient and surgeon. The patient wants to be healthy if surgery is performed, patients tend to be somewhat biased when being questioned regarding the surgical result at follow-up. I have personally met many patients who according to Hospital records were better after surgery, but when carefully questioned, in reality no change had occurred. If the surgical intervention has introduced a complication, the patient may develop both psychological and social dysfunction. Pain is the most typical complication of most operative procedures, including "simple" median nerve decompression.

Any nerve can be compressed but some nerves are specifically prone to entrapments. The most common nerve with entrapment symptoms is the median nerve at the wrist, resulting in the so-called carpal tunnel syndrome (CTS). [7, 28, 38, 39, 48, 58, 68, 93, 128].

History of peripheral nerve surgery for CTS

Paget mentions CTS in his original paper from 1865 followed by Marie and Foix who in 1913 suggested that the transverse carpal ligament could be the compressive agent resulting in proximal neuromas of the median nerve [48]. Brain discussed in 1947 – immediately after World War 2 – the pathophysiology of CTS [58, 93]. This was the time when standards of peripheral nerve surgery evolved rapidly [48, 58, 117] with the introduction of operative microscopes, microsutures, fibrin glue, intraoperative neurophysiology and nerve grafting whereby the concept of how to treat an injured nerve changed [29, 39].

Peripheral nerve anatomical structure

A peripheral nerve comprises nerve cells e.g. conducting axons, insulated by Schwann cells and surrounded by connective tissue (Fig. 1).

The neuronal structures are bounded together and bundled in fascicles by the perineurium. These fascicles have patterns that vary longitudinally in the nerve [117]. There is a natural sliding between fascicles and nerves can stretch 10–20% before structural damage occurs. Endoneurium encircles each myeli-

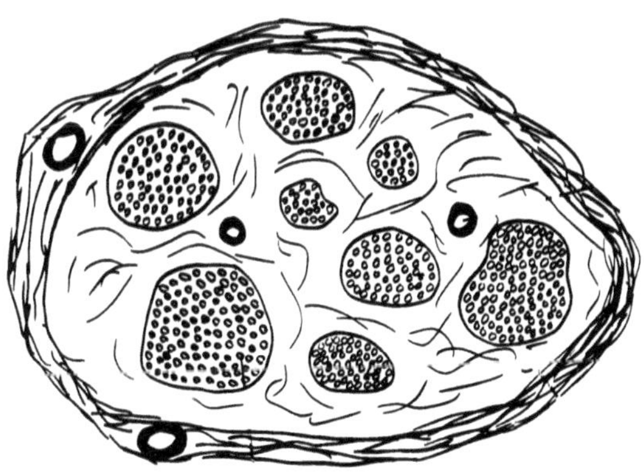

Fig. 1. Cross section of a peripheral nerve

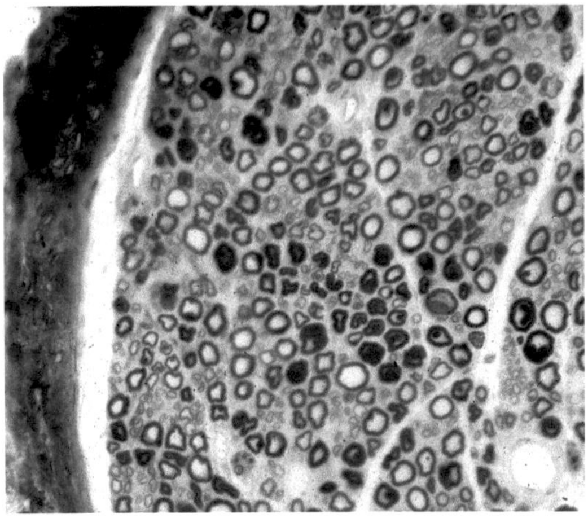

Fig. 2. Peripheral nerve histology

nated axon and groups of non-myelinated axons. Schwann cells provide the axons with lipoprotein coverage and some unknown trophic factors [120]. Outside the Schwann cells a basal lamina layer is found serving as a road for growing nerve fibers [66]. The cross section in Fig. 2 shows the micro histology of a peripheral nerve.

Connective tissue constitutes 50% component of a peripheral nerve. It consists of an external layer – the epineurium and an internal layer called the interstitial epineurium. Nerves close to a joint often have up to 85% connective tissue and only few fascicles. The connective tissue is made up of fibroblasts, fat, macrophages and blood vessels [117]. The vasculature of a nerve comprises both regional vessels entering the nerve obliquely at intervals along its course and an extensive longitudinal network of anastomotic vessels. Vessels traverse the perineurium and their sleeves close to the vascular walls of the nerve and thereby create a connecting channel. The major blood/nerve barrier is through the tight junctions of the perineurium [117, 120].

Carpal tunnel anatomy

Major anatomical variations exists within the carpal tunnel area [63]. Nevertheless, a general conception of this anatomy is important for surgeons.

An illustration of the wrist region is found in Fig. 3, where the skin has been removed. The transverse carpal ligament (TCL), the palmar aponeurosis, the tendon of the different flexor muscles and the nervous structures are outlined.

If we look further into the carpal tunnel it has a floor and walls created by the Navicular, Trapezius, Scaphoid, Hook of Hamate and Pisiform wrist bones as shown in Fig. 4.

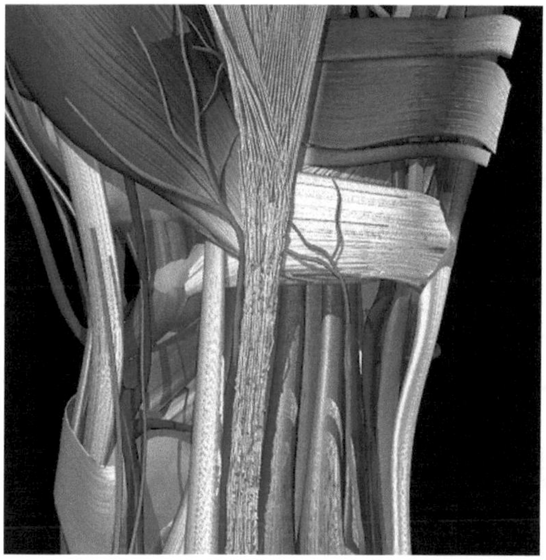

a

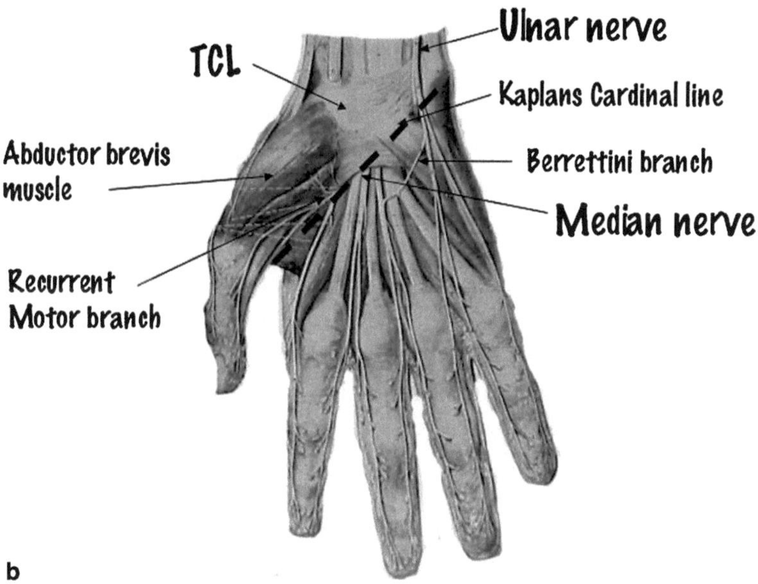

b

Fig. 3. View of wrist region with skin removed (a, b). 3D image courtesy of Primal Pictures Ltd., www.primalpictures.com

Transverse carpal ligament (TCL)

From the surface of the hand it is our surgical task to visualize the structures of our surgical target – the transverse carpal ligament (TCL). The TCL attaches to the Pisiform, Hamate, Scaphoid, and Trapezium bones and creates the carpal tunnel. Different lines, and landmarks will guide us to this TCL. One of these

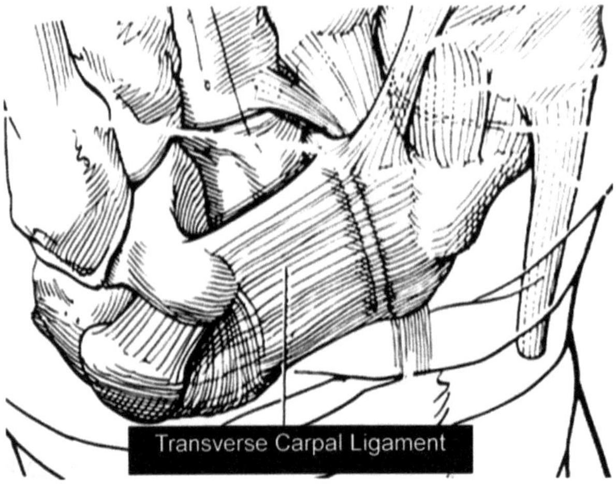

Fig. 4. TCL, wrist bones and ligaments

are Kaplan's cardinal line that is drawn from the apex of the first web space (between the thumb and index finger) toward the ulnar side of the hand, parallel with the proximal palmar crease (Fig. 3). The recurrent motor branch of the median nerve emerges at the intersection of Kaplan's cardinal line and a line through the axis of finger 2. The mean distance from the distal edge of the TCL to the recurrent motor branch of the median nerve is 2.7 mm (range 0–4.1 mm). The palmar cutaneous branch of the median nerve passes over the tubercle of the Scaphoid bone that can be felt in normal hands.

Entrance to the carpal tunnel is proximal and distal by the rim of the TCL. The size of the carpal tunnel can vary from 2 to 5 cm in length and is in a recent cadaver measurement a mean of 41 mm (35–45 mm) [49]. It is 2–3 cm wide and has a roof that is 0.5 cm thick with major variations [32, 33, 47, 49].

The mean distance from the radial aspect of the Pisiform bone to the radial border of Guyon's canal and the ulnar edge of the long palmar muscle tendon is 10.3 mm (range 9–12 mm) and 16.1 mm (range 12–22 mm), respectively. The mean distance from the distal portal of the carpal canal to the superficial vascular palmar arch and the ulnar artery is 10.4 mm (range 5–15 mm) and 7.6 mm (range 4.5–9 mm), respectively. The carpal tunnel has a rather steep descent into the palm as seen in Fig. 5.

The TCL serves as a trolley for the flexor tendons [58, 81]. The median nerve and the nine long flexor tendons of the digits pass through the carpal tunnel in synovial sheets. When we move our fingers or bend the wrist the tendons move up to 5 cm provided they are well lubricated. The eight superficial flexor- and the deep flexor tendons are in the same synovial sheet, whereas the long flexor tendon to the thumb has its own sheet radially placed in the carpal ligament (Fig. 6).

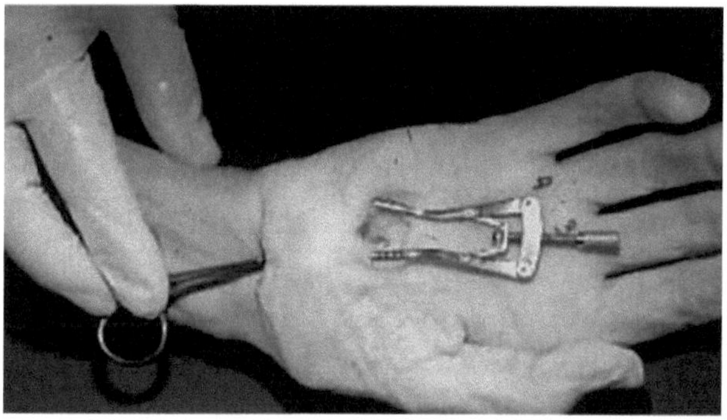

Fig. 5. Carpal tunnel, cadaver demonstration with instrument inside the tunnel

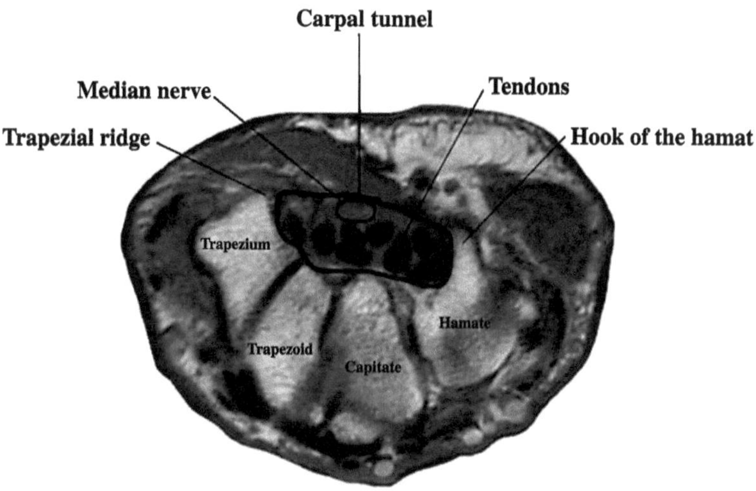

Fig. 6. Carpal tunnel, cross section, wrist bones, tendons and median nerve

Superficial to the TCL lies the palmar aponeurosis. Deeper transverse fibers of this fascial plane (volar carpal ligament), continues into the ante brachial fascia of the forearm that on the ulnar side of the wrist constitutes the roof for Guyon's canal. The radial edge of Guyon's canal contains the ulnar nerve and artery limited by the cooptation of the palmar aponeurosis with the TCL. The superficial longitudinal fibers of the palmar aponeurosis are in proximal continuity with the tendon of the long palmar muscle (Fig. 3). The abductor brevis muscle inserts from the radial side upon the TCL.

The median nerve

Variations in the anatomy of the median nerve at the wrist are of importance to the surgeon preparing to divide the TCL. The median nerve passes in the forearm radially to emerge between the tendons of the superficial long flexors and the radial flexor carpi (Fig. 6). It enters the carpal tunnel under the radial edge of the long palmar muscle tendon (Fig. 3). The median nerve consists of sensory and motor fibers to the radial part of the hand. The motor fibers are mainly located in one or two fascicles volar located in the median nerve [117]. The nerve passes through the carpal tunnel located volar close to the TCL and radial to the superficial flexor tendons between those to the middle finger and the radial flexor carpi tendon (Fig. 6). The median nerve dips under the TCL usually after having given off a cutaneous palmar branch that lies radial to the tendon of the long palmar muscle. This branch may also pierce the TCL and great variations of this superficial cutaneous branch exist. On the ulnar side of the palmar minimal muscle tendon the ulnar nerve gives off some smaller branches that can be found in the majority of variations.

The median nerve divides into five sensory branches at the distal end of the TCL. These five branches include:

1) A proper digital nerve to radial side of the thumb;
2) A short common digital nerve to the first web space that quickly divides into a proper digital nerve to the ulnar side of the thumb;
3) A proper digital nerve to the radial side of the index finger; and
4, 5) Two common digital nerves to the second and third web spaces [32, 119].

Within the carpal tunnel the median nerve gives off a recurrent motor branch radially and distally to the abductor brevis muscle with many variations. It is in 46% of patients leaving the median nerve freely extra ligamentous distal to the TCL. In 31% it is placed subligamentous and in 23% it passes through the TCL. In these two situations it is easily possible to injure this nerve during

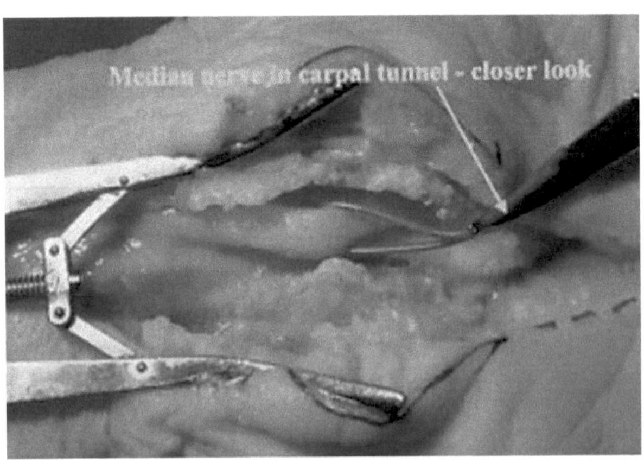

Fig. 7. Cadaver presentation of the median nerve with the TCL cut

surgery [32, 49]. Branches from the median nerve at the same level may also innervate the first interdigital- and lumbrical muscles.

Distal to the TCL the communication branch between ulnar- and median nerves (Berrettini branch) is found among 84%, always closely related with the distal vascular communication vessels [49].

The median nerve changes size and format according to the position of the wrist joint and with movements and elongation of the TCL. It is oval becoming more elliptical at the level of the Hamate bone. With the wrist extended it is found more anterior and deep to the TCL whereas it in flexion is pressed towards the TCL. It may move up to 2 cm during flexion/extension [53]. The median nerve is seen in the carpal tunnel in Fig. 7.

Cutaneous innervations of the palm

The palm derives its cutaneous sensation from branches of both the median and ulnar nerves. The cutaneous branch from the median nerve – already mentioned – is found 3–11 cm proximal to the wrist crease following the radial flexor carpi tendon, with penetration of the superficial layers of the TCL at the level of the Scaphoid bone [119]. The cutaneous branch from the ulnar nerve is found up to 16 cm proximal to the wrist crease. It innervates skin at the thenar eminence in approximately 50% of the patients. Short palmar branches originate proximal to the wrist crease penetrating the fanning fibers of the long palmar muscle tendon and terminate in the TCL [32].

The distal edge of the TCL

The superficial palmar arch lies in soft fat 2–26 mm from the distal edge of the TCL. It consists of the communicating branch between the ulnar and median nerves (Berettini branch), and the common digital nerve to the adjacent long and ring fingers. The superficial vessel connection between radial- and ulnar arteries lies together with these nerves. The hook of the Hamate marks the ulnar edge of the distal TCL, and the deep motor branch of the ulnar nerve passes around this hook (Fig. 6).

Carpal tunnel size – imaging

There is a great difference between measuring anatomical structures on cadavers and in the living [63]. Therefore with the introduction of Magnetic Resonance Imaging (MRI) we have received better information regarding the carpal tunnel. MRI is used to measure the transverse dimension of the carpal tunnel in neutral, flexed and extended positions among 16 normal subjects. In wrist extension the anterior–posterior (A–P) dimension and cross-section area (CA) decreased compared to neutral. Similar the transverse dimension (TD) increased at the level of the Pisiform bone and CA at the Hamate level. In flexion TD and CA decreased at Pisiform level. With wrist extension, the median nerve may be subject to significant pressure at the Pisiform level [131]. A plain radiographic study of 21 uninjured wrists in 12 volunteers defined the position of the distal wrist flexion crease (DWC) with respect to the hand. In 19 of the 21 wrists the DCW was within 2 mm of the proximal pole of the Capitate bone. Newer studies prove that the distal part of the tunnel is the narrowest in all these situations [49, 94]. The cross-sectional area of the carpal canal proximal and distal to the wrist flexion crease demonstrates on MRI a gradual increase in the area of the carpal canal moving proximal from its distal narrowest point. There is no significant increase in area until approximately 23 mm proximal to the narrowest point [78].

The dimensions of the carpal tunnel are slightly but not significantly smaller among patients with symptoms indicating CTS. These have thus a normal mean distal cross section of the carpal tunnel of 2.857 mm^2 [94].

Important to note is that this volume depends on the wrist position and decreases with wrist extension. The volume of a 400 mm long TCL is thus $2{,}857 \times 400 = 114.280\ mm^3$. The size of CTS symptomatic and abnormal carpal tunnels is a mean of $238{,}9\ mm^2 \times 400 = 95.560\ mm^3$. The difference is $114.280 - 95.560 = 16\%$. When cutting the TCL the size of the carpal tunnel should increase. In one series it changed only 6%, whereas other series have shown up to 24% increase [123].

The ulnar nerve and artery is located ulnar to the hook of the Hamate (Fig. 6). Radial flexion of the wrist joint causes in 30% the ulnar artery to move inside of Guyon's canal whereas ulnar flexion causes it to move radial toward the carpal tunnel [49].

What is a carpal tunnel syndrome?

"The Danish poet and storyteller Ludvig Holberg used in his play Erasmus Montanus the following circular argument – said to his mother by the clever student (Erasmus) that returned to Denmark from studies in a University abroad: "A stone cannot swim, You – mother – cannot swim – therefore You are a stone".

Despite what has been written in thousands of papers, we do not have a golden standard for what a CTS is [7, 79, 128].

In a patient with "symptoms" of Diabetes Mellitus, we will monitor blood–glucose levels and find them elevated. We know from pathophysiology that he lacks insulin. Now providing him with insulin he will feel better. His primary symptoms are soon relieved and simultaneously his blood–glucose level is lowered. Then we are now confident that the primary diagnosis was correct.

With CTS it is partly the same. We suspect CTS if patients are having certain "symptoms". Our problem here is that we do not know what parameters to monitor to find the "glucose" of CTS. When we surgically decompress the median nerve, and for example increase the volume of the carpal tunnel, most patients will recover. From that it is deducted that it is because the carpal tunnel volume was too small. We know from experimental science that an irritated median nerve will result in symptoms like paraesthesiae. Then we begin to look for pressure in the canal to prove our point. However it is still the neuropractic dysfunction of the median nerve that is the cause of the symptoms. Instead of monitoring pressure we seek simpler methods such as a better description of symptomatology (Hand-Diagrams). We start also to monitor nerve dysfunction with electrophysiology, and in both case we find many false positive and false negative results. We must evidently be careful in comparing results of treatment of CTS as the majority of papers describe "typical symptoms" of CTS and uses these "typical symptoms" in a circular argument, that when these symptoms are present, the patient harbours CTS – just like Ludvig Holberg did.

We have to add information on the population our patient is living in to decide which diagnostic tests we can rely on in the actual population. How to document an entrapment is therefore still today open to much debate – and often a very heated debate. How can we define CTS? Which test shall be used to diagnose a CTS? How shall we treat CTS? All these questions are some of the major issues for us as neurosurgeons. Most important for the future is that we try to answer our questions in evidence based way, and not just by "personal opinion" [104]. Following a personal screening of >2500 scientific papers dealing with CTS, I believe it is necessary to understand part of epidemiological basic statistics if we are to draw any conclusions regarding the true value of diagnostic and screening tests.

If one is interested, a check-up at the Cochrane Library [18] can be valuable for the understanding of how many unnecessary papers have been written on CTS problems through out the years.

For the remainder of this chapter we will accept that:

"*The most plausible reason is, that the median nerve is compressed in the carpal tunnel and that this is leading to the symptomatology of a CTS*",

and remember that the CTS based on symptoms alone are not just "one" disease, but possibly a combination of many [79, 97].

Pathophysiology of CTS

When a peripheral nerve is compressed this leads to immediate biochemical changes of the nerve and subsequent anatomical changes. The metabolism of a peripheral nerve was thoroughly studied by the Swedish scientist Lundborg

[66] and the deeper understanding of peripheral nerve biology gave a significant input to our understanding of entrapment treatment policies.

The carpal tunnel is to be considered as a closed hydrostatic space. An Italian group proved by continuous pressure monitoring, that daily fluctuating pressures occurs with a peak at 6 am – the time most patients are awakened shaking their hand. Lundborg [66] confirmed in his important work on blood circulation and vessels in peripheral nerves that a pressure of 30 mmHg leads to the first neurophysiologic changes and that a total blocked nerve conduction was found with pressures >50 mmHg. The normal pressure in the carpal tunnel is 2.5–15 mmHg and is highest distally [33]. The most compressed point is 10 mm distal to the wrist crease, with a pressure of 44.9 ± 26.4 mmHg. The correlation coefficient between the highest canal pressure and the latency was 0.393 and between highest canal pressure and duration of symptoms was 0.402. The most compressed part of the median nerve found in the carpal canal is 10 mm distal to the wrist crease and is related to the distal motor latency and to the duration of symptoms [51, 87]. Flexion/extension in the wrist reduces the carpal tunnel volume and increases consequently the pressure to around 30–50 mmHg – even up to 200 mmHg especially by wrist extension. Pressures measured with the wrists in three positions: neutral, full passive flexion and full passive extension showed that at each wrist position, the mean pre-operative pressures in a study group were significantly higher than in the control group. In both groups, the pressures were maximal with full passive extension and minimal in the neutral wrist position [33, 106].

The thick, myelinated fibres are more sensitive to hypoxia than the small thinner fibres [66]. An incremental loss of motor and sensory function of the median nerve occurs with increasing pressure [33] and a direct linear relation is found between electrical nerve conduction velocity and pressure in the tunnel.

This elevated pressure results at the same time in a slowing of the capillary circulation leading to a slight venous engorgement and further to hypoxia of nerve structures [66, 68].

A physical compression of the median nerve results also in further anatomical changes as distal axoplasmic flow is disturbed if the compression is static. Axonal membrane excitability is also altered and if the compression is continued, polarized distortion of the internodes is developed. The myelin lamella slips away from the site of compression and telescope through the node of Ranvier first described by Ochoa [3, 66]. Local demyelisation is found as a result of stretching and increased pressure, whereby blood flow is reduced and ischemia the result, but is reversible and recovery begins within hours. In cases of nerve compression, the proximal axons are distended and a decreased transport of nutritive substances and enzymes are found distally [66, 98]. A pseudoneuroma of the median nerve with distended vessels and cyanosis is developed and in 14% of operated CTS hands an hourglass deformity of the median nerve has been encountered [3]. The oedematous tissue facilitates proliferation of fibroblasts and in later phases internal long lasting compression of the median nerve even with scarring inside the fascicles. Fibrotic changes of the circumferential and interstitial epineurium are always found later in this process [66]. The longer the duration of/and amount of pressure – the more neural dysfunction is found.

The intermittent compression, stretching or dislocation of the nerve dictated by anatomical factors leads to development of an additional axon cylinder constriction [98]. These fibrotic changes affect the degree of free neural gliding [68]. The restricted nerve sliding may lead to increased strain, and possibly contributing to symptoms. Both among CTS patients and control patients longitudinal movements of the median nerve fascicles in the forearm averaged 2.62 mm. The nerve strain is thus not increased and should not contribute to symptoms. The CTS patients have in contrast to this a 40% reduction in transverse nerve movement at the wrist.

Tensile strength of a peripheral nerve is mainly determined by the perineurium and allows the nerves to stretch up to 20% before structural changes occurs [66].

When Fibrotic changes increases axonal degeneration will occur. Wallerian degeneration of the distal part of the axons is seen in the most severe degrees of compressions [117]. The neurophysiologic correlation to these changes is that only fast nerve conduction velocity will be reduced in the phases of documented clinical presenting CTS e.g. the more severe cases. Sensory fibers predominates in the median nerve, and therefore we find mostly sensory findings but we have no clues to why sensory fibers are more selectively injured following a compression of peripheral nerves [117]. Sensory nerve fiber dysfunction seems to start at larger fibers and gradually extend to smaller fibers [82]. The autonomic median nerve dysfunction not caused by vasoconstriction but increased sweating is often the first signs of CTS [88].

It is thus a combination of ischemic and mechanical factors that are involved in compression neuropathy. This suggests two mechanisms of the nerve entrapment, one with reversible dysfunction in nerve fibers due to simple lipid/myelin changes associated with some ischemia and one with more slowly developed structural changes in nerve fibers due to pressure.

In summary, the peripheral nerve reacts to pressure in a standard scenario. First stage is called neuropraxia being the physiologic, reversible functional disruption of a neuron. This first-degree injury is a reversible local nerve conduction block at the site of compression. In the second degree injury axonotmesis with loss of continuity of some axons is found with the endoneurium sheet being intact. These lesions tend also to recover but in a slower rate with axons sprouting from 0.7–2.7 mm per day. If fibrosis increases, further Wallerian degeneration develops and fixed nerved lesions is the result.

After denervation the muscle fibres undergoes fibrosis that will be maximal and permanent after 2 years [28, 117, 120].

Definition of carpal tunnel syndrome (CTS) for epidemiological purposes

The fact is that it is subjective symptoms that lead us neurosurgeons to validate patients. CTS is currently anticipated to be the most common peripheral nerve compression neuropathy affecting an estimated 1% (or more) of a given population so it seems important to develop a system that can be used for screening/diagnosing [4, 38, 39, 44, 72, 85, 93, 124, 128]. The golden standard for CTS diagnosis exists only if by consensus [38].

This consensus has not yet been achieved despite attempts [97].

How do we diagnose CTS in a scientific way?

Appropriate patient selection is extremely important for a successful outcome and inaccurate diagnosis of CTS is one of the most common causes of treatment failure of CTS [38, 39]. We know from history and experience, that a majority of patients claiming CTS-hand-symptoms will benefit from surgical decompressive treatment. As this treatment is linked with increasing the volume of the carpal tunnel we assume that the volume of the carpal tunnel plays a role. Anything that can decrease the size e.g. volume of the carpal tunnel or increase the contents of the carpal tunnel structures, may thus lead to increased pressure on and in the median nerve [4, 128]. Nervous structure size changes is not related to bodyweight as could be expected. The median nerve cross-sectional area was found to be equal in an obese and a thin groups (9.3 vs. 9.4 mm^2), as was the carpal canal pressure (16.2 vs. 15.5 mmHg), respectively [78].

We must as a consequence of this experience describe precisely how and when reduction of volume and increase of pressure in the carpal tunnel causes a functional reaction in the median nerve. Only then can we to make a firm objective diagnosis of CTS. Therefore we need to be able to screen know the population to be able to discuss prevalence or incidence of a specific disease e.g. CTS.

There are three types of anatomical problems in this context: The carpal tunnel is decreased in size due to:

1) External factors.
2) Intrinsic factors.
3) The carpal tunnel is smaller than "normal".

In all three situations, the possibility of developing symptoms from the median nerve is possible. To this anatomical information, we may add further scientific documentation of an actual median nerve injury at the wrist level using electrophysiology.

Incidence, prevalence and diagnostic epidemiology – important facts for diagnosing CTS

We use the terms specificity and sensitivity when we introduce a diagnostic procedure or disease [75, 79, 85]. These are linked with the terms incidence and prevalence used to compare groups of patients and are often mentioned in scientific papers. In many papers, quoted "incidence rates" are in reality prevalence rates. Thereby misunderstandings can easily occur because they relate to totally different populations.

Specificity and sensitivity of diagnostic procedures

"Description of a disease" is also called nosographic. Therefore a nosographic description of CTS differs from that being used when describing CTS by clinical evaluation. The nosographic specificity and sensitivity are irrelevant for clinical practice, but both terms are too often used in the literature called simply: "specificity/sensitivity". It is only valid to discuss the true value of a clinical test e.g. neurophysiology, if we know the clinical population we are dealing with.

Incidence

The number of new cases of a disease (CTS) that develop within a specified population over a specified period of time. The crude incidence is thus the mean number of cases found per year in e.g. Denmark per 100,000 inhabitants = the number of CTS-entrapment cases divided by number of person-years under risk, multiplied by 100,000. Incidence is therefore obviously dependent on the composition of what is usually a continuously changing population and that of the diagnostic parameters used.

Prevalence

Prevalence is in contrast the ratio (for a given time period) of the number of occurrences of a disease (CTS) to the number of people "at risk" for having the disease in the population. Therefore an entrapment syndrome like CTS must have a higher prevalence among patients with any type of e.g. polyneuropathy.

The prevalence should only be referred to in a well defined, and stable population – and this is usually not the case in our global world. In 1961–65 the prevalence of CTS in Rochester, USA was 88/100,000 and in 1976–80 it rose to 125/100,000 [114]. Either the frequency of the disease has increased in this part of the US or the diagnostics and general interest in the disease have increased or – perhaps (?) – the diagnostic criteria are not the same in the two time periods. An electrophysiological CTS prevalence study in the Netherlands showed that it was 5.8% among women and only 0.6% among males.

Scandinavian figures show almost equal representation with a marginal tendency of having more females harbour CTS than males [4, 68, 128]. Both statements cannot be true demonstrating this basic problem. The influence of diagnostic interest and general knowledge among Physicians may be found in the figures from Denmark. With a population of 5.3 million, we treated in year 2001: 7500, in 2002: 8860 and in 2003 10,700 patients with the diagnosis of CTS.

Diagnostic methods – and their validity

Diagnosing CTS is like asking, "What is a Duck?" My good friend and colleague James Steers often uses the following: We all know that a duck is a bird. If we add that it also has large feet, that it waddles, further that it can swim and finally that it quarks we are very close to have identified a duck and not a sparrow.

Carpal tunnel syndrome (CTS), or compression neuropathy of the median nerve at the wrist, is the one of the most common conditions encountered and is diagnosed with increasing frequency in the general population and among certain occupational groups [4, 85]. CTS is a frequent cause of morbidity in western societies and can have a profound impact on an individual's ability to perform their daily activities. There are a wide variety of predisposing factors and conditions that are associated with the development of CTS symptoms [68].

We may agree that clinical signs of median nerve neuritis e.g. paresthesia, sensory deficits, nightly painful paresthesia ("screening"), often leads to our proposed surgical interventions. Too often Medical Doctors assume that this symptomatology is synonymous with a true compression of the median nerve [104].

From a scientific point of view it is irrelevant to define CTS caused by compression from "clinical subjective symptomatology" alone, unless we know precisely the population structure – and then search for reasons hereafter. However this is generally the case when you review the literature.

The clinical picture alone is not sufficient to predict the diagnosis of CTS. A compressive lesion of the median nerve at the carpal tunnel can be present both among patients with no typical symptoms of CTS (asymptomatic individuals) and among symptomatic patients in which neurophysiologic studies are negative. In a general population a 0.7% prevalence of undiagnosed CTS is found. These patients have all symptom-severity similar to that of patients undergoing surgery. Therefore variable numbers of this group may be drawn into a "medical system" and thus account for variations in the rate of surgery performed [4, 37].

In this review I try to look at the history, anatomy, epidemiology, diagnosis and the key issues in the management of CTS.

CTS are usually diagnosed based on a combination of history taking that includes subjective signs combined with objective findings and objective measurable "imaging" of carpal tunnel and nerve [6, 30, 125]. The predominant classic symptoms are nocturnal painful paraesthesiae of the hand, and sensory disturbances within the distribution of the median nerve, both of which are characteristically relieved by hand movements (hand shaking). Ancillary tests are used to objectively document the problems at the carpal tunnel. These include imaging techniques and nerve conduction studies. Imaging tests (ultrasound/ sonography and MRI) are useful for demonstrating the structure of the carpal tunnel. In cases with persistent symptoms following surgical relief of the median nerve they may explain the reasons. These methods are still considered to have a lower diagnostic accuracy than neurophysiology, Neurophysiology with nerve conduction studies are specific less accurate in the early stages of CTS and among younger patients. Development of these imaging modalities and supplementary tests of small nerve fiber function and techniques of measurement the intra carpal pressure, may in the future improve early recognition of CTS [126].

Our present diagnostic methods includes a combination of the following:

1. History taking, e.g. symptomatology or "subjective" signs.
2. Clinical evaluation e.g. "objective" examination by a MD.
3. Diagnostic tests, by tradition but only partly objective and reliable.
4. Imaging of the median nerve and carpal tunnel.
5. Electrophysiology.

1. History taking – symptomatology

The following general medical conditions may often lead to a peripheral nerve symptomatology mimicking CTS. They can both be a part of the syndromes and by reducing the carpal tunnel volume lead to median nerve pressure.

A prominent example is thus rheumatoid arthritis, which reduces the carpal tunnel volume and simultaneously gives structural disturbances inside the median nerve. Obesity results in normal median nerve and carpal tunnel sizes, but endoneural oedema is found together with reduced SNCV [123]. Synovial engorgement is the result of fluid retention seen in pregnancy, and post menopause (PMS) with water retention and through increase of contents causes nerve symptoms simulating CTS. Renal failure and long-term haemodialysis, high blood pressure, and congestive heart failure may be associated with the build up of amyloid in the median nerve and increase in size.

Hormonal disorders such as acromegaly and hypothyroidism are commonly related to CTS for the same reasons.

CTS has been described together with persistent median artery, lipomatosis, gout, anomalous hand muscles, vascular tumors, collagen vascular diseases, inflammatory or septic tenosynovitis, lepra, tuberculosis, Fungal infection, Gout, De Quervain's disease, wrist fractures and dislocations including wrist bone luxations. Hemorrhages during anticoagulation therapy are another well-known cause of CTS [7, 58, 68, 93, 128].

Peripheral neuropathies (polyneuropathy) associated with Diabetes Mellitus, cancer and alcoholism are diseases that easily mimic CTS symptomatology. 5–25% of diabetic patients with polyneuropathy, may also have a "true" CTS = with a compression of the median nerve. Hereditary neuropathy with liability to pressure palsies (HNPP) is an autosomal-dominant peripheral neuropathy that results from deletion of a 1.5-Megabase pair (Mb) segment of the short arm (p) of chromosome 17. It should increase susceptibility of peripheral nerves to pressure and trauma and can be associated with symptoms at multiple anatomic entrapment sites. There is no evidence for an association between HNPP and patients who have multiple surgical releases for upper-extremity entrapment neuropathies [25, 105].

Significant vascular ischemia usually provoked by cold with subsequent Raynaud's phenomenon also causes paresthesia of the fingers [128].

More proximal upper extremity Median Nerve entrapment can also result in CTS symptoms. This has lead to a discussion on the possibility of a so-called double-crush syndrome. Cervical disc herniation, proximal median nerve entrapment and Dystonia are possibilities of entities with a Double-crush. According to this idea, nerve fibers that are injured proximal close to the spinal cord should become more sensitive to supplementary distal lesions [122]. The frequency and electrophysiological data of CTS analyzed according to cervical radiculopathy level do not support a neurophysiologic explanation of double crush syndrome so that it must be considered a highly hypothetical idea but not an actual existing entity [60]. If palsy of thumb flexion is found on clinical examination it is often caused by affection of the median nerve more proximal than the wrist. In this situation we will find sensory disturbances in the palm. Supplementary entrapments of other nerves exist and an ulnar nerve entrapment in conjunction with CTS is not uncommon.

We also know that patients often complain of nightly painful paresthesia. If this symptom is added to the previous, we are further tempted to conclude that the patient has CTS. Which weight we shall add to each symptom is difficult to assess. This has been tried by expert groups and in situations using Bayes theorem [38, 75, 84].

From a large case-control study using the UK General Practice Research Database [34] the relative contributions of the common risk factors for carpal tunnel syndrome (CTS) in the community were quantified. Cases were patients with a "diagnosis of CTS" and for each, four controls were individually matched by age, sex and general practice. The dataset included 3391 cases, of which 2444 (72%) were women, with a mean age at diagnosis of 46 (range 16–96) years. Multivariate analysis showed that the risk factors associated with CTS were previous wrist fracture (OR = 2.29), rheumatoid arthritis (OR = 2.23), osteoarthritis of the wrist and hand (OR = 1.89), obesity (OR = 2.06), diabetes (OR = 1.51), and the use of insulin (OR = 1.52), sulphonylureas (OR = 1.45), metformin (OR = 1.20) and thyroxine (OR = 1.36). Smoking, hormone replacement therapy, the combined oral contraceptive pill and oral corticosteroids were not associated with CTS. The results were similar when cases were restricted to those who had undergone carpal tunnel decompression [34].

With history taking we need to know more details as shown in the following:

1) Age and family history?

From literature studies it is concluded that CTS is most common in age group 30–60 years and with preponderance for the female gender [68, 128]. A family history is found among 20% of "proven" CTS patients especially if they have bilateral symptomatology [2]. Other authors have in contrast found an equal distribution among gender suggesting differences in screened populations. Interestingly it is shown that 14.4% of the Swedish population without any other signs of CTS complains of pain, numbness and/or tingling in the median nerve distribution [4, 5]. Increased occurrences of CTS near menopause and during last months of pregnancy emphasizes that secure information of the population screened is needed for a global discussion of gender preponderance. Male gender is not associated with poor outcome but many male patients are involved in heavy manual work activities, which is a poor prognostic indicator [5].

2) Is the history of symptoms short- or long lasting and work-related?

Did the symptoms start abrupt or were they as expected more continuous? Did we find a work history of force-presence, sustained or extreme vibration, awkward posture or repetition in work duties? A combination of personal and occupational risk factors is according to modern ideas the major determinant of CTS [12, 44, 100, 101]. Workers in cold environments e.g. butcher and poultry workers have higher frequencies of CTS than others [4, 101]. If the industrial work situation includes repetition, high force, awkward joint posture, direct pressure, vibration and prolonged constrained posture, including recently prolonged keyboard work, the risk for developing CTS is high. The diagnosis is best established using a combination of history and symptom distribution for screening for CTS in the industrial setting has questionable benefit [124]. Among blue-collar workers psychosocial factors seems more pronounced [5, 12]. By improving the consistency of the diagnosis of CTS these consensus criteria could lead to a more effective treatment and a better understanding of the effect of e.g. work place exposures in the development of this condition [38].

3) Does the history include subjective symptoms like numbness, tingling and/or burning sensations of the hand involving the distal median nerve distribution?

Sensory problems progressing gradually over months should be typical for CTS. They are affecting at least two of the first three digits and not involve dorsal- and palmar aspects of the hand should be typical for CTS [39, 58, 128]. Despite the fact that these first symptoms of a CTS may be pain in the wrist and hand and paraesthesia of the 3–4 radial fingers they can also involve the 5th finger. An explanation today is that extra-median spread of sensory symptoms is associated with higher levels of pain and paresthesia suggesting that central nervous system mechanisms of plasticity may underlie the spread of symptoms [133].

From a clinical history including 8223 patients with suspected CTS these were compared with the results with neurophysiologic findings [7]. Symptoms from the radial part of the hand and nocturnal exacerbation of symptoms showed the strongest individual correlations with positive nerve conduction studies. The regression model derived from the complete questionnaire achieved an overall sensitivity of 79% and specificity of 55% for the diagnosis of carpal tunnel syndrome. A simple regression model for evaluating the history compares favorably with the widely used clinical signs in its ability to predict the findings of nerve conduction studies. Similar fifty-seven clinical findings associated with CTS have been ranked previously in order of diagnostic importance using Delphi as a method of establishing consensus among a panel of expert clinicians. The 8 most highly ranked criteria were then placed into all possible combinations to create 256 unique case histories. Two new panels of experts rated these case histories. One panel made a binary evaluation as to whether the case history did or did not represent CTS. This allowed the development of a logistic regression model that had the probability of carpal tunnel syndrome as the dependent variable and the weighted diagnostic criteria as the independent variables. This model then was validated against the judgments of the second panel of clinicians who estimated the probability of CTS for each of the same case histories. The correlation between the probability of CTS predicted by the model and the panel of clinicians was 0.71. A methodology that emphasizes a rigorous approach to item generation and item reduction through expert consensus, followed by validation, may represent a template for establishing consensus among experts on controversial clinical issues [38].

4) What is the distribution and character of symptoms and are they worse with activity or at night?

Nocturnal painful paresthesia disrupting sleep being relieved by manipulation such as shaking of the hand should be linked with CTS [20, 118]. Patients with arthritis may also have the same symptoms but during daytime. The use of neurodynamic tests for CTS is perhaps able to differentiate the diagnosis from other wrist and hand pathologies [19].

5) Does the patient feel a weakness of the hand?

The patients note that they often drop items and sense that the hand is swollen. Hand clumsiness is thus a frequent symptom and many females may have stopped knitting or sewing, as symptoms increase with wrist/finger movements [128]. Decreased muscle power e.g. grip strength due to changed long flexor tendon pulley function is seldom described in neurosurgical literature but plays an important role in orthopedic literature [81, 128].

6) Is there a trauma?

If a history includes earlier fractures of the arm, wrist or hand, pain during daytime, other atypical symptoms (polyneuropathy), a Swedish study advocates a supplementary neurophysiologic examination [41].

7) Hand-diagrams – self-assessment

Median nerve neuropathy creates paresthesia (subjective information) that we as physicians try to convert into objective signs. Many attempts have been made to categorize symptoms [55, 62, 118]. Among these are the best known "Katz Self-administered Hand Symptom Diagram" [56]. Similar has been developed "Michigan Hand Outcomes- and Disabilities of the Arm, Shoulder and Hand" (DASH) questionnaire, Patient Evaluation Measure questionnaire (PEM) [46] and the Boston – Self Administered Score System (BO) being a disease-specific questionnaire [96].

"The Katz Hand-Diagram" [56] is a personal patient screening procedure that documents the distributions of (subjective) symptoms for the Physician rather than one used for diagnosing the disease [55]. A correlation between PEM and DASH shows that the combination of subjective information and objective measures are high in PEM and DASH [46]. In a prospective series of 323 hands undergoing surgery for CTS a Boston self-administered questionnaire was used 1 and 6 months after CTS surgery. By grading the clinical and electrophysiological severity, it was found to obtain a valid, precise, reliable, and straightforward comparison of results from different patient series and different operating techniques [96].

Szabo *et al.* [118] validated three groups of patients. One group with CTS based on history, clinical presentation and with improvement following CTS surgical release. Group two included a variety of upper extremity disorders. Group three were normal healthy volunteers. All were submitted for a self-administered Hand-Diagrams, including validation of nocturnal pain, symptom duration, Phalen, sign, Tinel sign, Durkan test and monofilament testing before and after a Phalen manoeuvre for 5 minutes. A uni-variate analysis of the first two groups showed that the most sensitive symptom predictor was the nocturnal pain. With a multivariate equation the probability to diagnose the CTS was 86% and that if all tests were normal there is only a 0.7% chance of having a CTS [118]. Patients under 40 years of age with normal or questionable Hand-Diagram ratings have thus a low risk of CTS [56].

A prospective study evaluated the DASH questionnaire by comparing it with the disease-specific Boston questionnaire (BQ). To measure responsiveness (sensitivity to clinical change), 57 patients with a clinical diagnosis of carpal tunnel syndrome completed the DASH and BQ preoperatively and again 3 months after open carpal tunnel decompression. A second group of 31 patients completed the questionnaires in the outpatient clinic and again 2 weeks later to assess test-retest reliability. The time to complete all questionnaires was recorded. Responsiveness of the DASH is comparable with the BQ with standardized response means of 0.66, 1.07 and 0.62 for the DASH, BQ-symptoms and BQ-function, respectively. Test-retest data show both questionnaires are reliable. Mean times to complete questionnaires were 6.8 minutes (DASH) and 5.6 minutes (BQ). The DASH questionnaire is thus a reliable, responsive and practical outcome instrument in carpal tunnel syndrome [40]. A combination of symptom diagrams, hypalgesia and thumb abduction strength testing were most helpful in diagnosis of CTS. All other signs (nocturnal paresthesia, Phalen and Tinel signs, thenar atrophy, 2-point-, vibratory- and monofilament sensory test) had little or no diagnostic value [20].

2. Clinical evaluation, "objective" signs

The clinical examination is linked with physicians evaluating the objective documentation of median nerve compression. Use of decreased sensibility findings will indeed increase the specificity of the disease CTS, but we will at the same time under diagnose CTS and exclude many patients with moderate CTS, who would benefit from treatment [79].

Clinical examination by an experienced medical doctor seems sufficient for screening purposes, if symptoms of CTS are found. Unfortunately many reports do not include methodology, which makes the results difficult to reproduce and thereby to apply to other populations [73]. It is in this context essential to standardize the clinical diagnostic criteria and develop a consensus for this testing [73, 92].

What are the most important objective signs?

1) Anatomical deformity of wrists and range of motion

Looking at the wrists, we may suggest that they are "square" meaning with an increased antero-posterior to medio-lateral wrist dimension, or long and thin. None of these mean anything significant for the diagnosis of CTS. Do we see a swelling or masses e.g. tumours, ganglia, arthritis at the wrist? How is the perfusion state of hand? Does the wrist present with visible erythema? When we touch the wrist is it warm, do we feel crepitus [132]? We are now as investigators close to be subjective. We need to define what tests we use for these and how to demonstrate them, otherwise they are only for personal use?

2) How is the sensibility?

Sensibility changes involves sensory loss/reduction to pin prick, light touch, Semmes-Weinstein monofilament evaluation [117] and reduced two-point discrimination [4] are all modalities of interest in this context. How do we compare them is our major problem.

Two statisticians (A and B) were at scientific meeting small talking. A's wife stands 20 meters away. B says to his friend: "What a beautiful wife you have". A responds: Compared to whom?

Bear in mind that distribution of sensory symptoms may vary in many aspects [111] and can have several degrees of seriousness including, intermittent subjective paresthesia in the median nerve territory, to severe lasting sensibility disturbances. The literature suggests that 2-point discrimination has low sensitivity for diagnosing CTS. If a decreased sensation in the median nerve distribution is the most helpful finding in making the diagnosis, it will mainly help to diagnose the more advanced CTS cases. Similar hypalgesia to pin prick is important in the more advanced cases [20]. Sensibility reduction at finger 1–3 is often biased, as the technique of investigation may not be the same from one Physician to the other [117]. It should be stressed that the position of the hand/wrist is essential during the examination. If the sensibility testing is carried out subsequent to a Phalen test with flexion of the wrist it tends to be more abnormal.

We need to customise our sensory sense tests and carry them out with the patients blinded [112]. Many patients with open eyes will try to please the examining Physician by saying: "Yes – I feel a difference" in the area of "paresthesia". The cortical representation of the sensory functions of hands is not symmetric, however a distinct difference between 3rd finger and 5th finger is demonstrable. There may also be differences between left and right (dominant) hand based on cerebral function. Many studies do not have sufficient detail or include methodology to allow repetition of the protocol by other researchers. The sensitivities and specificities reported for each can be compared with the quality criteria ratings they each received [73].

We can thus perhaps increase the specificity, but not the sensitivity of a CTS diagnosis by simple clinical sensibility examination.

3) Muscle function

Thenar atrophy

The abductor pollicis brevis muscle may be congenitally absent and can also be difficult to assess in thick hands. It is a sign only seen in connection with severe long-lasting cases of CTS.

Motor paresis

Thumb abduction strength test is maybe a useful indicator for ruling out CTS [20]. Weakness of abductor pollicis brevis muscle is tested by pressing the palms together and then tests the abductor strength of the thumbs. This is a very biased investigation.

Grip and Pinch strength measurements

Measurement of grip strength may be influenced by pain. Monitoring grip strength is not generally accepted by neurosurgeons as a diagnostic tool. It serves mostly as a method to follow the individual patients course. It is widely used by hand surgeons because they are much focused on the hand movements. For the postoperative evaluation it is essential to know that testing with the wrist in a flexed position decreases the strength further due to tendon bowing. A consensus on how to monitor muscle function is badly needed.

3. Objective diagnostic tests – by tradition – but only partly objective

If we look more detailed into the different objective signs we may receive further information for our personal diagnostic scenario:

Neuro-provocative tests

We also use provocative tests in our clinical work where we try to induce e.g. sensibility disturbances as an objective sign. Through Medline, Current Contents, and related readings a critical review were undertaken [73]. The use of clinical diagnostic tests for CTS was further compared with the results of neurophysiology. Criteria for systematically reviewing the studies were developed, tested for reliability, and applied to the studies. Many studies did not have sufficient detail to allow repetition of the protocol by other researchers. The sensitivities and specificities reported for each could be compared with the quality criteria ratings they each received. This literature review supports that the use of the wrist flexion (Phalen-test) and carpal compression test (Durkan-test) has a low sensitivity for diagnosing CTS [95].

The goal in recommending a clinical examination technique for the diagnosis of CTS is both high specificity and sensitivity. The carpal compression tests (Durkan- or Phalen test) is therefore not a markedly better way to achieve this goal. The more severe the nerve compression is, the less sensitive these provocative tests seem to be [77]. By validating the 5 clinical tests Tinel, Phalen, reverse Phalen, carpal compression and vibration sense none of these had a degree of specificity that they could serve as an indicator of a CTS.

The efficacy of provocative tests for diagnosing CTS was evaluated in a Dutch study. Each test and them all in combinations did not show the probability of patients harbouring CTS. The authors recommends as a consequence of this to use neurophysiologic examination to increase diagnostic specificity [21].

Phalen sign/test

Phalen himself stated: "Positive sign is pain and paresthesia in the median nerve distribution with prompt exacerbation of symptoms when the wrist is held in a flexed position and the production of tingling in the fingers by percussion over the Carpal tunnel" [45, 117]. Is this how all of you have been taught to interpretated this test? I guess is that the answer is: No!!. Phalen-test is positive in among 20% of normal people [4]. One of the reasons may also be that the test is not performed in a standard fashion by different clinicians. It is highly questionable whether a test that does not harbor a strong positive correlation among different investigators can be used for diagnosing a disease – also in our situation with CTS.

Tinel sign

Originally it is called Hoffman/Tinel sign as it was first described by Hoffman [117]. It is elicited by careful percussion on the nerve starting distally and moving the tapping centrally. Almost everyone can have a positive Tinel sign; it only depends on the degree of percussion. It can thus in the literature range from being positive in 8–100% and in control patients it is positive from 6 to 45%. So the same questions as with Phalen sign can be applied here.

Durkan test

Carpal compression test where the examiner applies direct pressure on the carpal tunnel leading to symptoms of pain and paresthesia. Durkan's compression test had a sensitivity of 89% in diagnosing CTS – but it is suggesting rather than diagnosing [118].

Closed fist test

Holding fist closed for 60 seconds reproducing median nerve paresthesia [128].

Positive signs from the contra lateral wrist

Is also considered to suggest CTS in this situation as some 20% have bilateral symptomatology [2].

Complementary findings

Myofascial findings

A common finding among these patients. Many CTS patients have been treated for cervical spondylosis for long periods of time. The pain is believed to be a referred pain from the median nerve and may resemble a C5 or C6 radiculopathy [122].

Psychological evaluation

These testing are used if a result of treatment is not turning out as expected and if the symptomatology and clinical findings are not clearly linked.

The psychological testing must include history of employment, interpersonal relationships, leisure activities current perception of the medical system, results of current treatment, perceive locus of control and childhood history including abuse and family history of disability [2].

Laboratory tests

Serum rheumatoid factor
TSH for hypothyroidism
Fasting glucose and/or loading test
Serum protein electrophoresis
SR
Serum calcium, phosphorus, uric acid, alkaline and acid phosphates
Liver and kidney function profiles

A combination of the above-mentioned self assessment tests (Hand-Diagrams), history taking and a thorough clinical examination and laboratory tests are best to exclude those patients without median nerve compression e.g. for screening.

For categorizing our diagnosed CTS patients, we must use imaging and/or neurophysiology.

4. Imaging of the median nerve and carpal tunnel

Mainly four methods are being used to evaluate the carpal tunnel size and contents using imaging such as: – Radiography/Computerized Tomography, MRI, Bone-scan and Sonography [6, 30, 94, 131].

Radiography and computerized tomography

An additional part of a general evaluation is radiographic imaging of joints. Axial x-ray with the hand in maximal dorsal flexion and with the beam parallel to 4th metacarpal bone and 30 degrees off a perpendicular line of the film have been used to demonstrate the size of the carpal tunnel and signs of previous fractures. Standard X-ray imaging is hardly used routinely anymore in Europe and has widely been replaced by CT scanning techniques [15, 132]. In the hand-surgeons outpatient clinic painful wrists diseases are common and it is therefore in these situations suggested to use a systematic approach including use of imaging modalities such as bone scans and CT imaging, when diagnosing painful wrists [132]. Standard CT scan will not reveal many of the soft tissue abnormalities. Helical CT is in this situation more sensitive and can give us information of minor bony trauma and 3-D models of the carpal tunnel.

These methods have no value for a general "diagnostic" screening for CTS among a normal population. However they are still important in the Hand Surgeons Outpatient clinic.

Magnetic resonance imaging (MRI)

With MRI we can measure the volume of the Carpal Tunnel and visualize intrinsic structures related to it. Pierre-Jerome *et al.* [94] tested two groups of patients with rheumatoid arthritis (thirty one) and carpal tunnel syndrome (sixty two), and a group of asymptomatic controls (fifty four). All underwent bilateral MR axial wrist imaging from the metacarpal bases to the distal radio carpal joint. The imaging techniques included spin echo (SE), turbo spin echo (TSE) and fast field echo (FFE) sequences, using 3 mm-slice thicknesses. Different anatomical variants including hypoplasia of the Hamulus or hook of the Hamate bone (4 cases), anomalous muscles (lumbricals) inside the carpal tunnel (2 cases), unusual location (5 cases) and double branching of the median nerve (14 cases), and aberrant median artery (one case) were detected. These variants, if unfamiliar to MR readers and neurosurgeons, may be misinterpreted as pathological features [94].

Quantitative MRI is a valuable method for assessing the anatomic characteristics of the carpal tunnel [94]. Carpal tunnel areas are largest in neutral and smallest at the distal end with wrist flexion. An extended wrist resulted in the smallest carpal tunnel and content volumes as well as the smallest carpal tunnel content volume to carpal tunnel volume ratios. While men had significantly larger areas and volumes than women for both the carpal tunnel and it contents, there were no differences in ratios between the contents and tunnel size [10].

Earlier papers have concluded that nerve compression in CTS is proximal located in the carpal tunnel. This is in contrast with our present knowledge, where we show that it is in the distal part of the tunnel that the compression takes place. Twenty-seven female patients with CTS and 28 asymptomatic female controls were examined with MRI of the wrists [94]. On the MRI axial images, the volume of carpal tunnels, the wrists and the thenar muscles were calculated bilaterally in all subjects. The values for the signal intensity of the median nerve from all wrists were also quantified. The carpal tunnel volume (CTV) and the wrist volume (MV)/CTV ratio were almost identical in both groups ($p = 0.36$ and $p = 0.45$, respectively). The focal narrowest point of the tunnel was located at its distal third, about 8 mm from the tunnel distal outlet. The median nerve in the patients were hyper-intense compared with the controls, $p = 0.037$. In another study bilateral MRI axial wrist images were obtained by means of turbo spin echo (TSE) and fast field echo (FFE) sequences. The mean (SD) length of the carpal tunnel, from inlet to outlet was 36.3 mm (SD = 3.4) [94]. The tunnel has a cone shape, with the proximal inlet constantly larger than the outlet distal in all subjects. The mean (SD) cross-sectional area of the tunnel inlet was found to be larger among women >45 years of age, compared to women <45 years of age ($p = 0.029$). The calculated mean (SD) volume of the tunnel also appeared significantly larger in the older group ($p = 0.023$) [10, 94].

MRI findings in 23 cases of CTS demonstrated perfect correspondence with MRI findings and operative views. Misalignment of the tendons was found in 20 cases and fibrous tissue deposits in 20 of a smaller series [13, 94].

What type of MRI images should be used? This is the decision for our Radiologists. The neurosurgeon must nevertheless be familiar with the different options. Inflammation of the Synovial sheets can be seen as low signal intensity on T1-weighted images and increased signal intensity on T2-weighted.

T1-weighted imaging with planes parallel and transverse along the nerve using phased-array coils defines the bony structures and the detailed anatomy of tendons and nerves (Fig. 6). Gadolinium enhanced T1 weighted imaging is used if we suspect nerve tumors. T2-weighted imaging defines pathology such as edema and ischemia of the median nerve [30].

The MR Neurography (MRN) is performed with high-resolution fast spin echo (FSE) and T2 imaging technique and often with suppression of the normal high signal intensity of fat (FLAIR chemical shift selection or inversion recovery). Flow sensitive sequences or dynamic contrast-enhanced MRI can detect circulatory disturbances within the median nerve where marked enhancement of the nerve is found with hypervascular edema and lack of enhancement if nerve ischemia. In later phases of CTS the internal nerve fibrosis will be shown as decreased intensity on both T1 and T2 images. Wrist flexion/extension can alter these patterns due to mechanical obstruction of blood flow. MRI imaging makes it a potential useful diagnostic tool for initial evolution and management but also for postoperative evaluation of patients with CTS [30]. If the patient is still symptomatic, we may see residual increase T2 signals of the median nerve and lack of complete section of the TCL.

MRI shows important changes in synovial tissue, excessive fat and lesions in the abductor pollicis muscle. In muscles that by electromyography have undergone severe denervation changes similar severe changes in the thenar muscles can be found using short tau inversion recovery sequences of MRI [13]. When dealing with apparent significant nerve dysfunction, the T2 weighted imaging of muscle fibers can be of interest, as they will remain normal if the lesion is neuropractic and show atrophy if we are dealing with axonotmesis.

Comparison with the other hand is not valid as bilateral CTS are common.

MRI documented disturbances and movements of tendons and median nerve can be found among patients with CTS. Patients with CTS will show proximal swelling, distal flattening and increased signal intensity of the median nerve combined with palmar bulging of the TCL at the level of the hook of the Hamate and Pisiform bone.

A Scandinavian study discussed the problems of validity and consistency of evaluations of MRI's in CTS. The conclusion was that better validated diagnostic criteria must be used in the future [91]. Modern techniques make it possible to specify location of nerve entrapments and muscle disturbances and it is only a question of time before MRI will be introduced in our diagnostic scenario.

Magnetic Resonance Imaging (MRI) is today less accurate than standard electro diagnostic testing as a diagnostic specificity test and is so far not directly recommended for diagnosing CTS in 2007 [13, 30, 57].

Nuclide bone scans

This includes injection of radionuclide that is absorbed by inflamed tissue e.g. connective/cartilage. It is sometimes used in the more complicated cases, but plays no role for the primary simple diagnosis or screening.

Sonography

The technique is simple, low-cost, non-invasive and easy to use (walker) with update equipment that include a high frequency transducer with a frequency of 7–13 MHz [6]. It may be an excellent adjunct in the diagnostic scenario. It can show exactly where the median nerve is placed which can be of interest for surgeons using endoscope methods for cutting the transverse carpal ligament. Transverse normal elliptical median nerve is visualized becoming more and more flat when moving distally. Sonography and MRI images were compared and it is concluded that sonography is acceptable for screening the carpal tunnel contents especially the shape of the median nerve was found to be equal demonstrable with sonography and MRI [15]. High-resolution ultrasound shows enlargement of the median nerve at the distal wrist crease in symptomatic patients and is a reliable modality for imaging the wrist in patients with CTS.

Nerve flattening in the distal tunnel, nerve swelling at the level of the distal radius and palmar bowing of TCL with a nerve cross sectional area greater than 9 mm^2 proximal is the best criterion for the diagnosis of CTS.

Median nerve cross-sectional areas were found to be larger in arthritic patients with CTS than in RA patients and healthy persons without CTS. This supports previous studies of idiopathic CTS in which increased cross-sectional areas have been found. Thus, as with idiopathic CTS, arthritic patients may be examined by US of the median nerve when CTS is suspected. Still today, sonography is mainly used for detecting space-occupying lesions in the tunnel [6].

Wrist arthroscopy

When the surgeon cannot identify where the wrist pain comes from it is possible to visualize inflammation and cartilage damages, to remove debris, ganglion cysts etc through minor endoscopes. This is a specialist investigation for Hand surgeons, not neurosurgeons.

5. Electrophysiology – neurophysiology

Neurophysiology serves both as a diagnostic categorizing factor and allows a possible prognostic validation for the neurosurgeon. It is a method that solely expresses the functional state of the median nerve alone within CT.

An electro physiologic or neurophysiologic examination consists of

1) Electromyography (EMG) testing muscle cell and end-plate zone function,
2) Electroneurography (ENG) testing nerve conduction and
3) Distal Motor Latency (DML)

For details the reader should consult textbooks on neurophysiology [61, 64].

1) Electromyography (EMG)

Describes the functional state of muscle cells. This is obtained by insertion of fine electrodes into the appropriate muscles. This may reveal a normal muscle cell function or show “Denervation potentials”. These small size denervation potentials are normally clear signs of previous or ongoing neurogenic lesions with axonal loss = Wallerian degeneration.

Following relief of nerve compression, a typical reinnervation pattern is found often earlier than that by clinical examination [64].

Muscle fatigue can mimic a CTS. Compound Muscle Action Potentials (CMAP) can occasionally be used when screening between occupational and primary care cases of CTS [5].

2) Electroneurography (ENG)

This is the most important for the CTS diagnosis. It consists of electric stimulation of the median nerve at one site and recording the traveling potential at another place along the nerve across the potential lesion site. Sex, diurnal variations and handedness have no significant influence on conduction velocities [61, 64]. For clinical work, males present with milder symptoms but often more severe electrophysiological changes than females.

This nerve stimulation may be carried out with needles or as today surface electrodes [61] (Fig. 8).

Knowing the distance between the electrodes, the spreading speed of potentials = conduction velocity, can be estimated and measured in m/s [61, 64]. We can monitor both motor nerve conduction velocity (MNCV) and sensory nerve conduction velocity (SNCV). Sensory neurography responses have much smaller amplitudes measured in microvolt compared with the larger motor responses measured in millivolt (mV).

Slowing of median nerve conduction is due to demyelization of neurons. With this focal nerve lesion demyelinization a temporal dispersion of the stimulus response is found. It includes a fall in signal amplitude, an increase in its latency or a drop in conduction velocity. Axonal loss is very likely to be present if the recorded signals have reduced amplitudes. Amplitudes of both sensory and motor responses also tell us something about the number and synchrony of the fibers being tested. Most important for the diagnosis of CTS is measurement of the sensory nerve conduction velocity (SNCV). Our problems here are that in many instances we cannot detect the sensory potentials. Electronic noise may be a problem when recording the small amplitude sensory nerve action potentials (SNAP's). It is heavily influenced by electrode placements, especially if they are too close to each other.

Therefore practicing neurologists/neurosurgeons often rely on DML monitoring. We know that in 25% of cases with abnormal sensory nerve conduction

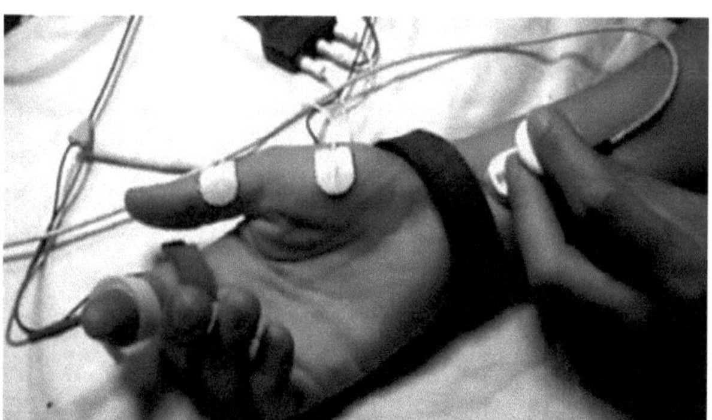

Fig. 8. Surface electrode set up for electrophysiological investigation of CTS

studies the motor studies are normal [61, 64]. It has been suggested that the following should be used as criteria for CTS syndrome: SNAP < 45 ms, however if conduction distance is >8 cm and SNCV is normal turn to new measurement over a shorter distance or compare with radial nerve SNCV or ulnar nerve SNCV [52]. Further the neurophysiology defines the median nerve involvement (A-fibres) more precisely and we can compare our neurophysiology-investigated patients in controlled prospective studies. Hand/arm temperature plays an important role as a change in temperature of 1 degree Celsius may lead to a change in sensory nerve conduction velocity of 1.2–2.4 m/s per degree Celsius [64]. Age also influences the nerve conduction velocity, which decreases after 60 years of age with 0.5–1.8 m/s per decade. Discussions on thresholds for abnormalities are different, but important for consensus [82].

Norwegian scientists uses photoplethysmography and laser Doppler fluxmetry in order to monitor autonomic nerve function [88]. They have showed that the micro vascular perfusion in fingertip skin and skin temperature are significantly reduced among patients with CTS in contrast to normal subjects.

Polyneuropathy is diagnosed by abnormalities in multiple nerves (ulnar nerve) and the presence of late F reflexes. F-waves monitoring occurs when a motor nerve is stimulated and impulses travel from the stimulation point to the neuron and back to the muscle. F-wave measurements reflect conduction along the entire nerve and are of general interest for diagnosing polyneuropathy and proximal lesions [61].

3) Distal motor latency (DML)

Distal motor latency (DML) estimates the traveling time of a stimulus potential from the site of stimulus to an electrode in/on a muscle. Therefore it includes measurement of the delay of impulses in the end-plate zones. Changes in DML can be found already as soon as one hour following operative decompression of a median nerve and it seems therefore to be a sensitive parameter.

In CTS cases DML is measured to the abductor brevis muscle. If DML preoperatively is >6 ms, the surgical results are good and fast. A mild improvement can be expected if DML is between 4–6 ms whereas nothing happens if it is <4 ms [102]. DML values in CTS cases have often been given with upper limits of 4.5 ms/8 cm, but the influence of distance between electrodes gives rise to a problems and interested readers should consult [64, 102] for further information.

Motor fibers are affected in CTS even when conventional electro diagnostic tests show normal motor conduction. Altered recruitment of motor axons could mainly be due to impairment of energy-dependent processes that affect temporal dispersion of the compound volley or axonal conduction block. In mild CTS, motor fibers are more often affected than was originally thought of.

If submaximal stimulus intensities are used, the sensitivity of wrist-to-APB motor conduction studies may be increased and used to document a beginning CTS.

Benefits and critical observations obtained from the use of neurophysiology

Clinical neurophysiologic investigations play a role in describing, defining and document whether a nerve irritation exists or not! – the latter perhaps being the most important. If a patient claims persisting symptoms following CTS decompression, the neurosurgeon can only deal with the question of potential insufficient operation if a preoperative electrophysiological evaluation is present.

Neurophysiology may – depending on who is referring physician – primarily be used for differential diagnostic purposes. When General Practitioners are referring patients it is mainly for diagnostic purposes, while neurological specialists are more interested in whether they may deal with polyneuropathy.

Additionally the correct (consensus) tests should be used [52, 62]. It is suggested that over 1/3 of Medicare patients treated for CTS in Washington State, US had an inappropriate electro diagnostic workup before surgery [115].

Single electrodiagnostic findings are therefore not recommended for routine use [97, 98].

Supporters of routine preoperative neurophysiologic investigations forget their shortcomings: lack of standardization, absence of population-based reference intervals, and lack of sensitivity and specificity. Only controlled trials, in which patients are randomized to receive treatment either with or without nerve conduction studies, will determine whether this investigation improve the outcome in patients with a firm clinical diagnosis of carpal tunnel syndrome. The influence of demographics is huge. The value of electro diagnosis has been challenged by Lee Dellon who stated: "There is no reason to deny surgery to a patient with a normal preoperative electrical study or to require all patients to have such a study, if the history and physical examination of the patient are themselves consistent with . . . . 'The dispute between WF Brown – a devoted neurophysiologist- and Lee Dellon, can be consulted in the discussion about the "WOG" syndrome (Word of God Syndrome) [14]. Therefore, if the neurosurgeon asks the neurophysiologist: "Do we have neurophysiologic indication for "surgery"? – They can only answer: "Yes and No".

In a patient group of normal youngsters we may not need neurophysiology to document a clinical CTS while it must be demanded if we are dealing with an outpatient clinic of hand surgery. 504 people from a "general population" were tested and it was found that 50 (10%) of these were awakening by nocturnal paresthesia in 93 hands (bilateral symptoms) [21]. Only 44 (47%) of these hands had neurophysiologic signs of CTS. So with these false negative results we have again to accept that we have no precise definition of what the "general population" was.

Why use electroneurography at all the reader may ask faced with series of papers on the great value of Hand-Diagrams etc? The answer is clear; we need to document objectively what the causes of CTS symptoms are.

Our electrophysiological results can only be used in conjunction with the clinical situation [17]. The highly myelinized fibre lesions are rather easy to document. Neurophysiologic changes are definitely not significant nor specific in the milder cases of CTS unless special techniques are used [110, 115].

One of the key features of using neurophysiology is to make it possible to monitor median nerve function. Problems are also that all electrophysiological values obtained are based on local laboratories, local equipment and may occasionally include/exclude monitoring of hand temperature [64].

With this in mind, it must be accepted that a testing of the same person will show a 5% deviation by interpreter bias alone. For a given nerve conduction test value, post-test probability of CTS can be determined from the estimated pretest probability (derived from clinical data), interval likelihood ratios, and Bayes theorem [75].

Neurophysiology is possibly not needed if the chances of harbouring CTS are high. This in contrast to the situation where it is doubtful or low. Electrophysiological test data should be interpreted in a Bayesian context using the output of the diagnostic instrument as an estimate of pretext probability. The ability to report the electro diagnostic test results as a post-test probability may improve their precision beyond the current standard of establishing the CTS diagnosis based on comparison with a threshold for nerve conduction velocity [38]. Nerve conduction (NC) tests, using rigid cut-offs separating normal from abnormal test values, are commonly used to confirm CTS.

The authors [84] studied patients with clinically defined mild CTS and a normal median DML to determine: 1) How much sensory mixed NC test results increase (or decrease) the probability of CTS and 2) The NC test values required to confirm (or exclude) CTS for the range of pretest probabilities of CTS. Palmar, digit 4 (D4), and digit 2 (D2) median NC tests were reviewed in 125 hands with mild carpal tunnel syndrome (CTS) and 100 control hands with musculoskeletal pain. Receiver operating characteristic curves and interval likelihood ratios were plotted for the three tests. Using Bayes theorem, post-test probability of CTS was then determined for the range of pretest probabilities and NC test values. Receiver operating characteristic curves showed that for a set specificity of 97%, palmar and D4 studies had higher electrodiagnostic utility than D2 studies with cut-off test values (sensitivities of 0.3 ms, 64.0%; 0.4 ms, 71.2%; and 50 m/s, 44.8%). However, Bayesian analysis showed that to confirm CTS more conservative cut-off values (palmar 0.5 ms, D4 0.7 ms,

D2 44 m/s) were required for pretest probabilities 50%, whereas borderline abnormal values (palmar 0.4 ms, D4 0.5 ms, D2 48 m/s) sufficed when pretest probabilities were 75%. Conversely, normal test values could exclude CTS only for pretest probabilities <25%. For a given NC test value, post-test probability of CTS can be determined from the estimated pretest probability (derived from clinical data), interval likelihood ratios, and Bayes theorem. Use of rigid cut-off values to confirm CTS is problematic, because more conservative cut-offs are required for low pretest probability. Conversely, NC tests with sensitivity <95% cannot exclude CTS when pretest probability is high [84].

In a British study a scored questionnaire was used and an electrophysiological assessment given by two independent observers assessing a group of patients. The patients with CTS on either one or on both type evaluations were operated upon and the result e.g. symptom relief used as a standard for having treated a "true CTS". The predictive positive value of the questionnaire was 90% and for nerve conduction 92% [55].

Hand-diagram from questionable patients may witch an added positive nerve conduction velocity study, make the diagnosis more likely. Combined with a negative nerve conduction velocity-study there can remain a high percentage of possible minor CTS syndromes as we do not monitor the thin c-fibres [50].

How MRI data are correlated with pressure increase and neurophysiology is not yet completely solved, except for the fact that the more electro diagnostic abnormalities is found in CTS cases, the more severe disease can be expected in the nerve using MRI [30, 94].

Many attempts have been made for classification of types of CTS and include neurophysiologic findings, usually without lasting effect on our global discussion:

A *mild CTS* is often said to include a prolonged median sensory or mixed action potential distal latency. This may be so – but is not to me an absolute indication for surgery. However these are often operated upon because the results will be "good".

A *moderate CTS includes* usually abnormal median sensory latencies and prolongation of median motor distal latency both in both absolute- and relative values, comparing these with the asymptomatic "normal" hand. With clear-cut symptoms this supports the surgical indication because we have documented a nerve lesion.

Severe CTS shows both prolonged median motor and sensory distal latencies with absent sensory or palmar potentials and or low amplitude or absent thenar motor action.

Similar to this, CTS patients were described and combined with neurophysiologic values [59]. It was suggested that four degrees or stadiums of "CTS-disease" exists.

Summarized they are as follows:

Stadium 1

From a pathophysiological point of view, intermittent ischemia of sensory neurons is the basic feature of this initial stage of the disease.

Clinically these patients experience acroparesthesia, nightly painful paresthesia and pain provoked by handwork. By clinical examination and neurophysiologic investigations, we find no abnormalities. These are the so-called symptomatic but neurophysiologic negative cases!

Stadium 2

Clinical it is found that these patients' presents with added minor hypoesthesia. If the decreased capillary flow continues for longer periods of time more permanent changes of the endothelium will develop with secondary protein leakage from the capillaries, resulting in oedema within the nerve fascicles. The intra fascicular pressure will therefore increase, leading to a further internal compression to the nerve structures and a circulus vicious has developed. Chronic ischemia of sensory highly myelinized axons is the bases. This will result in a focal reduction of sensory nerve conduction velocity (SNCV) due to paranodal demyelization.

Direct mechanical distortion is the major factor underlying these more severe long lasting forms also seen following tourniquet paralyses.

In these early stadiums (1 & 2) of entrapment it is thus probably mainly a biochemical lesion caused by a shock like injury that leads to anatomical changes. Recent evidence suggests that ischemia may be primarily responsible for the milder type of reversible entrapment nerve lesions.

These findings suggest a stadium 3 leading into a stadium 4 with more significant structural disturbances inside the median nerve mainly involving the highly myelinized fibres.

Stadium 3

Clinical examinations reveal sensory disturbances and beginning of muscle atrophy and palsy of abductor pollicis brevis muscle and in the thenar muscle denervation potentials in the abductor pollicis brevis muscle is present. The developed axonal degeneration resulting in both decreased amplitude of sensory nerve potentials and a reduced SNCV. The painful paraesthesias are less pronounced in this stadium.

Stadium 4

Clinical examination reveals a persistent hypoesthesia/anesthesia in the distal median nerve distribution. Consistent with this less clinical pain and lack of the nightly painful paresthesia is found. The loss of many axons and subsequent a significant reduced SNCV may end in a stadium with no functioning fibers at all.

Accepting these suggestions makes it even more confusing and difficult to make comparisons.

Conclusion

The neurophysiological investigation is a concrete attempt to monitor electric function in peripheral nerves. Use of electro diagnosis remains an important part of the objectification and evolution of peripheral nerve injuries [52]. It is not valid for screening patients with clinical symptoms of CTS unless very special information is needed.

We have to very carefully describe our findings and use them based on a universal consensus. Only in that case can we compare different patient groups. If we compare operations among patients with specific documented neurophysiologic disturbances with groups of patients with clinical "typical" symptomatology, it is not two populations defined the same way and it is like comparing apples and pears and no firm conclusions on treatment efficacy can be drawn.

Among patients presenting with hand paresthesia – the most common symptom – they must therefore for scientific purposes be divided in two groups of patients:

1) A neurophysiologic positive-group and
2) A neurophysiologic negative-group.

So when is neurophysiology needed? First and foremost neurophysiology is used for differential diagnostic purposes e.g. to document or exclude polyneuropathy. Secondly it serves for the clinician to be able to grade the degree of nerve affection both pre- and postoperatively.

Combination of electro diagnostic study findings and symptom characteristics provides us the most accurate information for classification of CTS syndromes as it may document the median nerve involvement [97] and thereby compare valid groups of CTS patients in the future.

Treatment of CTS

"*We may discus glioma treatment and aneurysm surgery but whenever you try to discuss the carpal tunnel, however, people get up and start hitting each other over the head with chairs. As always, this kind of emotionalism denotes a lack of data. If there is clear-cut data, there is no need to get emotional*".

Allan Hudson
Toronto Canada

1. Non-operative or conservative treatment

What is "conservative treatment of CTS"?

This is usually not clearly outlined in the literature, nor is the effects proven. From a Dutch Cochrane study it is evident that very little is known about the efficacy of most conservative treatment options and that high quality trials are needed to show their benefits [36]. By adding a conservative treatment such as splinting or rest or "wait and see" to a treatment protocol, the fluctuating symptomatology of CTS may "cure" the patient spontaneously through time. Another problem is that roughly 50% of CTS may be occupational and related to forceful grasping of pinching tools, awkward position of wrist, and vibrating hand-held tools [35, 72, 100, 101, 124].

The most important conservative treatment is therefore perhaps simply to avoid situations that provoke symptoms – prevention. Prevention is important if symptoms evidently are provoked by use of vibrating tools, or other working conditions that should of course be changed first. If a patient stops using e.g. vibrating tools = prevention, and simultaneously add another "conservative treatment modality" e.g. yoga or splinting at the same time, it is difficult to tell which these that is the essential. Among patients treated conservatively only 40% remained free of symptoms after 12 months [33]. Similar among milder cases – but all with an abnormal SNCV – only 35% were symptom free after 6 months.

In a resent Cochrane review [33] it was shown that patients did not obtain effect on their disease course from steroids, splinting, ultrasound, yoga or carpal bone mobilization [86].

Which are the conservative treatment options?

Job site alterations

Occupation with forceful grasping of pinching tools, awkward position of wrist, vibrating hand-held tools relates in approximately 50% of CTS. If vibrating tools is the cause, it is easy to reduce the use of them. If bicycling (Mountain Bike) with compression on the wrist is the cause, change posture so that the wrists are not loaded on the handlebar.

Ergonomics

Many CTS patients claim they have shoulder and arm pain too developed while they perform repetitive work tasks. Therefore it has often been advised that frequent break periods should be benefited but it has never been documented. Among normal people changing the sequence of active muscle fibres carries out these repetitive movements. Some patients cannot change their sequences as normal persons do and this leads to muscle-fatigue and pain. They are the so-called "Repeaters" and they tend to use the same muscle pattern for the repetitive movements, whereas normal persons the "Replacers" change pattern. Much of the pain these patients develops based on repetitive movements is thus caused by changes in the muscles and not within the median nerve.

The frequency of carpal tunnel syndrome among computer users at a medical facility was 10.5% if they had the clinical diagnosis of CTS, which is almost the same as in a normal population [114]. When discussing CTS this fact may also influence our figures, as those patients that come to evaluation could easily be overrepresented by "Repeaters".

Nerve gliding promotion exercises

Athletes and swimmers seem to have a lower risk for developing CTS. Therefore it has been suggested that exercises may be benefited in preventing symptoms of CTS. These exercises include isometric- and stretching for both hands, and exercises for neck and rest of the upper extremity. They involve wrist circles, finger exercises are thus advocated but randomized trials are lacking and we have no scientific proof of its value.

Manual therapy

Can be used providing there is no contraindication. No controlled series exists.

Orthotics

Immobilization with splinting may have a short-term effect in milder cases of CTS [33, 86]. Splinting including nighttimes splints seems of some initial benefit. However this could also be a documentation of the known fluctuation of symptomatology among patients with CTS.

Yoga techniques

A group of patients treated with yoga were compared with a control group treated with simple splinting. The yoga group improved grip strength, reduced the wrist pain and normalized the Phalen sign whereas nothing happened in the control group. However the set up was not scientifically acceptable and there is still no scientific proof that yoga helps [60].

Medications

Vitamin B6 has often been advocated but no documented benefit is found. NSAID medication is also without scientific proven effect. In a CTS book you can find advises on how cream/jelly may help, just documenting how unscientific much of the actual advises on the Internet are.

Ultrasound

In a prospective trial ultrasound were CTS patients were compared with “sham” patients showed a possible short-term significant benefit. However we need more investigation before we can use ultrasound routinely. The effect postulated can easily be pure placebo function.

Acupuncture

Acupuncture with and without electrical stimulation has been suggested for treating CTS. How acupuncture functions is still not clearly understood. It influences central “pain” perception and this is therefore possibly the reason for some success for this treatment. We need controlled studies in the future for documentation.

Biofeedback

No scientific documentation of its value.

Micro-current TNS

Similar there exists no scientific proof of benefit.

Botulinum A (Botox®, Dysport®) injections

Resent information seems to indicate a direct effect on the muscle function, but a controlled study is needed before it can be recommended. If muscles are tense and painful it may be a choice. However we need again controlled studies to prove this point.

Corticosteroid injections

Local steroid injections are said to be effective and affordable as early treatment of CTS. Best results are obtained among mild cases whereas hands with severe symptoms will not respond sufficiently [33, 38]. With a follow up of 6–26 months, 22% were symptom free at the end after steroid injections and splinting for three weeks at best. Local injection of corticosteroids is better than oral intake and gives a 1–3 month benefit [71]. The major complication is direct injection of corticosteroids into the median nerve leading to severe axonal and myelin degeneration. Avoiding repetitive movements in combination with steroid injections helps less than 50% and relapse rate is 60% e.g. an overall efficacy <20% – but which one is the key to this effect?

Local anaesthetics injections

The most severe complication is direct injection on the nerve, which can lead to nerve necrosis.

2. Surgical – operative treatment

In the US with 285 million inhabitants a total of 400,000 CTS hands are operated upon each year equivalent to figures from Scandinavia [4, 5, 24, 38, 80, 107, 114]. These high figures make it therefore relevant to discuss the surgical techniques, as complications are possible with all types of surgery.

The aim of surgery consist – in our cases of documented median nerve compression – of the following:

"There is only one step in surgery for carpal tunnel syndrome – cut the transverse carpal ligament completely – and do not injure the nerve in any way" [48].

During a trip to Europe Allan Hudson observed that many of the surgical details he thought of as being mandatory was not that in Europe – so he concluded that we are all biased by traditions [48].

This TCL cutting can be obtained by three different methods e.g.

1) Open surgery with and without the use of magnification (OCTR), or by
2) Using an endoscope to cut the TCL (ECTR) or by
3) Performing TCL section blindly/openly.

The major surgical problem is not whether the surgeons use an endoscope or not. Most important to all kinds of surgery is the question: "Will the procedure relieve symptoms and are the complication rate low and insignificant"?

The major difference between an OCTR and ECTR procedure is that with microsurgical techniques we cut the TCL from outside the carpal tunnel viewing all structures in a normal 3-Dimentional (3-D) fashion. This is in contrast to the endoscope method where we cut the TCL from inside the carpal tunnel viewing it in a new 3-D fashion that first must be learned through regular practice.

Fundamentally all surgical methods lead to the same result, but the complications of the methods are different apparently being more severe among the endoscope- or blind methods. The complication rate and severity is essential when evaluating any surgical technique [1, 3, 7, 8, 16, 23, 109, 116, 121, 122]. When carrying out surgery we need some kind of anaesthesia and complications to this must be added to the surgical technique.

In surgery, the surgical-methods and the education of the surgeons are closely linked to each other. If the surgeons have been working with the microscope he/she may suggest the use of microsurgical techniques because he is used to it. If he/she works with endoscopes e.g. for knee surgery, a tendency to test how endoscope techniques apply to CTS is equally natural. Many OCTR series have proven the benefit of with a success rate of close to 95–99%. The general problems of the ECTR techniques are that we do not always visualize the nerve perfectly in the tunnel during surgery, and that we only partly view the TCL. No endoscope surgeon can therefore be 100% confident to cut the ligament completely with these techniques [122].

My biggest concern – being educated in a Scandinavian country – is that if the surgeon is working in a private scenario he/she may be tempted to operate more than if he/she is in a community hospital.

So before we look into the different surgical techniques, we shall focus on the neurosurgeon and his/her level of education.

Surgical training for handling CTS surgery

Although we all may believe that we (personally) do know what a good neurosurgeon is, it cannot be commented further than to: "A healthy, intelligent, tenacious, dynamic, psychologically intact and sincere candidate with manual dexterity, resistant to psychological and psychiatric stress" (Gilsbach, personal note).

Learning curves and the importance of learning surgical techniques

Anatomical knowledge of the region is naturally mandatory for the success of surgical procedures. Primarily the senior experts must therefore first dwell on anatomy and neurophysiology techniques so called declarative knowledge. That mistakes in interpretation of anatomy do occur is clear even from well-established journals (J Hand Surgery (Br)) demonstrating, for example, e.g. a drawing of the TCL erroneously being placed proximal to the hand wrist creases [27].

Secondly the seniors must also teach our residents to obtain the skills of surgery [65]. This includes in most curricula that we seniors supervise this "simple CTS operation" being carried out by our trainees. The trainee fills out a logbook and documents in this way that he/she has performed e.g. 5 or 10 CTS cases.

The serious complications must be regarded as the result of: "Careless or inexperienced surgery and the established principle of surgery under direct vision has provided reliable protection against disaster". In a non-published series from the Department of Neurosurgery, Aalborg University Hospital from 1997 we tried to document our departmental complication rate. We found to our surprise several complications in all operated by junior staff. Among 85 openly operated CTS hands we had 11 complications =13%, with the majority of complications being incomplete sectioning of the distal part of the TCL.

Proper formal training in both open and endoscope techniques must be obtained [27, 43, 65]. Steep learning curves within both microsurgery and endoscopy. The endoscope surgeon needs to become thoroughly familiar with the actual anatomy and anatomical relationships viewed within the carpal tunnel through the endoscope. The 3-D Vision in an endoscope is different from that of obtained from the operative microscope that is like normal 3-D vision.

Part of the endoscope training may take place in a virtual scenario [42] besides using cadavers. Two groups of endoscope surgeons were examined, the one being trained in a virtual environment. The experienced virtual trained group completed the procedures faster ($p > 0.001$). Similar they had less errors ($p = 0.006$) and a higher score on economy of movements ($p = 0.005$) than the inexperienced group. A 17% complication rate for 12 hand surgeons learning the endoscope technique on cadaver specimens illustrates these problems.

"Endoscope surgical technique requires rigorous training in order to avoid dangerous pitfalls: it must be performed by experienced hand surgeons". Chow and Papachristos [16] emphasizes that we need well-trained surgeons to perform these endoscopy operations. Many of the potential complications that occur during CTS surgery can be avoided if the surgeon has a good grasp of the anatomy of the carpal tunnel and its possible anomalies. The learning curve is important and the fact that one great Endoscope surgeon or similar micro neurosurgeon can carry out CTS without a complication does not invariably indicate that the rest of the younger lesser experienced surgeons will do the same.

Surgical techniques are being developed through training and time [43]. For microsurgery fatigue is important and some of us may be able to operate for hours without fatigue, others will not.

The more experienced surgeons "seniors" giving lectures and writing papers telling young trainees about new techniques – because we "invented" them. Many published surgical series are thus "personal" by neurosurgical experts and are thus not suited for generalizing – which is always happening even today. Complication rates for both open (OCTR) and endoscopy carpal tunnel release (ECTR) procedures are usually low in these "expert" papers.

Training courses in endoscope decompression are many – in open surgery few, probably because "it is so simple". Release of the median nerve for the treatment of carpal tunnel syndrome (CTS) can be one of the most straightforward and satisfying procedures performed by a neurosurgeon.

The new UEMS charter [113] emphasizes this and training surgical techniques is soon an integrated part of all surgical programs and is today part of the formal EANS training courses today (www.EANS.org).

Anesthesia used for CTS surgery

Performing surgery to day demands some type of anesthesia.

Anesthesia may be

1) Local infiltration anesthesia (LA),
2) LA or intravenous (IV), with and without use of tourniquet and
3) General anesthesia (GA).

1) Local anesthesia

Where the skin cut is to be made 4–5 cc Lidocain 1% infiltration is used. Be careful not to inject the anesthetics directly into the nerve as this may result in interstitial nerve necrosis [45]. Applying topical anesthetic cream reduces the pain of infiltration if patients are nervous.

During surgery haemosthasis is obtained by the local anaesthetics and by using bipolar coagulation [70]. All bleeding vessels must be carefully occluded whereby postoperative blood oozing is very seldom experienced. Using LA, the patient and surgeon can communicate during surgery and any abnormal feeling from the patient's side alerts the surgeon on a potential complication [16].

Postoperatively a small bandage will be sufficient and active movement of fingers instituted.

It is standard in hand surgery to recommend that the patients should keep the hand high e.g. above the heart for the first days but there is no documented proof of its value.

2) Intravenous anesthesia, or local anesthesia eventually combined with tourniquet

Hand surgeons traditionally use intra venous anesthesia combined with extremity exsanguinations necessary for a bloodless field. An Esmarch bandage is used to empty the extremity of blood, followed by inflation of a tourniquet above systolic pressure. This method is absolutely mandatory for dissecting tendons and synovial tissue. Regarding dissection of nerves, it is – to me – a lesser good idea. Why? The nerve will appear pale during surgery with the same color as the tendons and vessels. Thereby cyanotic color changes of the nerve or distended vessels on the nerves caused by the entrapment cannot be visualized. Mauer *et al.* [74] found by Visual impression of the median nerve among 1.420 open CTS operations that 1.312 (92.4%) had a clear nerve compression and that 85 (34.2%) of these had color changes = cyanosis of the nerve (Fig. 9).

As with the development of a neuropathy, bear in mind that tourniquet also leads to ischemic disturbances in nervous tissue, changes that increase with the time tourniquet is used. It is suggested that a tourniquet should only be maintained for 30–60 minutes = the "safe-time period". If the patient harbors a polyneuropathy this "safe time period" may not apply and reperfusion will not always lead to restoration of nerve damage caused by the tourniquet [76, 83]. Patients with significant increased pressure in the carpal tunnel before the operation and patients with polyneuropathy have therefore a greater chance that tourniquet lead to a secondary iatrogenic nerve lesion.

Postoperative hemorrhages in the operative field are more common following use of tourniquet. If the tourniquet pressure drops during the operation,

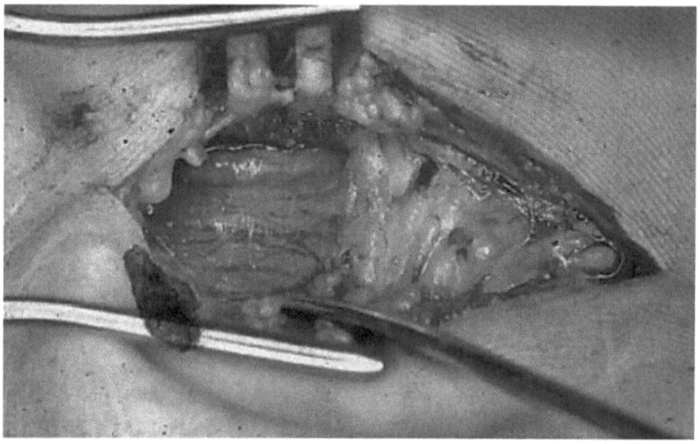

Fig. 9. Cyanosis of a compressed median nerve in the carpal tunnel

venous blood oozing may be a problem especially with endoscope techniques. Comparing blood oozing by the use of tourniquet and local adrenaline infiltrations simple infiltration of skin with adrenalin was superior to tourniquet [11].

So for neurosurgeons – a personal view – please forget all about using tourniquet. Our micro neurosurgical techniques and use of bipolar coagulation are sufficient for all types of open CTS surgery.

3) General anesthesia

"Virgin" operations can be carried out with simple local anaesthesia, but general anaesthesia may be indicated in cases of re-operations with significant scarring or if the patients are very nervous.

It is perhaps wise to begin with general mask anesthesia (Propofol® only) before attempting to perform the procedure with the patient receiving a local anesthetic as a supplement. Dealing with endoscopy surgery, the patients sense a certain degree of discomfort (and occasionally arm movement) when the obturator (endoscope) is inserted into the carpal tunnel. For this reason, many hand surgeons prefer general anesthesia with endoscope approaches.

Surgical techniques

1a) Open surgery (OCTR)

Many types of open surgery exist although they are traditionally thought of and classified as "one" in most clinical papers.

When correlating published surgical series, open surgery is often by mistake considered to consist of only "one procedure" despite that there is significant enough variation to classify open surgery as being several different procedures. Similar we always believe that patients with CTS are a uniform category. As you understand from the previous this is not the case. Open surgical section of the TCL has been the gold standard surgical treatment for patients with carpal tunnel syndrome over the past 50 years. Cutting the TCL with a scalpel under direct vision produces reliable symptom relief in the vast majority of cases. However – despite this high clinical success rate – transient post-operative symptoms such as "pillar pain," scar tenderness, or hand weaknesses are known to occur [45, 48, 99, 109].

1b) The minimal open technique – "Safeguard"

Limited open techniques with single and double incisions were introduced in 1993/1994 [134]. They involve both simple types and those with supplementary instruments to secure safe division of the TCL. A prospective study revealed that the single incision method gave better results in respect of grip and pinch strengths, whereas functional and symptom scores were not different. The Safeguard method seems promising. Another type of minimal open technique is the "Carpaltone" method. Basically this is just an OCTR with smaller skin incisions [134].

Before we discuss the different techniques please see my personal open technique description:

1c) The author's personal surgical technique
(learned and developed through a period of 40 years)

The goal for the surgery is viewed in Fig. 10.

The author uses local infiltration of the skin distal to the wrist creases with 4–5 cc of 1% Lidocain with noradrenalin. A 3–4 cm long incision is made with a 15 blade from the distal crease of the hand/wrist towards the interdigital space 3/4 (Fig. 11).

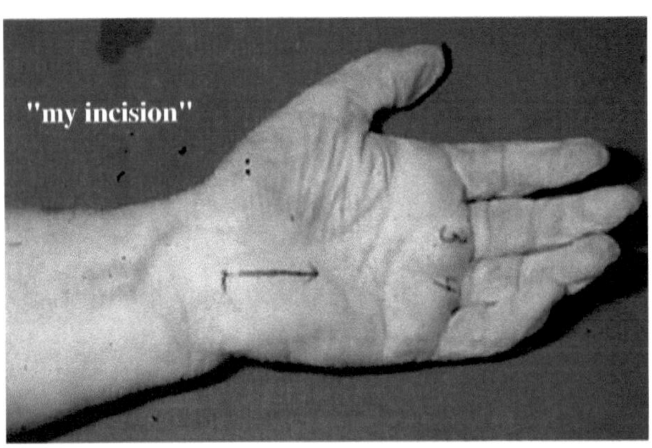

Fig. 10. "My incision" for CTS

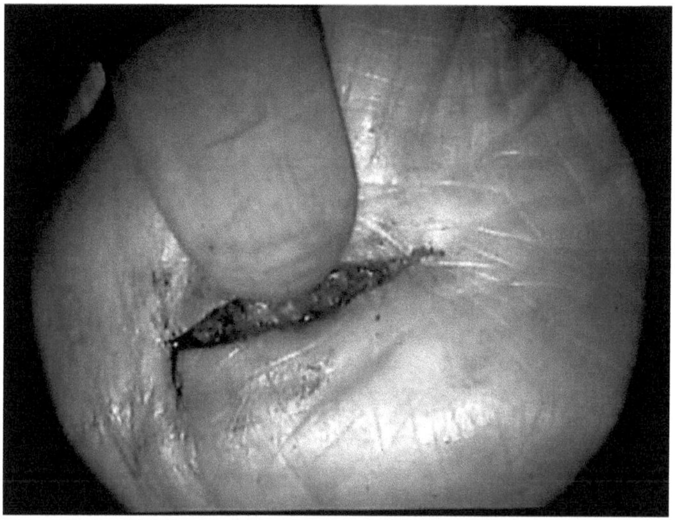

Fig. 11. Size of "my incision"

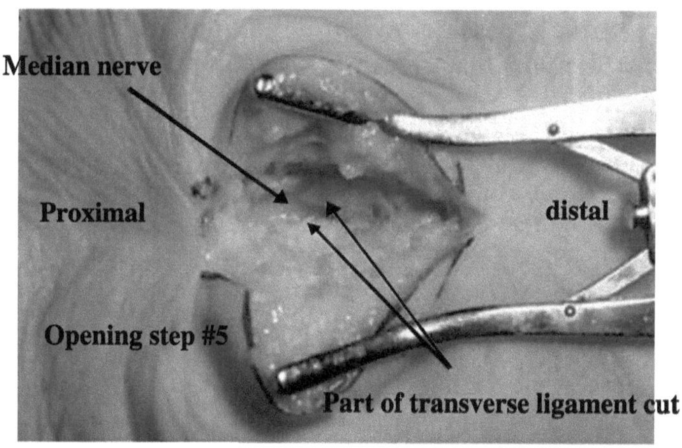

Fig. 12. The cadaver demonstration of the incision for CTS

Using the operative microscope and with a small self-retaining retractor, the palmar aponeurosis is visualized (Fig. 12).

Do not use too much power to spread the skin edges. The "safe zone" for incision of the aponeurosis and TCL is the ulnar part of the aponeurosis as the motor branch to the abductor brevis muscle usually leaves the median nerve from the radial side. The aponeurosis is cut longitudinally at the ulnar area. The

TCL is now found with its white transverse fibers. The TCL is opened with a fresh 15 blade.

When the contents of the carpal tunnel is encountered, the incision is carried further distally to the rim of the ligament whereby the normal fat in the hollow of the hand is visualized (Fig. 12). I do not touch the median nerve and do not try to se the recurrent branch of the median nerve. When the distal rim of the TCL is cut the palmar fat will protrude further and occasionally you may see the transverse vascular arcade pulsating. Then the proximal part of the ligament is cut and eventually part of the ante brachial aponeurosis – still keeping ulnar to the midline. You may lift the skin to observe this part of the cutting better (Fig. 13).

The palmar cutaneous branch of the median nerve is usually never seen with this approach. The palmar cutaneous branches of the ulnar nerve may be found and spared. Cyanosis of the median nerve is often visible where it is compressed (Fig. 9).

The use of internal neurolysis of the median nerve is to be abandoned.

Movements of the flexor tendons and the median nerve are then tested and observed. The end of operation is seen in Fig. 7.

The ligament edges are coagulated with low current bipolar coagulation and the skin closed in one layer with single 5–0 nylon sutures. There is no significant difference between using non-absorbable and nylon sutures for any of our outcome measures at the final follow-up. The wound is covered with a

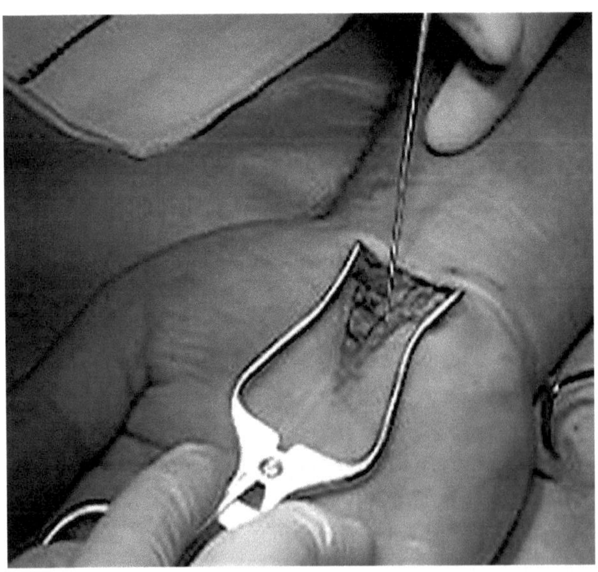

Fig. 13. The end of the operation, a hook is lifting the distal skin edge for better visualization of the antebrachial fascia

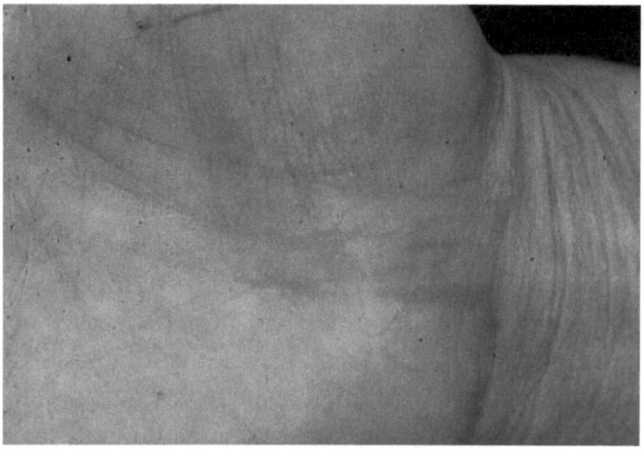

Fig. 14. Scar following OCTR after 6 months

band-aid and the hand bolstered leaving the fingers free for immediate active movements after surgery. The patient is instructed in using finger movements from day one. Skin sutures are removed after 12–14 days and movements of wrist begun after this, as early mobilization seems relevant.

End-result of CTS is not influenced whether immobilization or no-immobilization is used in the immediate post-operative period.

The scar will be minimal after 6 months as demonstrated in Fig. 14.

In a non-published consecutive series of 96 hands operated upon by two senior neurosurgeons at Aalborg University Hospital, Denmark in 1998, no complication was encountered with this technique.

2. Endoscope techniques (ECTR)

Application of endoscopy techniques to CTS treatment has not decreased operative expense, increased operative efficiency, or improved intraoperative visualization (compared with conventional OCTR). Despite these shortcomings, ECTR has many proponents who cite the potential benefits of faster patient recovery time, less incision pain, and improved grip strength recuperation [1, 14, 16, 24, 26, 45, 54, 80, 87, 90, 103, 108].

The first endoscope procedure for transecting the TCL was introduced in 1987 and many modifications have been described since that [16, 48].

Single-portal techniques are those in which a single skin incision is made in the proximal wrist crease. Dual-portal techniques are those in which a second small incision is made in the palm when the endoscope/obturator has reached this area. Both methods require some degree of hyperextension and fixation of the hand during surgery.

Visualization of anatomical structure is of course of paramount importance when performing endoscope procedures. Blood obscures vision and extremity exsanguinations with an Esmarch bandage followed by inflation of a tourniquet above systolic pressure is necessary to obtain a bloodless field. Even with perfectly planned endoscope surgery the surgeon must be prepared to change to an open type of surgery if anatomical landmark identification is not possible. If synovial tissue is prominent it may also hinder endoscope technique. As mentioned previously, the learning curve for endoscope surgery is very steep and it takes relatively long training to obtain mastery of endoscopes. Detailed knowledge of the complex anatomy of the anatomy of the carpal tunnel with respect to the related neurovascular structures is essential to perform safe endoscopy carpal tunnel release. Staying at the ulnar side of the long palmar tendon keeps the superficial palmar branch of the median nerve at a safe distance from the instruments. The "fat drop sign" is also a useful guide for the placement of the distal margin of the transverse carpal ligament, keeping the distal portal away from the superficial palmar arch. Synovial adhesions can usually cover the inferior surface of the transverse ligament, and they need to be removed for clear endoscopy identification of the transverse fibers before the ligament is cut [130].

We are basically dealing with 2 types of endoscope surgery (ECTR):

a) *One-port technique* includes those described by Okutsu, Agee, Menon, Worseg, and Jimenez [1, 16, 54, 80, 90, 121]

The original Okutsu technique was modified in 1989 so that the endoscope was inserted directly in the carpal tunnel on the ulnar side of the long palmar muscle tendon instead of starting extrabursal. A retrograde hook knife is introduced alongside the ulnar aspect and used – under direct visualization – to incise the TCL cutting from distal to proximal. Agee *et al.* [1] introduced in 1990 a technique with a pistol grip endoscope seen in Fig. 15.

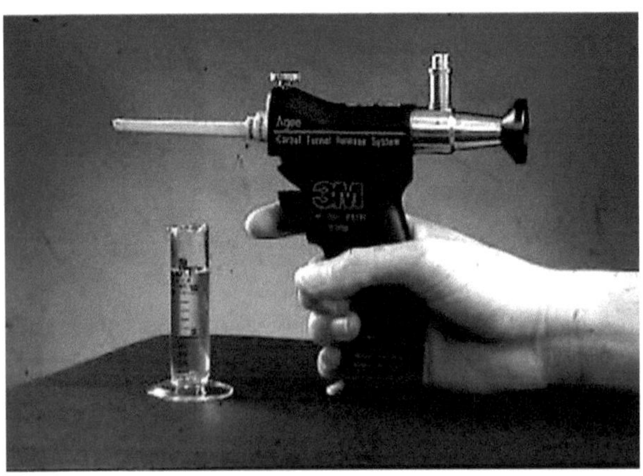

Fig. 15. 1 pistol grip one-port endoscope

A window near the tip of the system made it possible to view the undersurface of the transverse carpal ligament through the endoscope when inserting it. A small 2 cm transverse skin incision is used positioned ulnar to the palmar tendon at the distal wrist crease. The ante brachial fascia is incised and the endoscope is passed into the carpal tunnel till the distal edge of the ligament is viewed. A cutting blade is then inserted and cutting of the ligament takes place from distal to proximal viewing the ligament but not the median nerve with this technique, the cutting blade cannot always be visualized when cutting [1].

The success rate of one-port techniques reported in published papers was 96.2%, with a complication rate of 1.83% and a failure rate of 1.44% [90].

b) *Two-port technique*: includes lesser different types

With the two portal techniques the introducer/obturator is passed somewhat blindly through the carpal tunnel through a similar small transverse cut in the skin crease and a supplementary contra incision is made in the hand palm where the tip of this introducer pushes the skin from the inside. The original Chow technique included an extrabursal approach to the carpal tunnel with gentle retracting the flexor tendons. The canal is visualized and it is secured that no tendons or nerve are in the field view. Then the endoscope and a probe are inserted in the inserter from the distal end of the carpal tunnel in order to cut the ligament with a forward movement. The custom designed instrumentation protects the median nerve and flexor tendons, and positioning of the slotted cannula through the two portals ensures a stable surgical environment [16]. This technique was modified so that the surgeon inserts a hook knife via the proximal port and advances it behind the distal end of the TCL. The TCL is caught by the knife and the ligament is cut in a backwards pull [14].

The option for all types of CTS operations is to reduce pressure in the carpal tunnel by increasing its size. In order to obtain e.g. a 6% increase of carpal tunnel volume [94], you introduce an endoscope. The size of an abnormal carpal tunnel (length 4 cm) is $238.9 \times 400 = 95.560\,\text{mm}^3$. A 6% change in this volume is $5.734\,\text{mm}^3$. The size of this endoscope of 3 mm diameter is: $400 \times 2 \times 3.14 \times 1.50 = 3.768\,\text{mm}^3$. So we actually introduce a devise that has a volume close to what we want to obtain in reduction and we do that in a situation where the pressure in the canal is increased. How will pressure in the canal be influenced by ECTR? 20 patients had surgery for idiopathic CTS by one-portal Agee endoscopy section of the TCL (MicroAire, Charlottesville, VA). With a special transducer pressures were measured and were all elevated initially. The pressures were maximal (mean 93 mmHg) with full passive wrist extension. Peaks of high pressures, on average 97 mmHg, were recorded with the Agee endoscopy device in the canal. Release of the endoscopy TCL resulted in a marked decrease of the pressures [108]. The single-portal ECTR does not seem to influence the median nerve excursion for the wrist positions studied in patients with carpal tunnel syndrome. The results from an in vivo study showed longitudinal gliding of the median nerve being twice as great as in vitro studies.

Although the potential decreased palmar tenderness, better preservation of grip strength, and earlier return to work associated with ECTR are very noteworthy, these advantages may still be negated by the risk of neurovascular and tendon injury. Many surgeons remain skeptical about the safety and reliability of ECTR. Today >5.000 patient hands have been treated with the 2-port technique with an average success rate reported of 98.3%, a complication rate of 1.87% and a failure rate of 1.44%.

If the surgeon is unfamiliar with the actual technique or the anatomy he/she may easily injure the nervous structures and create severe failures [27] According to recent studies, the overall complication rate is in the range of 1–2% in experienced hands for both ECTR and OCTR surgery [122, 127, 129].

For the author it is still philosophically difficult to accept that despite we base our surgical indication on an increased pressure in the tunnel (small space). We add hyperextension e.g. reduces this carpal tunnel volume and simultaneously increase pressure even more performing endoscope surgery.

3. The blind "Paine" retinaculum technique

This was introduced with the purpose of cutting the TCL without opening the skin in a broad manner. After opening the ante brachial fascia ulnar to the palmar tendon, a retinaculatome instrument is blindly passed down the carpal tunnel with its foot under the ligament cutting the ligament simultaneously [89]. Its movement leads to a "characteristic sound" telling the surgeon when the ligament is cut. In 0.3% of cases an incomplete divisions of the TCL was found. In another 4 cases a palmar haematoma were discovered. Supplementary technique is – after having cut the ligament – to pass a light source down the carpal tunnel and watch light passing through the skin indicating whether a complete cutting has been achieved. This method is hardly in use to day in Europe.

Complications to surgical treatment of CTS

Complications to CTS surgery are frequent [1, 7, 14, 45, 67, 90, 96, 99, 122]. Despite that the complication rates sited in the literature seems significantly underestimated. Complications are many and rank from simple postoperative wound infections to median nerve laceration. The main advantages of the ECTR techniques are considered to be minor postoperative pain and a more rapid postoperative recovery. The rate of other complications (reflex sympathetic dystrophy, haematoma, wound problems, etc.) was about the same with endoscopy as with open release [8].

Disadvantages are thought to be the impossibility of a direct median nerve neurolysis and a higher and more severe surgical complication rate, including injury to the median nerve and vascular structures with profound physical and psychological sequel [32, 45].

The frequency and severity of complications have increased since endoscope release began [24]. This is not based on the technique used, but mainly on the lack of education in new surgeons.

Most common complications are incomplete release of the TCL or postoperative scarring with both OCTR and ECTR [23].

A survey of the most common and serious complications to open surgery (OCTR)

The operative mistakes/complications using open surgery are mainly:

1) Recurrent CTS due to inadequate cut of the transverse ligament.
2) Erroneous decompression of the ulnar nerve instead of median nerve.
3) Direct surgical lesion of the median nerve.
4) Direct surgical lesion of the recurrent motor branch of median nerve.
5) Lesion of the palmar cutaneous branch of median nerve.
6) Reflex Sympathetic Dystrophy (RSD).
7) Hypertrophy scar.
8) Hypersensitive scar.
9) Pillar pain.
10) Dysaesthesia.
11) Injury to superficial vascular arch.
12) Wound infection.
13) Decreased grip strength.
14) Decreased wrist movements.

Supplementary complications to the endoscope methods (ECTR)

The same as with the open method +

15) Lesion of the motor branch of ulnar nerve,
16) Lesion of ulnar nerve in Guyon's canal.
17) Lesion of the Berrettini branch between ulnar and median nerves.
18) Pseudo aneurysm on superficial arch.
19) Cutting of median nerve.
20) Significant lesions of digital nerves.
21) Lesions of tendons to the superficial digital flexor 4–5 muscle.
22) Deep hand space infections.

Discussion on surgical techniques

Many reasons for inadequate surgical results are found – incorrect diagnosis, inadequate decompression, iatrogenic compression or direct nerve injury. Most clinical papers on CTS results are unfortunately typical retrospective studies without necessary precise pre- and postoperative information. They simply do not give us a possibility to neither validate results by time nor by precision of the used operative techniques. When we read these papers information is found regarding "good" results.

What is a "good" result?

When we discuss results of CTS operative treatment we must decide what we in fact mean by a "good" result?

Most patients will be operated upon due to significant painful paraesthesiae. Relief of these will be "a good result". Shapiro [109] found that the mean time before patients returned to work was 6 weeks e.g. also good results, just a different way of looking upon results.

How do we handle information of transient paraesthesiae as the referral symptom?

If symptoms disappear fast the overall prognosis is "good". However, if this result is based on a lesion of the median nerve with subsequent absent sensibility, it seems to be a "good result" with some reservations. Total relief of pain and nightly paresthesia is generally obtained within the first postoperative 24 hours in close to 90% of cases.

If the patient becomes free of pain very fast, but that these returns 6 months later? So we also need exact information on follow-up periods. Among patients with hard hand labour postoperative problems are found in up to 80% – but it is important to remember that "time heals". After 6 months only 2% had pain and hypersensitive scars and 5% pain in hand and wrist after OCTR. Pagnanelli and Barrer [89] found what he called good results among 90% of patients operated upon but only 81% among a group of diabetic patients. Again we lack information on the demographics in this paper.

What about age? "The surgical results among elderly patients had significant better results among men >70 years of age compared to non-surgical treatment". What shall we do with a statement like this?

If the primary symptom is atrophy of thenar muscles, is it the normalization of muscle function? Patients in later states of CTS with significant loss of sensation due to axonal injury cannot expect full recovery in years [3, 4, 8, 16, 24, 67, 74, 99, 103, 109, 121, 122].

So, we must accept that the multitude of symptoms and dysfunction makes it very difficult to decide what a good result is e.g. we need a consensus, and we need well designed prospective studies in the future to deal with these questions.

Similar we may ask:

What is a surgical "failure"?

Surgical failure rates are reported to be from 2–31% and in conservative series from 1–50%. These huge variations indicate to me that we have no firm consensus definition of what a failure is.

Major, if not devastating, complications can and do occur with both OCTR and ECTR [90]. Surgically treated CTS complications of endoscopy and open carpal tunnel release over a 5-year period were sent to members of the American Society for Surgery of the Hand to assess and compare major complications of the 2 procedures [24]. The 708 respondents treated a total of 455 major complications from ECTR. These included a total of 100 median nerve lacerations, 88 ulnar nerve lacerations, 77 digital nerve lacerations, 121 vessel lacerations, and 69 tendon lacerations. There were similar 283 major complications from OCTR treated by 616 respondents, including 147 median nerve lacerations, 29 ulnar nerve lacerations, 54 digital nerve lacerations, 34 vessel lacerations, and 19 tendon lacerations. The conclusion was: That there is no difference in complication rate between open and endoscope surgery. Although this is a retrospective voluntary study with resultant methodological flaws, the data support the conclusion that carpal tunnel release, be it endoscopy or open, is not a safe and simple procedure. Only 15% OF CTS operations in this 5-year time periode in New York were ECTR. Never the less they resulted in 46% of the nerve laceration complications in the whole series. This implies that ECTR surgery in fact had more severe complications than OCTR [50].

A surgical failure is it just a situation where an expected result is not reached? Have we in all these cases before treatment was instituted defined the symptoms and the expected result? I doubt it. Is it a so-called "bad result"? or is a failure a case with a direct complication? – Something unexpected happening?

In a prospective series of 378 patients 97% improved their motor weakness and only one patient showed worsening [109]. Is this worsening a failure or a complication? If the recurrent motor branch was cut resulting in the worsening of muscle power it is a surgical complication and not a failure of the operation.

Two large, prospective, randomized, multicenters, clinical trials compared OCTR and ECTR methods emphasize the potential benefits of ECTR [1, 14]. Agee *et al.* [1] showed in a randomized, prospective, multicenter study of 147 hands (65 OCTR patients vs. 82 ECTR patients) that the median time to return to work was 21 days shorter in the ECTR group than the OCTR group. In this series it was said that the best predictors of return to work were lack of incision tenderness and good return of grip strength. In the ECTR group three complications were found: one incomplete release of the ligament and two transient ulnar nerve neuropraxia. In the OCTR group four complications were described: two wound dehiscence, one bowstringing of the flexor tendons, and one injury to the deep motor branch of the ulnar nerve. Brown *et al.* [14] found in his randomized, prospective, multicenter study of 160 hands (82 OCTR patients vs. 78 ECTR patients) that the median return to work time was 14 days shorter in the ECTR group than the OCTR group [45, 90, 121, 127].

An analysis of 54 publications, reporting a total of 9516 endoscopy and 1203 open releases showed the rate of irreversible nerve damage to be 0.3 and 0.2%, respectively. Reversible nerve problems were more common after ECTR [8].

How can we scientifically compare these results? We lack besides demographics with precise definition of working conditions, information on social structures, and consensus on what we base our "good" results on.

How to avoid the most common and serious complications?

Direct complications can be related to the skin incisions, inadequate sectioning of TCL and injuries to tendon, nervous and vascular structures. There may also develop scar tissue in and around the median nerve. Pain symptoms may develop locally or as part of a RSD.

Problems with skin incisions

What type of skin incision should be used?

The skin incision used in order to reach the TCL, can have many shapes and lengths [45, 48]. Most important is that it allows full visualization of the entire carpal tunnel contents and the whole TCL ligament. The length of the skin incisions may vary between 2 and 8 cm. The skin incision can be located from the forearm crossing the distal wrist crease and end at the midpalm. The incision is positioned along the axis of the third web space, towards the third or fourth finger or along the thenar crease. The most common longitudinal incision is aiming towards the interspace between the 3rd finger, and 4th finger. The shape of the incision may be curved, straight, sigmoid, or any combination thereof. The skin incision should not cross the wrist flexion creases as this may lead to hypertrophy scarring. Six months postoperatively only 2% have hypersensitive scars. If a painful hypertrophic scar should occur a complicated revision with a Z-plasty may be needed.

If the incision is placed towards the ulnar territory of the hand, the surgeon can easily by mistake enter Guyon's canal with the ulnar nerve and artery. If it is placed too radial a lesion of the palmar cutaneous branch of the median nerve may happen and severe neuromas pain and reflex sympathetic dystrophy (RSD) may be the result. The Palmar cutaneous branch of the median nerve emerges some 6 cm proximal to the wrist and runs parallel and on the radial side with the median nerve and the long palmar tendon, some 2 cm proximal to the proximal border of the transverse carpal ligament [119] (See Fig. 3). With any incision made in the palm it is likely to injure the small terminal cutaneous branches of the palmar cutaneous nerves. Even though an incision based on the axis of the ring finger may reduce the incidence of this nerve lesion, there is no true "inter-nervous plane" that will completely avoid all cutaneous palmer branches, whether of median or ulnar origin. Injury to the large palmar cutaneous branch is probably the second most commonly cited complication in OCTR. After section of this nerve a subsequent neuroma formation occurs. The result is a reduced sensibility in palm and persistent neuromas. We are now faced with inferior treatment options, burying the neuromas in the forearm muscles or to cut it. Neither of these options have had a high success rate [67].

Hands are very different and very large, bulky hands are found among acromegalics and hard working people. In this context, the Kaplan Cardinal Line is used by hand-surgeons for identification of the distal part of the TCL. Testing hand-surgeons knowledge of this line it was shown that it varied where they thought it to be. Kaplan's cardinal line does not locate the deep structures of the hand accurately but may assist in making palmar incisions. Before the surgeon reaches the TCL the palmar aponeurosis and palmar minimal muscle tendon is found and cut longitudinally. Persistent minimal incision tenderness is present in 61% of OCTR patients versus 36% of ECTR patients at 12 weeks follow-up.

Transverse incisions are abandoned as the surgeon will injure the palmar cutaneous branch and give an inferior view of the operative field. It was popular many years ago but forces the surgeon to cut the TCL blindly and injuries to vessels and nerves were common. Analysis of the OCTR CTS literature reveals thus great variability regarding the location, length, and shape of the skin incision [45, 48].

The incisions used for ECTR are as invalidating as the small used for open surgery. The proximal incision for the 1-port techniques may also injure cutaneous branches. Its length is roughly 1.5–2 cm. In the 2-port technique we must ad the distal incision of 1.5 cm so the total length is 3–3.5 cm. The length of the standard incision I use for OCTR is about 3–4 cm (Fig. 11) and it cannot be seen after 6 months (Fig. 14). In an attempt to minimize openings, a short (approximately 2 cm) incision may be used as part of a mini OCTR operation technique [134]. No statistical difference in scar length, scar tenderness, rate of complications, or length of time before return to work was found in a prospective series of 71 patients undergoing OCTR surgery through an average 2.1-cm incision versus 66 patients in whom an ECTR two-portal technique was used. The minimal-incision OCTR technique can thus achieve the same low incidence of incision tenderness [47, 134].

These historical types of incisions have all been discussed in details by Hudson *et al.* [48].

Visualization of carpal tunnel – use of magnification

With a long microsurgical experience I cannot understand why all surgeons performing CTS do not use magnification. Even loupes are better than normal vision. I always use an operative microscope as seen in Fig. 16. The use of visual magnification during the operative procedure is optional to prevent complications occurring due to anatomical variations of the recurrent motor branch. Chances for recognizing a wrong dissection, aberrant nerve structures and vessels are greater using an operative microscope and lesions of larger cutaneous nerves are seldom found with microsurgical techniques.

In addition to general better vision it is far easier to make precise bipolar coagulations and thus obtain perfect haemostasis.

The better visualization has the benefit of demonstrating the TCL far better before we cut it. The main reason for incomplete operations with postoperative pain and unchanged symptoms is from all series incomplete sectioning of the TCL distally. Because of the potential for neurovascular and tendon injury, most endoscopy surgeons agree that if the transverse fibres of the TCL cannot be visualized along its entire length, the endoscopy procedure should be converted into an open one. Inferior visualization of the anatomical structures leads to a similar problem.

Haemostasis

Blood oozing is controlled by bipolar coagulation at a low setting. Postoperative hemorrhage is virtually never seen [70]. Whether this is a problem or not

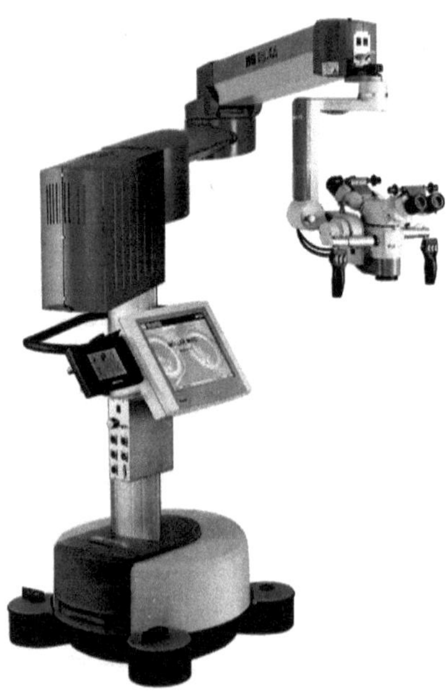

Fig. 16. Möller-Wedel operative microscope HiR 700; www.moeller-wedel.com

can be discussed, but the hand surgical wide use of exanguation working in a bloodless field is not only a tradition but also serves to reduce blood oozing. Braithwaite *et al.* [20] examined the use of tourniquet and local adrenaline infiltrations and found that simple adrenalin was much better than tourniquet to prevent blood oozing from skin. Postoperative hemorrhages are more common following use of tourniquet. If the tourniquet pressure drops during the operation, venous blood oozing may be a problem [11]. A lesion of vascular structures may lead to wound haematomas and in one OCTR series 1.4% haematomas was found [14]. The major problem besides inferior surgical vision is that blood can result in tendon and median nerve adhesions.

TCL cutting

Most common complication in all types of CTS surgery is inadequate cutting of the TCL. The cut in the TCL is usually straight [48]. It is appropriate to transect the ligament over 4 mm apart from the lateral margin of the hook of the Hamate without placing the edge of the scalpel toward the ulnar side. We would also recommend not transecting the TCL in the ulnar flexed wrist position to protect the ulnar neurovascular structure [53]. A cut like a flap with secondary reconstruction of the ligament has been tried but failed. Similar there is no identifiable benefit in lengthening the TCL when decompressing the carpal tunnel. The TCL can then be cut by a knife or by scissors. Many surgeons insert a Mickey probe in the carpal canal and cuts the TCL using this probe as a protection of the median nerve. In some cases an injury to the recurrent motor branch to the abductor muscle can occur especially if the distal part of the ligament is cut "blindly" with scissors [67]. Cut of the vascular arcade by mistake is also possible if the cut is made blindly. If, in an attempt to avoid the median nerve, the surgeon cuts through the ulnar side of the TCL, the motor branch of the ulnar nerve may be injured. Similarly, if the surgeon blindly cuts the distal fibres of the TCL in a radial direction, the third common digital nerve may be injured.

Immediately after surgical release of the TCL, there is a marked decrease of the carpal canal pressure. During the second postoperative month and persisting after 12 months the pressure arises again but stay inside normal ranges. These findings suggest that the TCL reconstitutes by normal scar formation, but with some lengthening [106]. This is also visualized on MRI where the carpal tunnel contents may show significant postoperative alterations including displacement of flexor tendons [94].

The potential for neurovascular and tendon injury, most endoscopy surgeons agree that if the transverse striations of the TCL cannot be visualized along its entire length, the endoscopy procedure should be converted to an open one. This is in accordance with the fact that incomplete section of the TCL is the most common complication to OCTR and ECTR. With OCTR twelve cases of incomplete release of the ligament, constituting 35% of the total 34 complications were found in 186 patients [67]. In another series 67% of patients with persistent symptoms had incomplete section of the TCL. Two hundred patients with recurrent symptomatology were reoperated during a 2 years follow-up period. In 108 cases (54%) the TCL had been incompletely sectioned and among these 46 (43%) the median nerve was fixed by simple scar tissue and with circumferential scarring among 17 (16%) of these [116].

With ECTR we are dealing with three types of incomplete release:

1) release of Guyon's canal,
2) incomplete distal ligament release (as in OCTR), and
3) incomplete central (superficial) ligament release.

It is thus somewhat more complicated to cut the TCL with ECTR than the simple OCTR. Incomplete ligament release in ECTR ranges from 5% to as high as 50% in cadaver studies.

Infection

Superficial skin infections occur as in all types of surgery and should be treated accordingly. They are seldom constituting some 0.5% to 6%. Deep infections is also found especially if surgical drainage is used, with prolonged operative time and if attempts to perform tendon synovectomy is undertaken. In the endoscope surgery, deep infections are serious and have been reported.

Pillar pain

Linked with the skin incision is "Pillar pain" an ill-defined pain in the thenar and hypothenar eminences aggravated by gripping.

Its etiology remains obscure. Cutting of the sensory nerve fibers supplying the palmar brevis fascia and resulting micro neuroma formation is one explanation. Other possible mechanisms include widening of the carpal arch and realignment of the carpal bones. It has been stated that pillar pain is more common if incising openly in the palm but has never been proven in a randomized prospective trial. Moderate or severe pillar and scar pain is common in literature, occurring in 25% of hands after surgery, but only in 4% by the 12th week and 2% by the 25th week of follow-up [96]. Sometimes this pillar pain may hinder functions among workers with heavy hand loading jobs. Among patients with hard hand labour postoperative problems are thus in some series found in up to 80% – but it is important to remember that "time heals".

Tendon adhesions

Tendon adhesions are not common in a neurosurgical practice. Tendon adhesions may result from poor haemostasis or bleeding from tenosynovectomy.

Resection of the synovium is usually only indicated in cases of extremely bulky synovium as we see it with Rheumatoid Arthritis.

Physical therapy with range-of-motion exercises and dynamic splinting rather than tenolysis surgery is the best treatment, but not randomized, prospective studies exists.

Lesion of vascular structures

It is most common with ECTR and among untrained surgeons. The lesions are of the superficial arch distal to the TCL and the ulnar neurovascular bundle injured at the proximal port by inadvertent entry into Guyon's canal. Similar occasional lesion of the ulnar artery has been published by failed OCTR dissection of Guyon's canal. Proper use of open surgery with microscope magnification and avoidance of working in a bloodless field reduces the chances of injuring the vessels during surgery.

Nerve lesions

A skin incision directly over the median nerve rather than toward the ulnar side may result in postoperative nerve adherence to the skin.

Intra- and perineural median nerve scarring may be the results of long term CTS and of surgery. It leads often to disabling dysaesthesias, severe local pain, and hypersensitivity of the skin. Proper haemostasis is as already stated, important to prevent perineural scarring. Internal neurolysis, epineurotomy or epineurectomy is not indicated and no series has proved benefit from such attempts.

Two hundred and seventy-three patients with CTS without advanced neurophysiologic changes (DML below 11 ms) were randomized to treatment by OCTR with – or without – epineurotomy. Patients were examined clinically and by nerve conduction studies preoperatively and at 3, 6 and 12 months postoperatively. No statistically significant difference between simple decompression and decompression combined with epineurotomy with regard to either the clinical or the neurophysiologic outcome were found [9].

If a median nerve adhesion is encountered it may be isolated from the skin using:

1) Rotation of a hypothenar fat-pad flap or
2) Rotation of local muscle pedicle with a pronator quadratus/abductor digiti 5 flap.

A Z-plasty with underlying temporary silicone sheeting to prevent scar adherence has also been advocated, but is not used today.

Direct cutting of the recurrent motor branch of the median nerve results in thenar atrophy and loss of opposition. Due to the many variations of the median nerve and its branching all surgery performed without perfect visualization carries a risk of nerve-branch lesions. Especially with ECTR lesions of the ulnar nerve and other nerve branches have been reported. Most common nerve branch lesions are: Injury to the: median nerve, ulnar nerve, digital nerves, communicating branch between ulnar and median nerve (Berretini branch). The radial digital nerve of the fourth finger can be injured at the distal port [14, 45]. Lesions of the common digital nerve to the adjacent long and ring fingers have all been reported using ECTR techniques but very seldom with OCTR [32]. Irreversible nerve damage is uncommon in either technique; however, there is an increased susceptibility to reversible nerve injury that is three times as likely to occur with endoscopy carpal tunnel release than with open carpal tunnel release.

The ulnar nerve and artery lie radial to the hook of the Hamate and volar to the ulnar aspect of the TCL in 15% of individuals something that predisposes them to injury during inadvertent release of Guyon's canal.

Grip and Pinch strength

We are dealing with the general "Grip of the whole hand" and the "Pinch grip" where we use our thumb and index finger [128].

One of the drawbacks of normal open technique is that we cut both skin and the palmar aponeurosis in order to reach the transverse carpal ligament. The subsequent volar displacement of the long flexor tendons leads to bow stringing. This may thus change the whole grip strength as the pulley function of the ligament is reduced. In the endoscope technique the palmar aponeurosis is kept intact and prevents perhaps the bowstringing of the flexor tendons to some degree. Bowstringing of the flexor tendons is found with clinical symptoms in a limited frequency. Postoperative evaluation showed that grip strength was reduced to some extent among 35% of patients. Some immediate postoperative loss of grip strength can be anticipated in all patients persisting in up to one-third of patients. Grip strength is most decreased in wrist flexion than in wrist extension. It normalizes fully only in 47%. In another series grip strength was 28% of normal 3 weeks postoperatively. It was 73% by 6 weeks and became as preoperative by 12 weeks. After cutting the TCL we may therefore anticipate a possible changed grip strength that normalizes after at least 12 weeks. Grip strength is less in wrist flexion possible due to prolapsed flexor tendons out of the carpal tunnel. Grip and pinch strengths were measured in different groups with and without ligament transposition. At 6 weeks after surgery in the group that underwent transposition flap repair exceeded preoperative grip strength values. All groups surpassed preoperative grip strength measurements at 12 weeks. By 6 weeks after surgery, all pinch measurements for 3 groups equalled or exceeded preoperative pinch measurements [81]. Grip and thumb key pinch strength were measured pre- and immediately postoperatively in another 30 patients with CTS. It was estimated both while the wrist was in flexion and when in extension. The CTS was performed under local infiltration with 1% lidocaine. Grip strength decreased postoperatively more in wrist flexion than in wrist extension. No difference was found in thumb pinch strength. The authors conclude that some of the immediate postoperative loss of grip strength in wrist flexion can be attributed to bow stringing of prolapsed flexor tendons out of the carpal tunnel in this position [58]. In these cases reconstruction of the TCL with lengthening may be considered and undertaken.

Pain

Long-term persistent "pain" is a major determinant of the success or failure of the open CTS release. The pain-complications of long-term persistent pain may arise from any of the following causes: hypertrophy skin scarring, intra- and perineural scarring, adherence of the nerve to the skin, subcutaneous tender nerve secondary to superficial position, adhesions between flexor tendons and the median nerve, Pillar pain at the thenar and hypothenar eminences, and reflex sympathetic dystrophy (RSD). It is considered a nociceptive pain in most cases. The median nerve carries approximately 70% of the sympathetic nerves to the hand. With every CTS operation nervefibres (skin, TCL) are cut and will result in some nociceptive pain. RSD is thus a possible complication of CTR but in most series it is very infrequent. In one serie [67] it was surprisingly found in 12% of cases. Here again we miss a precise definition/and common understanding of what we are discussing as RSD has many stages.

RSD develops through three stages. The first stage is characterized by swelling, hyperesthesia, skin that is warm and dry, and movement aggravates persistent pain. In the second stage proximal spread of pain and edema is found and a cool and pale shiny skin with atrophic changes, and joint stiffness. In the third stage a progressive degree of atrophy with joint contractures is found and the patient claims "intractable pain".

Treatment in the first stages is physical therapy and corticosteroids. Many attempts have been made to solve the patient's problem including use of sympatectomy. All papers on sympatectomy are based on a blend of poor quality, lack of evidence, being uncontrolled studies and based on "personal experiences" and have no evidence-based effects [69].

Failed tract – false road

Optimal clinical outcomes are obtained in ECTR when attention is paid to critical technical aspects with correct positioning of the portals, familiarization with the endoscopes and endoscopy carpal anatomy, and maintenance of clear visualization into the carpal canal [16]. The small openings for endoscope surgery carry higher risks of introducing false tracts especially if the patient has big hands. We can easily reach the Guyon's canal and injure the ulnar nerve/ artery by mistake [49, 83]. A 35% complications rate is found with the transbursal endoscope approach compared to 3.7% with the extrabursal endoscope technique [26].

With open surgery it occurs if the surgeon cuts the TCL too ulnar. Hereby the surgeon can easily slip into the Guyon's canal and will eventually release the ulnar artery – by mistake. Again it is benefited to be able to view our operative field with pulsating vessels. The size of the ulnar artery is so large that it will be obvious that you are in the wrong position for the more experienced surgeons.

The neurosurgeon who perform ECTR section of TCL must be aware of all the iatrogenic complications that potentially occur because of inadequate training or experience. Conversion of an ECTR procedure to an open procedure should be done whenever either an anatomic variation or a technical difficulty occurs [16].

Conclusion

For detailed validation of the generally used open surgical techniques, the reader is referred to the review in Surgical Neurology regarding "Carpal Tunnel" [48].

The fact is that populations from which we find our patients vary and the diagnostic methods that should only be used for screening are also used – erroneously – for diagnosing CTS. We can use the Hand-Diagram to validate the subjective symptoms and add our own "objective" tests in order to better categorize the patients.

Most important still is that we need a valid information about the carpal tunnel structure and the degree of nerve involvement. Neurophysiology adds to this latter if used in a scientific way. The simple DML monitoring favoured by many surgeons, as a screening method performed by surgeons is possibly completely unnecessary as the same information is obtained through Hand-Diagram and questioning.

The patients have today access to the Internet. They prepare their visit in the MD's office by consulting the www. The quality of Internet information about CTS obtained e.g. from "Google" is still today rather poor with much non-evidenced information = "Gaff" [31]. When we as neurosurgeons have to decide the operative technique we will be faced with numerous question from the Internet! Commercial views promote newer techniques e.g. use of endoscope and sales techniques and advertisement may have the surgeon feel that it is necessary to use the new method to "keep abreast of modern developments". Further a warning: "We should be wary about yielding to pressure to use endoscope carpal tunnel release from instrument makers, medical supply houses, insurance companies and patients" [22].

Are there situations where endoscope is favored or not? Endoscope technique with wrist extension is neither ideal for 78-year-old women with severe degenerative wrist arthritis nor for a patient with significant synovial reactions or for a patient with polyneuropathy? May be endoscope techniques are not suited for thin wrists or big hands? Similarly the preservation of handgrip is more important for some patients working with heavy handwork than others.

We must validate these problems in the future, instead of fighting between "endoscope versus open surgery" issues.

What about costs of the two methods? The ECTR is more costly if the complication rate of endoscopy surgery exceeds 6.2% (best case estimate, 5.0%). The ECTR is also more costly if the risk of career ending injury exceeds 0.001 (best case estimate, 0.0004) and if the average works absence following a complication exceeds 15.5 months (best case estimate, 12 months) [129].

Return to work is also important for estimation of costs. Return-to-work status followed in 291 cases (199 non-worker's compensation cases and 92 worker's compensation cases) showed that the worker's compensation patients returned to work in an average of 57 days, compared with 22 days for non-worker's compensation patients [80]. In these cases the ECTR technique would be in favor compared to the OCTR? With the endoscope technique [121] and double open incision technique [134], the palmar aponeurosis is left intact and prevents perhaps this bowstringing to some degree? Loss of grip strength, scar tenderness, and persistent pillar pain are late sequel of the OCTR procedure and has provided much of the impetus to switch to the alternative of ECTR. However, long-term satisfaction seems lower in an ECTR group, attributable to a 5% (or more?) rate of re-operation. Potential benefits of ECTR predominate in the 1st several postoperative weeks but diminish significantly beyond this time period.

In many series social function e.g. compensation is a strong indicator for the development of complications. Patients treated with endoscope techniques seem to recover strength faster. It is also stated that following endoscope decompression the time until return to work is shorter than with the open techniques. However no controlled series exist to prove that statement. In a recent review the problems of return was found related to type of work and eventual workers compensation [72]. In a US series no differences could be found while in Scandinavia workers tend to stay longer out of the work than blue-collar people [5]. This may indicate a difference in society cultural structure that makes it difficult to compare series from different countries.

The increasing very high number of operative procedures carried out in the US and Scandinavia may indicate that our diagnostic criteria are uncertain and used without critically accepting the epidemiological factors. As we assume that changes in the carpal tunnel are responsive for some of the CTS we need to agree on the final diagnostic methods for evaluation of the tunnel, which include MRI and sonography. Neurophysiology is in this scenario used to confirm the degree of neuronal degeneration and for differential diagnostic purposes.

It seems unethical to accept a complication rate above 1% with these operations – whatever technique being used. Proper endoscope or microsurgical training in techniques is a must. It is likely that most of the nerve injuries incurred during endoscope release have remained unreported, but sooner or later the medical defense associations will become aware of them [30].

We can now conclude that carpal tunnel release seems to be a widely underestimated procedure and revision surgery could be largely avoided by reducing technical errors during the primary operation [116].

What we need for the future is a protocol with a systematic prospective validation of symptoms and tests – a protocol to be used universally.

The optimal CTS operative technique would be one, which incorporates the decreased incision tenderness, increased preservation of grip strength, and earlier return to work provided by ECTR with the lower incidence of serious neurovascular and tendon injuries found in OCTR. According to a Cochrane review there is no evidence to support that endoscope surgery (ECTR) is better that open surgery (OCTR) [107].

The Year 2005 was the year of H. C Andersen, the famous Danish storyteller. Every one knows the story about the ugly duckling that turned into a beautiful swan. The ducks treated the ugly duckling badly despite they thought it was one of their own and only because it looked "ugly" e.g. different. They did not realise their mistake until very late when the young unhappy swan saw its brothers and sisters and understood that he himself was a swan and not a duck and suddenly he felt great and happy.

It is close to the same story that has happened with neurophysiology contrary to hand-diagrams or endoscopy surgery contrary to open surgery.

The goal of this chapter was to give the readers the possibility to achieve better results in the future remembering that this – for us neurosurgeons – simple operation for the patient is still a major event in life. The neurosurgeon treating these patients should be as cautious as if it were patients with complicated intracerebral aneurysms being treated.

The statement

"I have had to cope with damage, inexperienced surgeons have caused by doing, what I consider to be an unnecessary operation" (Allan Hudson, Toronto, Canada)",

tells me how we should treat these patients in the future. It also encourages us to take training of surgical techniques up to a review and increase global collaboration in designing prospective studies.

References

1. Agee JM, McCarroll HR, Tortosa RD, Berry DA, Szabo RM, Peiner CH (1992) Endoscopic release of the carpal tunnel: a randomized prospective multicenter study. J Hand Surg (Am) 17: 987–995
2. Alford JW, Weiss AP, Akelman E (2004) The familial incidence of carpal tunnel syndrome in patients with unilateral and bilateral disease. Am J Orthop 33: 397–400
3. Arons JA, Collins N, Arons MS (1999) Results of treatment of carpal tunnel syndrome with associated hourglass deformity of the median nerve. J Hand Surg (Am) 24: 1192–1195
4. Atroshi I (1999) Carpal tunnel syndrome: prevalence, electrodiagnosis and outcome instruments. Thesis Lund University, Sweden
5. Atroshi I, Larsson G-U, Ornstein E, Hofer M, Johnsson R, Ranstam J (2006) Outcomes of endoscopic surgery compared with open surgery for carpal tunnel syndrome among employed patients: randomized controlled trial. BMJ 332: 1473–1478
6. Beekman R, Visser LH (2003) Sonography in the diagnosis of carpal tunnel syndrome: a critical review of the literature. Muscle & Nerve 27: 26–33
7. Bland JDP (2005) Carpal tunnel syndrome. Curr Opin Neurol 18: 581–585
8. Boeckstyns MEH, Sorensen AI (1999) Does endoscopic carpal tunnel release have a higher rate of complications than open carpal tunnel release. J Hand Surg (Br) 24: 9–15
9. Borisch N, Haussmann P (2003) Neurophysiological recovery after open carpal tunnel decompression: Comparison of simple decompression and decompression with epineurotomy. J Hand Surg (Br) 28: 450–454
10. Bower JA, Stanisz GJ, Keir PJ (2006) An MRI evaluation of carpal tunnel dimensions in healthy wrists: Implications for carpal tunnel syndrome. Clin Biomechanics 21: 816–825
11. Braithwaite BD, Robinson GJ, Burge PD (1993) Haemostasis during carpal tunnel release under local anaesthesia: a controlled comparison of a tourniquet and adrenaline infiltrations. J Hand Surg (Br) 18: 184–186
12. Braun RM, Doehr S, Mosqueda T, Garcia A (1999) The effect of legal representation on functional recovery of the hand in injured workers following carpal tunnel release. J Hand Surg (Am) 24: 53–58
13. Britz GW, Haynor DR, Kuntz C, Goodkin R, Gitter A, Kliot M (1995) Carpal tunnel syndrome: correlation of magnetic resonance imaging, clinical, electrodiagnostic and intraoperative findings. Neurosurgery 37: 1097–1103
14. Brown WF, Lee Dellon A, Campbell WW (1995) Electrodiagnosis in the management of focal neuropathies: the "Wog" syndrome. Muscle & Nerve 17: 1336–1342
15. Buchberger W (1997) Radiologic imaging of the carpal tunnel. Eur J Radiol 25: 112–117
16. Chow JCY, Papachristos AA (2006) Endoscopic carpal tunnel release: Chow technique. Techn Orthopaedics 21: 19–29
17. Chung KC (2003) Commentary: severe carpal tunnel syndrome. J Hand Surg (Am) 28: 645–646
18. Cochrane: www.cochrane.com
19. Coppieters MW, Alshami AM, Hodges PW (2006) An experimental pain model to investigate the specificity of the neurodynamic test for the median nerve in the differential diagnosis of hand symptoms. Arch Physical Med Rehab 87: 1412–1417
20. D'Arcy CA, McGee S (2000) The rational clinical examination. Does this patient have carpal tunnel syndrome? JAMA 283: 3110–3117

21. De Krom MCTFM, Knipschild PG, Kester AD, Spaans F (1990) Efficacy of provocative tests for diagnosis of carpal tunnel syndrome. Lancet 335: 393–395
22. De Smet L, Fabry G (1995) Transection of the motor branch of the ulnar nerve as a complication of two-portal endoscopic carpal tunnel release: a case report. J Hand Surg (Am) 20: 18–19
23. Dodds SD, Trumble TE (2006) Management of complications related to carpal tunnel release. Techn Orthopaedics 21: 75–83
24. Duncan KH, Lewis RC Jr, Foreman KA, Nordyke MD (1987) Treatment of carpal tunnel syndrome by members of the American Society for Surgery of the Hand: results of a questionnaire. J Hand Surg (Am) 73: 384–391
25. Elstner M, Bettecken T, Wasner M, Anneser F, Dichgans M, Meitinger T, Gasser T, Klopstock T (2006) Familial carpal tunnel syndrome: further evidence for a genetic contribution [1] Clin Genetics 69: 179–182
26. Erdmann MWH (1994) Endoscopic carpal tunnel decompression. J Hand Surg (Br) 19: 5–13
27. Evans D (1994) Endoscopic carpal tunnel release – the hand doctor's dilemma (Editorial). J Hand Surg (Br) 19: 3–4
28. Fernandez E, Pallini R, Lauretti L, Scogna A, La Marca F (1997) Carpal tunnel syndrome. Surg Neurol 48: 323–325
29. Fernandez E, Pallini R, Lauretti L (1997) Neurosurgery of the peripheral nervous system: injuries, degeneration and regeneration of the peripheral nerves. Surg Neurol 48: 446–447
30. Filler AAG, Kliot M, Howe FA, Hayes CE, Saunders DE, Goodkin R, Bell BA, Winn HR, Griffiths JR, Tsuruda JS (1996) Application of magnetic resonance neurography in the evaluation of patients with peripheral nerve pathology. J Neurosurg 85: 299–309
31. Fricke M, Fallis D, Jones M, Luszko GM (2005) Consumer health information on the Internet about carpal tunnel syndrome: indicators of accuracy. Am J Med 118: 168–174
32. Friedman AH (1997) Surgical anatomy of the carpal tunnel. Neurosurg Focus 15: 31–41
33. Gelberman RH, Rydevik BL, Pess GM, Szabo RM, Lundborg G (1988) Carpal tunnel syndrome. A scientific basis for clinical care. Orthop Clin North Am 19: 115–124
34. Geoghegan JM, Clark DI, Bainbridge LC, Smith C, Hubbard R (2004) Risk factors in carpal tunnel syndrome. J Hand Surg 29: 315–320
35. Gerritsen AA, de Vet HC Scholten RJ, Bertelsmann FW, de Krom MCTFM, Bouter LM (2002) Splinting vs surgery in the treatment of carpal tunnel syndrome: a randomized controlled trial. JAMA 288: 1245–1251
36. Gerritsen AA, de Krom MC, Struijs MA, Scholten RJ, de Vet HC, Bouter LM (2002) Conservative treatment options for carpal tunnel syndrome: a systematic review of randomized controlled trials. J Neurol 249: 272–280
37. Gomes I, Becker J, Arthur Ehlers J, Bocchese Nora D (2006) Prediction of the neurophysiological diagnosis of carpal tunnel syndrome from the demographic and clinical data. Clin Neurophysiol 117: 964–971
38. Graham B (2006) The diagnosis and treatment of carpal tunnel syndrome. BMJ 332: 1463–1464
39. Grant GA, Goodkin R, Kliot M (1999) Evaluation and surgical management of peripheral nerve problems. Neurosurgery 44: 825–840

40. Greenslade JR, Mehta RL, Belward P, Warwick DJ (2004) DASH and Boston Questionnaire assessment of carpal tunnel syndrome outcome: what is the responsiveness of an outcome questionnaire? J Hand Surg 29B: 159–160
41. Gunnarsson LG, Amilon A, Hellstrand P, Leissner P, Philipson L (1997) The diagnosis of carpal tunnel syndrome. Sensitivity and specitficityspecificity of some clinical and electrophysiological tests. J Hand Surg (Br) 22: 34–37
42. Haase J, Musaeus P, Boisen E (2004) Virtual reality and habitats for learning microsurgical skills. Virtual applications. Applications with virtual inhabited 3D worlds. In: Andersen P, Qvortrup L (eds) Springer, Berlin Heidelberg New York, pp 29–48
43. Haase J (2007) Learning surgery. Surg Neurol (in press)
44. Harris I, Mulford J, Solomon M, van Gelder JM, Young J (2005) Association between compensation status and outcome after surgery: a meta-analysis. JAMA 293: 1644–1652
45. Henkin P, Friedman AH (1997) Complications in the treatment of carpal tunnel syndrome. Neurosurg Focus 15: 10–16
46. Hobby JL, Watts C, Elliot D (2005) Validity and responsiveness of the patient evaluation measure as an outcome measure for carpal tunnel syndrome. J Hand Surg 30: 350–354
47. Huang JH, Zager EL (2004) Mini-open carpal tunnel decompression. Neurosurgery 54: 397–400
48. Hudson AR, Wissinger JP, Salazar JL, Kline Dg, Yarzagary L, Danoff D, Fernandez E, Field EM, Gainsburg DB, Fabri RA, Mackinnon SE (1997) Carpal tunnel syndrome. Surg Neurol 47: 105–114
49. Hung JT, Lee SW, Han SH, Son BC, Sung JH, Park CK, Park CK, Kang JK, Kim MC (2006) Anatomy of neurovascular structures around the carpal tunnel during dynamic wrist motion for endoscopic carpal tunnel release. Operative Neurosurg 58: 127–133
50. Idler RS (1996) Persistence of symptoms after surgical release of compressive neuropathies and successive management. Ortop Clin North Am 27: 409–416
51. Ikeda K, Isanyra B, Tomita K (2006) Segmental carpal canal pressure with carpal tunnel syndrome. J Hand Surg 31: 925–929
52. Jablecki CK, Andary MT, Floeter MK, Miller RG, Quartly CA, Vennix MJ, Wilson JR (2002) Practice parameter: electrodiagnostic studies in carpal tunnel syndrome: report of the American Association of Electrodiagnostic Medicine. Neurology 58: 1589–1592
53. Jae TH, Sang WL, Seung HH, Byung CS, Jae HS, Choon KP, Chun KP, Joon KK, Moon CK (2006) Anatomy of neurovascular structures around the carpal tunnel during dynamic wrist motion for endoscopic carpal tunnel release. Neurosurgery 58 Suppl 1: ONS-127–ONS-13
54. Jimenez DF, Gibbs SR, Clapper AT (1998) Endoscopic treatment of carpal tunnel syndrome: a critical review. J Neurosurg 88: 817–826
55. Kamath V, Stothard J (2004) A clinical questionnaire for the diagnosis of carpal tunnel syndrome. J Hand Surg (Br) 29: 95–99
56. Katz JN, Simmons BP (2002) Clinical practice. Carpal tunnel syndrome. N Engl J Med 346: 1807–1812
57. Kleindienst A, Hamm B, Hildebrand G, Klug N (1996) Diagnosis and staging of carpal tunnel syndrome: comparison of magnetic resonance imaging and intra-operative findings. Acta Neurochir (Wien) 138: 228–233
58. Kline D, Hudson A (eds) (1995) Nerve injuries. WB Saunders, Philadelphia

59. Kremer M, Gilliatt RW, Golding JSR, Wilson TG (1953) Acroparaesthesia in the carpal-tunnel syndrome. Lancet 265: 590–595
60. Kwon HK, Hwang M, Yoon D-W (2006) Frequency of carpal tunnel syndrome according to level of radiculopathy. Double crush syndrome? Clin Neurophys 117: 1256–1259
61. Lehman RM (2004) A review of neurophysiology. Neurosurg Focus 16: 1–16
62. Levine DW, Simmons BP, Koris MJ, Daltroy LH, Hohl GG, Fossel H, Katz JN (1993) A self-administered questionnaire for the assessment of severity of symptoms and functional status in carpal tunnel syndrome. J Bone Joint Surg (Am) 75: 1585–1592
63. Lindley SG, Kleinert JM (2003) Prevalence of anatomic variations encountered in elective carpal tunnel release. J Hand Surg 28: 849–855
64. Liveson JA, Ma DM (1992) Laboratory reference for clinical neurophysiology. F. A. Davis Company, Philadelphia
65. Long D (2004) Competency based training in neurosurgery; the next revolution in medical education. Surg Neurol 61: 5–14
66. Lundborg G (2000) A 25-year perspective of peripheral nerve surgery: evolving neuroscientific concepts and clinical significance. J Hand Surg (Am) 25: 391–414
67. MacDonald RI, Lichman DM, Hanlon JJ, Wilson JN (1978) Complications of surgical release for carpal tunnel syndrome. J Hand Surg (Am) 3: 70–76
68. Mackinnon SE (2002) Pathophysiology of nerve compression. Hand Clin 18: 231–241
69. Mailis A, Furlan A (2002) Sympatectomy for neuropracthic pain. The Cochrane Database Syst Rev CD002918
70. Malis LI, Apuzzo ML (2006) Electrosurgery and bipolar technology. Neurosurgery 58 Suppl 1: ONS-1–ONS-11
71. Marshall S, Tardif G, Askwarth N (2002) Local corticosteroid injection for carpal tunnel syndrome. Cochrane Database Syst Rev CD001554
72. Masear VR, Hayes JM, Hyde AG (1986) An industrial cause of carpal tunnel syndrome. J Hand Surg (Am) 11: 222–227
73. Massy-Westropp N, Grimmer K, Bain G (2000) A systematic review of the clinical diagnostic tests for carpal tunnel syndrome. J Hand Surg 25: 120–127
74. Mauer UM, Raath SA, Richter HP (1993) Intraoperative anatomic and pathologic findings in 1.4200 initial operations in carpal tunnel syndrome. Handchir Mikrochir Plast Chir 25: 124–126
75. McNeil BJ, Keeler E, Adelstein SJ (1975) Primer on certain elements of medical decision making. New Engl J Med 293: 211–215
76. Mohler LR, Pedowitz RA, Myers RR, Ohara WH, Loopez MA Gershuni DH (1999) Intermittent reperfusion fails to prevent post-tourniquet neuropraxia. J Hand Surg (Am) 24: 687–693
77. Mondelli M, Passero S, Giannini F (2001) Provocative tests in different stages of carpal tunnel syndrome. Clin Neurol Neurosurg 103: 178–183
78. Morimoto KW, Budoff JE, Haddad J, Gabel GT (2005) Cross-sectional area of the carpal canal proximal and distal to the wrist flexion crease. J Hand Surg 30: 487–492
79. Myers KA (2000) Utility of the clinical examination for carpal tunnel syndrome. CMAJ 163: 605–610
80. Nagle DJ, Fischer TJ, Harris GD (1996) A multicenter prospective review of 640 endoscopic carpal tunnel releases using the transbursal and extrabursal Chow techniques. Arthroscopy 12: 139–143

81. Netscher D, Mosharrafa A, Lee M, Posen C, Choi H, Steadman AK, Thornby J (1997) Transverse carpal ligament: its effect on flexor tendon excursion, Morphologic changes of the carpal canal, and on pinch and grip strengths after open carpal tunnel release. Plast Rec Surg 100: 636–642
82. Nishimura A, Ogura T, Hase H, Makinodan A, Hojo T, Katsumi Y, Yagi K, Mikami Y, Kubo T (2004) A correlative electrophysiological study of nerve fiber involvement in carpal tunnel syndrome using current perception thresholds. Clin Neurophys 115: 1921–1924
83. Nitz AJ, Dobner JJ (1989) Upper extremity tourniquet effects in carpal tunnel release. J Hand Surg (Am) 14: 499–504
84. Nodera H, Herrmann DN, Holloway RG, Logigian EL (2003) A Bayesian argument against rigid cut-offs in electrodiagnosis of median neuropathy at the wrist. Neurology 60: 458–464
85. Nora DB, Becker J, Ehlers JA, Gomes I (2005) What symptoms are truly caused by median nerve compression in carpal tunnel syndrome? Clin Neurophysiol 116: 275–283
86. O'Connor D, Marshall S, Massy-Wentropp N (2003) Non-surgical treatment (other than steroid injection) for carpal tunnel syndrome. The Cochrane Database of Systematic Rev CD003219
87. Okutsu I, Ninomiya S, Hamanaka I (1989) Measurement of pressure in the carpal canal before and after endoscopic management of carpal tunnel syndrome. J Bone Joint Surg (Am) 71: 679–683
88. Orlin JR, Stranden E, Slagsvold CE (2005) Effects of mechanical irritation on the autonomic art of the median nerve. Eur J Neurol 12: 144–149
89. Pagnanelli DM, Barrer SJ (1991) Carpal tunnel syndrome: surgical treatment using the Paine retinaculatome. J Neurosurg 75: 77–81
90. Palmer AK, Toivonen DA (1999) Complications of endoscopic and open carpal tunnel release. J Hand Surg (Am) 24: 561–565
91. Pasternack II, Malmivaara A, Tervahartiala P, Forsberg H, Vehmas T (2003) Magnetic resonance imaging findings in respect to carpal tunnels syndrome. Scan J Work Environ Health 29: 189–196
92. Peabody JW, Luck L, Glassman P, Dresselhaus TR, Lee M (2000) Comparison of vignettes, standardized patients and chart abstraction a prospective validation of 3 methods for measuring quality. JAMA 283: 1715–1722
93. Pécina MM, Krmpotic-Nemanic, Markiewitz AD (eds) (2001) Tunnel syndromes, 3rd edn. CRC Press
94. Pierre-Jerome C, Bekkelund SI, Mellgren SI, Nordstrom R (1997) Quantitative MRI and electrophysiology of preoperative carpal tunnel syndrome in a female populations. Ergonomics 40: 642–649
95. Priganc VW, Henry SM (2003) The relationship among five common carpal tunnels syndrome tests and the severity of carpal tunnel syndrome. J Hand Ther 16: 225–236
96. Reale F, Ginanneschi F, Sicurrelli F, Mondelli M (2003) Protocol of outcome evaluation for surgical releases of carpal tunnel syndrome. Neurosurgery 53: 343–351
97. Rempel D, Evanoff B, Amadio PC, de Krom M, Franklin G, Franzblau A, Gray R, Gerr F, Hagberg M, Hales T, Katz JN, Pransky G (1998) Consensus criteria for the classification of carpal tunnel syndrome in epidemiologic studies. Am J Public Health 88: 1447–1451
98. Rempel D, Dahlin L, Lundborg G (1998) Pathophysiology of nerve compression syndromes: response of peripheral nerves to loading. J Bone Joint Surg (Am) 81: 1600–1610
99. Rodner CM, Katarincic J (2006) Open carpal tunnel release. Techn Orthopaedics 21: 3–8

100. Roquelaure Y, Mechali S, Dano C, Fanello S, Benetti F, Bureau D, Mariel J, Martin YH, Derriennic F, Penneau-Fontbonne D (1997) Occupational and personal risk factors in industrial workers. Scand J Work Environ Health 23: 364–369
101. Rossignol M, Stock S, Patry L, Armstrong B (1997) Carpal tunnel syndrome: what is attributable to work? The Montreal study. Occup Environ Med 54: 519–523
102. Rotman MB, Enkvetchakul BV, Megerian JT, Gozani SN (2004) Time course and predictors of median nerve conduction after carpal tunnel release. J Hand Surg (Am) 29: 367–372
103. Russell SM (2006) Dual-portal endoscopic release of the transverse ligament in carpal tunnel syndrome: results of 411 procedures with special reference to technique, efficacy, and complications. Commentary Neurosurg 59: 3–8
104. Sackett DL, Straus SE, Richardson WS *et al* (2000) Evidence-based medicine. How to practice and teach EBM, 2nd edn. Churchill Livingstone, Edinburgh
105. Sander MD, Abbasi D, Ferguson AL, Steyers CM, Wang K, Morcuende JA (2005) The prevalence of hereditary neuropathy with liability to pressure palsies in patients with multiple surgically treated entrapment neuropathies. J Hand Surg 30: 1236–1241
106. Sanz J, Lizaur A, Sánchez del Campo F (2005) Postoperative changes of carpal canal pressure in carpal tunnel syndrome: a prospective study with follow-up of 1 year. J Hand Surg 30: 611–614
107. Scholten R, Gerritsen A, Uitdehaag B, Geldere D, Vet H, Bouter L (2004) Surgical treatment options for carpal tunnel syndrome. Cochrane Database Syst Rev 18: CD003905
108. Schuind F (2002) Canal pressures before, during, and after endoscopic release for idiopathic carpal tunnel syndrome. J Hand Surg 27: 1019–1025
109. Shapiro S (1995) Microsurgical carpal tunnel release. Neurosurgery 37: 66–70
110. Sheu JJ, Yuan RY, Chion HY, Hu CJ, Chen WT (2006) Segmental study of the median nerve versus comparative tests in the diagnosis of mild carpal tunnel syndrome. Clin Neurophys 117: 1249–1255
111. Skre H (1972) Neurological signs in a normal populations. Acta Neurol Scand 48: 575–606
112. Spindler HA, Dellon AL (1982) Nerve conduction studies and sensibility testing in carpal tunnel syndrome. J Hand Surg (Am) 7: 260–263
113. Steers J, Reulen H-J, Lindsay KW (2004) UEMS charter on training of medical specialists in the EU – the new neurosurgical training charter. Acta Neurochir Suppl 90: 3–11
114. Stevens JC, Sun S, Beard CM, O'Fallon WM, Kurland LT (1988) Carpal tunnel syndrome in Rochester, Minnesota 1961–1980. Neurology 38: 134–138
115. Storm S, Beaver SK, Giardino N, Kliot M, Franklin GM, Jarvik JG, Chan L (2005) Compliance with electrodiagnostic guidelines for patients undergoing carpal tunnel release. Arch Phys Med Rehab 86: 8–11
116. Stütz NM, Gohritz A, van Schoonhoven J, Lanz U (2006) Revision surgery after carpal tunnel release – analysis of the pathology in 200 cases during a 2 year period. J Hand Surg 31: 68–71
117. Sunderland S (1969) Nerve and nerve injuries. Livingston ES, London
118. Szabo RM, Slater RR Jr, Farvr TB, Stanton DB, Sharman WK (2000) The value of diagnostic testing in carpal tunnel syndrome. J Hand Surg (Am) 25: 183–184
119. Taleisnik J (1973) The palmar cutaneous branch of the median nerve and the approach to the carpal tunnel. An anatomical study. J Bone Joint Surg (Am) 55: 1212–1217

120. Taniuchi M, Clark HB, Schweitzer JB, Johnson EMJ (1988) Expression of nerve growth factor receptors by Schwann cells of axonotomized peripheral nerves: ultrastructural location, suppression by axonal contact and binding properties. J Neurosc 8: 664–681
121. Trumble TE, Diao E, Abrams RA, Gilbert-Andersen MM (2002) Single – portal endoscopic carpal tunnel releases compared with open release – a prospective randomized trial. J Bone J Surg (Am) 84: 1107–1115
122. Urbaniak JR, Desai SS (1996) Complications of nonoperative and operative treatment of carpal tunnel syndrome. Hand Clin 12: 325–335
123. Werner RA, Jacobson JA, Jamadar DA (2004) Influence of body mass index on median nerve function, carpal canal pressure, and cross-sectional area of the median nerve. Muscle & Nerve 30: 481–485
124. Werner RA (2006) Evaluation of work-related carpal tunnel syndrome. J Occup Rehab 16: 207–222
125. Wiesler ER, Chloros GD, Cartwright MS, Smith BP, Rushing J, Walker FO (2006) The use of diagnostic ultrasound in carpal tunnel syndrome. J Hand Surg 31: 726–732
126. Wilder-Smith EP, Seet RCS, Lim ECH (2006) Diagnosing carpal tunnel syndrome – clinical criteria and ancillary tests. Nature Clin Pract Neurol 2: 366–734
127. Wong KC, Hung LK, Ho PC, Wong JM (2003) Carpal tunnel release, a prospective, randomized study of endoscopic versus limited-open methods. J Bone Joint Surg (Br) 85: 863–868
128. Wright PE (1998) Carpal tunnel syndrome. In: Canale TS (ed) Campbell's operative ortopaedics, 9th edn. Mosby, St Louis
129. Vasen AP, Kuntz KM, Simmons BP, Katz JN (1999) Open versus endoscopic carpal tunnel release: a decision analysis. J Hand Surg 24: 1109–1117
130. Vasiliadis HS, Tokis AV, Andrikoula SI, Kordalis NV, Beris AE, Xenakis T, Georgoulis AD (2006) Microsurgical dissection of the carpal tunnel with respect to neurovascular structures at risk during endoscopic carpal tunnel release arthroscopy. J Arthroscop Rel Surg 22: 807–812
131. Yoshioka S, Okuda Y, Tamai K, Hirasawa Y, Kodda Y (1993) Changes in carpal tunnel shape during wrist joint motions. MRI evaluation of normal volunteers. J Hand Surg (Br) 18: 620–623
132. Young VL, Higgs PE (1996) Evaluation of the patient presenting with a painful wrist. Clin Plast Surg 23: 361–368
133. Zanette G, Marani S, Tamburin S (2006) Extra-median spread of sensory symptoms in carpal tunnel syndrome suggests the presence of pain-related mechanisms. Pain 122: 264–270
134. Zyluk A, Strychar JA (2006) Comparison of two limited open techniques for carpal tunnel release. J Hand Surg (Br) 31: 466–472

Author Index Volume 1–32

Advances and Technical Standards in Neurosurgery

Subject Index Volume 1–32

Advances and Technical Standards in Neurosurgery

SpringerNeurosurgery

Advances and Technical Standards in Neurosurgery

Volume 29

2004. XIV, 304 pages. 101 figures, partly in colour.
Hardcover **EUR 125,–**
ISBN 978-3-211-14027-7

Advances: • Disorders of Consciousness: Anatomical and Physiological Mechanisms (J. L. Valatx) • Advances in Craniosynostosis Research and Management (J. Guimarães-Ferreira, J. Miguéns, C. Lauritzen) **Technical Standards:** • Preoperative Clinical Evaluation, Outline of Surgical Technique and Outcome in Temporal Lobe Epilepsy (A. Immonen, L. Jutila, R. Kälviäinen, E. Mervaala, K. Partanen, J. Partanen, R. Vanninen, A. Ylinen, I. Alafuzoff, L. Paljärvi, H. Hurskainen, J. Rinne, M. Puranen, M. Vapalahti) • Motor Evoked Potential Monitoring for Spinal Cord and Brain Stem Surgery (F. Sala, P. Lanteri, A. Bricolo) • Motor Evoked Potential Monitoring for the Surgery of Brain Tumours and Vascular Malformations. (G. Neuloh, J. Schramm) • Functional Neuronavigation and Intraoperative MRI (C. Nimsky, O. Ganslandt, R. Fahlbusch) • Surgical Anatomy of the Insula (M. Guenot, J. Isnard, M. Sindou)

Volume 28

2003. XIV, 360 pages. 80 figures, partly in colour.
Hardcover **EUR 167,95**
ISBN 978-3-211-83803-7

Advances: • Recent Advances in Stem Cell Neurobiology (T. Ostenfeld, C.N. Svendsen) • Mapping of the Neuronal Networks of Human Cortical Brain Functions (S. Momjian, M. Seghier, M Seeck, C.M. Michel) **Technical Standards:** • The Management of Brain Abscesses • (S. Livraghi, J.P. Melancia, J. Lobo Antunes) • Respective Indications for Radiosurgery in Neuro-otology Surgery for Acoustic Schwannoma • (W. Pellet, J. Regis, P-H. Roche, C. Delsanti) • Commentary • (R. Macfarlane, D. Moffet) • Cerebral Revascularization • (H.J.N. Streefkerk, A. Van der Zwan, R.M. Verdaasdonk, H.J. Mansveld Beck, C.A.F. Tulleken) • Surgical Anatomy of the Temporal Lobe for Epilepsy Surgery • (M. Sindou, M.Guenot)

All prices are recommended retail prices
Net-prices subject to local VAT.

SpringerWienNewYork

P.O. Box 89, Sachsenplatz 4–6, 1201 Vienna, Austria, Fax +43.1.330 24 26, books@springer.at, **springer.at**
Haberstraße 7, 69126 Heidelberg, Germany, Fax +49.6221.345-4229, SDC-bookorder@springer.com, springer.com
P.O. Box 2485, Secaucus, NJ 07096-2485, USA, Fax +1.201.348-4505, service@springer-ny.com, springer.com
All errors and omissions excepted.

SpringerNeurosurgery

Advances and Technical Standards in Neurosurgery

Volume 25

1999. XIV, 241 pages. 54 figures, partly in colour.
Hardcover **EUR 106,–**
ISBN 3-211-83217-3

Advances: • Treatment of Diseases of the Central Nervous System Using Encapsulated Cells (A. F. Hottinger, P. Aebischer) • Intracranial Endoscopy (G. Fries, A. Perneczky) • Chronic Deep Brain Stimulation for Movement Disorders (D. Caparros-Lefebvre, S. Blond, J. P. N'Guyen, P. Pollak, A. L. Benabid) **Technical Standards:** • Recent Advances in the Treatment of Central Nervous System Germ Cell Tumors (Y. Sawamura, H. Shirato, N. de Tribolet) • Hypothalamic Gliomas (V. V. Dolenc) • Surgical Approaches of the Anterior Fossa and Preservation of Olfaction (J. G. Passagia, J. P. Chirossel, J. J. Favre)

Volume 24

1998. XIII, 310 pages. 57 figures, partly in colour.
Hardcover **EUR 134,95**
ISBN 978-3-211-83064-2

Advances: • The Septal Region and Memory (D. Y. von Cramon, U. Müller) • The in vivo Metabolic Investigation of Brain Gliomas with Positron Emission Tomography (J. M. Derlon) • Use of Surgical Wands in Neurosurgery (L. Zamorano, F. C. Vinas, Z. Jiang, F. G. Diaz) **Technical Standards:** • The Endovascular Treatment of Brain Arteriovenous Malformations (A. Valavanis, M. G. Yasargil) • The Interventional Neuroradiological Treatment of Intracranial Aneurysms (G. Guglielmi) • Benign Intracranial Hypertension (J. D. Sussman, N. Sarkies, J. D. Pickard)

All prices are recommended retail prices
Net-prices subject to local VAT.

SpringerWienNewYork

P.O. Box 89, Sachsenplatz 4–6, 1201 Vienna, Austria, Fax +43.1.330 24 26, books@springer.at, **springer.at**
Haberstraße 7, 69126 Heidelberg, Germany, Fax +49.6221.345-4229, SDC-bookorder@springer.com, springer.com
P.O. Box 2485, Secaucus, NJ 07096-2485, USA, Fax +1.201.348-4505, service@springer-ny.com, springer.com
All errors and omissions excepted.

Springer-Verlag
and the Environment

MIX
Papier aus verantwortungsvollen Quellen
Paper from responsible sources
FSC® C105338
FSC
www.fsc.org

If you have any concerns about our products,
you can contact us on
ProductSafety@springernature.com

In case Publisher is established outside the EU,
the EU authorized representative is:
Springer Nature Customer Service Center GmbH
Europaplatz 3, 69115 Heidelberg, Germany

Printed by Libri Plureos GmbH
in Hamburg, Germany